Suicide in Modern Literature

Josefa Ros Velasco
Editor

Suicide in Modern Literature

Social Causes, Existential Reasons, and Prevention Strategies

Springer

Editor
Josefa Ros Velasco
Department of Philosophy and Society
Complutense University of Madrid
Madrid, Madrid, Spain

ISBN 978-3-030-69391-6 ISBN 978-3-030-69392-3 (eBook)
https://doi.org/10.1007/978-3-030-69392-3

This Springer imprint is published by the registered company Springer Nature Switzerland AG
The registered company address is: Gewerbestrasse 11, 6330 Cham, Switzerland

Preface

From the turn of the twentieth century to the present, debates over the meaning of suicide became a privileged site for efforts to discover the reasons why people commit suicide and how to prevent this behavior. Since the French sociologist and philosopher Émile Durkheim published *Suicide: A Study in Sociology* in 1897, a reframing of suicide took place, giving rise to a flourishing group of researchers and authors who wanted to understand better the causes of suicide, as well as to the formation of suicide prevention organizations. A century later, we still keep on trying to reach such an understanding of suicide, the nature and nuances of its modern conceptualization, to prevent suicidal behaviors.

The question of what suicide means *in* and *for* modernity is not an overcome one. Suicide is an act that touches all of our lives and engages with the incomprehensible and unsayable. In fact, since the turn of the millennium, a fierce debate about the state's role in assisted suicide has been adopted. Beyond the discussion as to whether physicians should assist in the suicide of patients with unbearable and hopeless suffering, the scope of the suicidal agency is much broader concerning general people wanting to die.

To explore the place where reasons end, in addition to traditional and clinical suicidology studies, we count on fictional literature as an invaluable resource to address this issue and achieve the following aims: i) To shed light on the social, existential, and psychological causes of suicide, and ii) to explore innovative strategies to prevent suicidal behavior. In searching for solutions to make life valuable, modern neuropsychiatric research alone is not able to offer such a chance to people after all. On the contrary, self-reflection and self-analysis through fictional literature seem a good alternative.

This is a book in which some well-known experts in the field of Suicide Studies worldwide—including David Lester (Stockton University), Jared Stark (Eckerd College), Katrina Jaworski (University of South Australia), Anita Virga (University of the Witwatersrand, Johannesburg), Barbara Hawellek (Beta Clinic Bonn), Michelle Falkoff (Northwestern University), Andrew Bennett (University of Bristol), and Jeffrey Berman (University at Albany, State University of New York), among others—analyze the social and contextual causes of suicide, the existential, philosophical, and psychological reasons for committing suicide, and the prevention strategies that modern fictional literature places at our disposal. They go through the review of modern fictional literature, in the American and European geographical framework, following the rationales that modern narratives based on fiction can serve the purpose of understanding better the phenomenon of suicide, its most inaccessible impulses, and that has the potential to prevent suicide.

In this book, modern literature based on fiction, from American to European writers along the last century, is the tool to facilitate such reflection and analysis, especially considering that the selection of works—including those of Edith Wharton, Jeffrey Eugenides, Joyce Carol Oates, Susan Glaspell, Luigi Capuana, Giovanni Verga, Margarita Nelken, Guido Morselli, Walker Percy, William Styron, Paulo Coelho, Joost Zwagerman, or Yiyun Li, to name a few—is fraught with social, philosophical, psychological, and pedagogical narratives.

Agency in suicide is more than human and depends on non-human materiality, that is to say, suicide is a social fact, a by-product of every society. For that reason, this book starts paying attention to social and cultural determinations that might cause suicide in different settings presented in fictional literature. The first part of the book, entitled "Social Causes of Suicide in Modern Fictional Literature," is divided into two virtual groups of four chapters each: One devoted to exploring the social and cultural reasons of suicide in modern American literature based on fiction, and another devoted to analyzing the same causes in European modern fictional literature. Both virtual sections show their respective approaches chronologically and thematically.

The American literature context mainly puts into question the decisive role that suicide plays in modern visions of the ethical subject and the ethical society, paying attention to the social ills that prompt suicide in North America. This part highlights the role of gender that literature based on fiction enlightens. On the one hand, some contributions deal with the difficulties of being a woman in the last century and currently. The authors demonstrate, by making use of new materialist feminist writings, that being vulnerable to a society that objectifies women and little understands and respects female creativity, beauty, and genius is one of the top reasons for women to commit suicide.

According to the works analyzed, the power of the masculine gaze on feminine expectations often contribute to women to live by obeying strict rules for fear of shame and social punishment. In sum, these chapters show the political claims that women were/are making for feminist purposes and point out that suicide is sometimes the only way out for them. On the other hand, the authors do not ignore that suicide is a phenomenon with enormous political implications that affect both women and men. As they discuss, skewed life chances, limited access to health and education, incarceration, and impoverishment are strong reasons for people to commit suicide too.

On the basis of the above, the book starts with an introduction by suicidologist David Lester to the nature of psychological studies on suicide, the emergence of the sub-discipline of Suicidology, and the role of literature to represent suicide imaginary and its background.

From this historical and methodological approach, we move towards Jared Stark's chapter, "Suicide and the Interpretation of Modernity: Edith Wharton's Early Fictions." Stark (Eckerd College, Florida) focuses on the modern conceptualization of suicide in the works of American writer Edith Wharton. Her complete oeuvre, from the first poem she ever published pseudonymously in 1879, to the last novel, *The Gods Arrive*, released in 1932, weaves a thread of reflection on the question of modern suicide. Through a detailed examination of Wharton's fictional suicides, this chapter investigates how the author exposes and grapples with a double imperative. On the one hand, to bear witness to social and other determinations that might cause suicide and, therefore, demand a public response and acknowledgment of responsibility. On the other hand, to bear witness to the ineluctable and perhaps ultimately indeterminate agency of the one who takes their own life. In Wharton's writings, moreover, this double-bind pertains not only to the theme of suicide, but illuminates the author's situation, as a writer, as a woman, and as a woman writer in turn-of-the-century America. Wharton's writings thus both exemplifies and puts into question the decisive role that suicide plays in modern visions of the ethical subject and of the ethical society.

The next chapter, by Noelia Hernando-Real (Autonomous University of Madrid, Spain), is about suicide in modern and contemporary theater. "Suicide Across the Waves: On the Feminist Possibilities of Dramatic Suicide in Plays by Susan Glaspell, Marsha Norman, and Naomi Wallace" closely looks at plays that deal with suicide to reveal a consistent gender bias and the ways and reasons male and female protagonist commit suicide. From a feminist perspective, Hernando-Real uses three plays by three different authors as case studies: Susan Glaspell's *Bernice* (1919), Marsha Norman's *'night, Mother* (1983), and Naomi Wallace's *And I and Silence* (2011). Placed within their Feminist Waves, this chapter examines the reasons that lead female protagonists to commit suicide—its social implication—and how this can be transferred to broader political claims that women were/are making at the time. Hernando-Real takes into account the theatrical and dramatic techniques these playwrights employ to make audiences see suicide not just as the conflict, climax, or end of their plays—that is, as a mere element of their plots—but as a personal phenomenon with enormous political implications that, in theater, teaches and requires the active role of the audience to reflect upon and amend social ills that prompt such suicides.

Katrina Jaworski (University of South Australia) thinks about the assumption that the agency of suicide is entirely human because of the individual desire and intention to die. However, she asks in her chapter, "The Gendering of Suicidal Agency in Jeffrey Eugenides' *The Virgin Suicides*," *what if the exercise of human agency depends on something else in the course of materializing the act of suicide?* Jaworski's chapter responds to this problem by analyzing the gendering of suicide in *The Virgin Suicides* (1993), written by Jeffrey Eugenides. She begins by discussing the cultural context in which the plot of the novel unfolds and the way this context influences the interpretation of the suicides of the teenage Lisbon sisters—Cecilia, Bonnie, Therese, Lux, and Mary. She then focuses on the power of the masculine gaze and the way it frames and reframes the five suicides. She also goes through the gendering of feminine embodiment and sexuality. Finally, Jaworski considers the significance of the landscape, material culture, and affect as key to understanding suicidal agency. Drawing on new materialist feminist writings, she argues that agency in suicide is more than human because that, which is human, depends on nonhuman materiality. She also argues that the feminine, traditionally interpreted as reactive and passive in suicide, is, in fact, agentic.

"*Magic Friend, Beggar Maid* and *The Fair Princess, Method Actress* and *Loving Mother*: Fantasies of Love, Loss, and Desire in Joyce Carole Oates' Fictional Account of Norma Jeane's Reality," by Gail Shanley Corso (Neumann University, Pennsylvania), is on Oates' fictional writings (2009) about the American iconic film star and beauty Marilyn Monroe. Oates reveals much about the psychological needs of such a woman—the need to be understood and to be unconditionally loved. Her *magic friend* in the mirror allows her to transform from the ordinary orphan or the lonely woman into the expected Marilyn identity, America's pin-up and sensational star. The fairytale script of her evolution, from a "Beggar Maid" into a "Fair Princess," surfaces throughout her relationships with many men over time. With numerous attempts at suicide throughout her life, Marilyn's death, in the end at age 36, as Oates describes, shows her vulnerability to a society that objectified her as a human being according to Corso's proposal.

Beyond the American fictional literature, the European literature context covers another group of social reasons to commit suicide—including similarly those of people belonging to the lower classes of society and living in a hypocritical society, one in which appearances are the most important—especially those related to historical events in the Europe of the last century. Literature, in this case, introduces political and economic factors as responsible for suicide through fictional representations of life under the surveillance of the State Apparatus in socialist regimes and military dictatorships that resemble those of Spain and Germany, for example. Suicide, following the authors' approaches, might be the result of regional, international, and generational particularities around the social division, ideological underpinnings, social contradictions, social impositions, tensions among private and public property, modern social relations, circumstances of production, and economic and moral crisis that generate the impression of a false life.

Anita Virga (University of the Witwatersrand, Johannesburg) analyzes suicide in the two Italian writers Luigi Capuana and Giovanni Verga. Leading exponents of the Italian Realism—known as *verismo*—in the second half of the nineteenth century, both aimed to narrate the reality objectively in their fictional works. According to Virga's research in "Suicide Is Not for the Poor: Self-death in *Veristi* Authors, Luigi Capuana, and Giovanni Verga," the lower social classes—especially peasants, fishermen, and servants—forcefully enter their stories and sometimes become protagonists. At the same time, Virga thoroughly investigates the reality in all its diverse facets, including suicide. Self-death, however, is not typically associated with the lower classes; on the contrary, it remains the prerogative of the rich and noble. As this chapter shows, even when it is a character from the lower strata of society who commits suicide, yet the final gesture tells more about an existential condition than about their social struggle. Virga considers the two novels *Giacinta* (1879) and *Il Marchese di Roccaverdina* (1901) by Luigi Capuana, and the novels *Una peccatrice* (1865) and *Eros* (1875), and the short story "L'ultima giornata," in the collection *Per le vie* (1883), by Giovanni Verga. She aims to analyze suicide as an option for wealthy people in *Giacinta*, *Una peccatrice*, and *Eros*, and as an existential reason for poor people in *Il Marchese di Roccaverdina* and "L'ultima giornata." It is clear that suicide, in both Capuana and Verga, is not deployed as a social critique of the society and does not intend to denounce inequities, but it is instead a privilege for a few.

"Irony, Suicide, and Social Criticism in Margarita Nelken's Short Novel: *Mi suicidio* (1924)," by Juan A. Godoy Peñas (University of Cincinnati), engages in the short story *My Suicide* by Margarita Nelken, in which after a supposed suicide attempt by the main character and with a tremendous satirical charge, the Madrilenian writer creates a work of fiction that allows us to see a hypocritical society marked by social division, appearances, and economic interests. A love relationship of convenience, a promising career, and a world of interwoven social relations begin to flourish after the suicide attempt. In this way, this chapter aims to explore the use that Nelken makes of suicide to make the more humble reader aware of the social situation of Spain in the 20s, which also paints the worlds of folklore and the publishing revolution of the time. Also, Godoy Peñas analyzes the use of irony because it is the suicide itself that marks the beginning of a successful career in the publishing market for the main character. In short, he focuses on how Nelken uses such a macabre episode as suicide to shed light on the darkness of Spanish society, a society in the midst of one of its most difficult periods of the twentieth century.

Angelika Potempa (The University of Texas Rio Grande Valley) writes "The True Life in the False One (*Das wahre Leben im falschen*). Suicide Attempts of Literary Heroes in Eastern German Literature." This chapter studies suicide in texts of Eastern German writers such as Plenzdorf (1972), Braun (1977), Görlitz (1978), Wolf (1979), Zinna (1981), Hein (1982), and Muthesius (1982), in the context of the German Democratic Republic, a political and economic unit with Soviet-influenced but specifically Eastern German determined *socialist* socialization. Literature in this period ascribes the role of a participant in an educational dictatorship to form well-rounded socialist personalities. Consequently, seen as educators of the people (*Volkserzieher*), writers had to walk a fine line when thinking publicly about the chances of realizing the high ideals (*hehre Ideale*) of socialism in their home country. Under the umbrella of debating suicide, Potempa investigates the concerns of the writers such as the intolerable circumstances of political oppression or a critique of the conventional notion of literary heritage. For this research, however, the focus is on value interpretations and philosophical and ideological underpinnings of what it means for the literary character to live a meaningful life until the end and how sociopolitical conditions interweaves themselves into the decision to end their lives.

Also focused on the German scope, Ricardo Gutiérrez Aguilar (Complutense University of Madrid) delves around the social contradiction implicit in the intricacies and stern duties of living under the surveillance of the State Apparatus in the 80s' East Berlin, and the experience of having to cope with those imposed social conditions. In his chapter, "*The Life of Others.* Marx and Durkheim on Suicide and Social Good(s)," he focuses on the *Filmbuch* titled *Das Leben der Anderen* (2006) by Florian Henckel von Donnersmarck. There is an inner logic all through the *Filmbuch* that confronts devotion and passion, altruism and egoism, with its relative weight in the service to the

Common Good. Is it life—*each one's life*—Gutiérrez Aguilar asks himself, the lives of others, some goods we possess, an amenity? At the peak of the *Filmbuch*, suicide makes its entrance into the plot. The concept officiates as a dialectical reminder of the tensions among private-public property. With the help of the short text that Marx published in January 1846 "Peuchet on Suicide" and Durkheim's *magnum opus* on the same issue in 1897 *Le Suicide*, this chapter aims to stress the argument that makes out of life a class of belonging which ownership is in social dispute. For the former, it is in the very essence of the suffocating modern social relations and circumstances of production where we can find the apparent cause that explains Peuchet's statistical account. For Durkheim, instead, society is the final recipient referred to in such a sacrifice. Suicide is a social fact, a by-product of every society. Sometimes it reinforces bonds with the others, the community. Michaël Foessel serves as a final contrast. His concept of intimacy offers the third articulation to the previous two that clarifies what a special kind of goods life could be beyond its relation to the common.

This first section serves as a means to claim for the public response and acknowledgment of responsibility to address the problem of suicide. However, society is not the only cause of suicide. A more compassionate understanding of death by suicide than that of the social stigma requires going through the existential and psychological reasons for committing suicide in modernity. In the second part of this book, titled "Existential and Psychological Reasons for Suicide in Modern Fictional Literature," the contributors analyze the plots of some works in which suicidal behavior in the main characters is related to our most profound and unfathomable instincts and impulses. Following philosophical and psychological theories, the chapters in this part delve into the indeterminate and moral agency of persons who commit suicide to reveal some internal and subjective causes of suicide. From the most recurrent psychological causes of suicide in the fictional characters, experts conclude that libidinous instincts such as primary aggression and defended aggression (which turns into auto-aggressive behavior), and an extreme susceptibility to narcissistic injury in a person, are responsible for the suicide. Apart from this, on many occasions, suicide is just a matter of immaturity, weakness, psychological vulnerability, social isolation, and loss of cultural origin. Suicide might be, also, the result of being suffering from severe depression and meaningless sensation. Nevertheless, maybe suicide is just a means to cope with a life of grief. Understood as an anthropocentric phenomenon, some contributions to this book demonstrate that suicide might be a consequence of the struggle for existence. The image of the solitary intellectual, who possess a high sensibility as well as high reflection levels, who is continuously struggling with self-analysis and philosophical and psychological speculations, and who feels the absurdity of life, on the one hand, and longs for a deeper sense and transcendence, on the other, might get caught up in an existential crisis that leads to suicide. The behavior of many of the characters in the works the authors analyze is the consequence of becoming excessively aware of the central paradox of human existence. For some, suicide is, after all, an act of personal liberation.

Coming back to Spain, "Desire of Death, Suicide, and Salvation: Problems with Eternity in Miguel de Unamuno," by Rodolfo Gutiérrez Simón (Complutense University of Madrid, Spain), shows that death has a permanent presence in the work of Miguel de Unamuno, both novelistic and philosophical. His conception of mortality can only be understood from the *hunger of eternity* and a search for salvation that may be contradictory with a rationality that in no way is the specific human attribute. Gutiérrez Simón intends to develop not only Unamuno's conception of death but of self-induced death and the desire to die, as well as its relationship with the Catholic dogma that would prevent the salvation of suicides. To get this task, he approaches the question from a double perspective. On the one hand, he develops the philosophical elements of Unamuno's thought related to this topic fundamentally in three works: *The Life of Don Quijote and Sancho* (1905), *Tragic Sense of Life* (1913), and *How to Make a Novel* (1927). The consumption of human life, as an indispensable condition to understand the development of it and its outlet in death, and the question of the conservation of the individual (if possible), vertebrate the first part of his research. He also considers Unamuno's conception of the hero as *sinner by ambition* and the concept of transcendental egotism. Naturally, the assumptions that Unamuno inherits from authors such as William James are duly explained here. Secondly, he addresses the question of death and, in particular, suicide (consummated or not) in the novels of the Basque author. Thus, *Love and Pedagogy* (1902), *Mist* (1914), and *Aunt Tula* (1921) are especially relevant and, with some emphasis, some passages by *San Manuel Bueno, mártir* (1931), in which the problem of salvation and suicide is explicitly considered.

From Italy, ""The End of the World? Let Me Die." Guido Morselli's *Dissipatio H. G.* between Suicide and Mankind's Dissolution," by Roberto Risso (Clemson University, South Carolina), presents a hybrid narration, half philosophical pamphlet and half literary, of what comes after the end of humanity he novel by Guido Morselli *Dissipatio H. G.* (1977). The book tells the story, in the first person, of a man who tries to commit suicide in a cave, fails, goes back home, and finds out that the whole of humanity has dissolved. The protagonist finds himself living in a world deprived of humans in a crescendo of short travels, meaningless actions, and a profusion of philosophical and psychological speculations, quoting and antagonizing Durkheim, Hegel, Freud, Marcuse, and mentioning an array of Italian and other foreign writers. This chapter seeks to reconstruct the historical and cultural background of Italy from the late 60s and early 70s, when the reflux of the *Italian economic miracle* put the country in an economic and moral crisis. In this troubled context, Risso analyzes *Dissipatio H. G.* as the narration of a struggle with the temptation of suicide and the international tradition of the post-disaster narration.

Barbara Hawellek (Beta Clinic Bonn, Germany) conducts a psychological analysis of the behavioral and understanding patterns of suicide in the work of Percy. In "The Existential and Suicidal Crisis in the Work of Walker Percy," Hawellek reveals an in-depth insight into and a broad perception of this phenomenon beyond traditional/clinical suicidology in the literary work of Percy. She tries to point out the personal perspective of his protagonists, their present interpersonal/social context and the ruling *Zeitgeist*, and identifies multiple releasing factors of existential crisis and suicidal ideas/behavior. The major one is the central paradox of human existence, involving the feeling of absurdity on the one side, and an intense longing for a more profound sense and transcendence on the other. In particular, Hawellek highlights, Percy teaches us that people with a high sensibility, as well as with high reflection levels, notice this conflict of intense ambivalence and, in consequence, despair. Hawellek claims that Percy's literary protagonists under this process can get intensified and reach its entire depth about the symbolic existential crisis with the option to projective identification.

To put an end to this part, Robyn R. Gaier (Youngstown State University, Ohio) notes the moral component of suicide in "What *Darkness* Reveals: A Look at Depression and Suicide in the Works of William Styron." In *Darkness Visible: A Memoir of Madness* (1989), William Styron criticized the practice of attributing moral wrongdoing to persons who either died by suicide, attempted suicide, or, otherwise, experienced suicide ideation. He also criticized the attribution of moral wrongdoing to such persons because he saw it as a gravely mistaken accusation that contributes to the social stigma of death by suicide. Drawing upon Styron's first-person account of depression as a mental illness along with his suicide ideation, the aim of this chapter is three-fold. First, to establish that some of the difficulties that arise in determining what constitutes suicide rest upon ambiguities in moral agency. Understanding a person's degree of intentionality towards death is imperative concerning suicide, even if it remains elusive. Second, to show that a fragmented sense of moral agency may characterize the experiences of persons who suffer from severe depression, primarily by appealing to insights from Styron's narrative. Such insights are also illustrated through the portrayal of a few characters in his writings, and so this chapter notes those relevant similarities as well. Third, to explain why an integrated form of moral agency is necessary for moral accountability. Since such integration was compromised in Styron's experience of depression, this chapter ultimately aims to show how Styron's battle with severe depression, in conjunction with the depictions of a few characters in his writings, advances a more compassionate understanding of death by suicide than what social stigma permits.

The consequent next step in this book, after revealing some causes and reasons of suicide through the literary analysis of modern fictional narratives across the globe, is to examine the power of literature itself and concrete literary works as preventive tools for suicide ideation. The last part of this book, "Suicide Prevention Strategies of Modern Fictional Literature," aims to show how we can use fiction to make things up and the way that fiction becomes us, becomes our lives, our stories. Especially among teenagers and young people, the readers have developed a seemingly inexhaustible thirst for novels that address the topic of suicide. In this sense, the authors of this part demonstrate, by paying attention to fictional works, that engaging in conversations with characters of modern literature is useful for avoiding suicidal ideation resulting from loss, trauma, anger, guilt, sorrow, or regret. In the same vein, fictional narrations based on the relationship between psychiatrists and patients is also truly educative and teaches why hopes are vital in life. Sometimes, the metaphors with which the writers address suicide are significant for people to cope with their frustrations and suicidal ideation.

As an example of the latter, Fazila Derya Agis (Independent Scholar, Turkey) studies, in "Ecological Metaphors: Suicide Versus Life in Paulo Coelho's *Veronika Decides to Die*," the ecological metaphors dealing with depression and hope based on the suicidal thoughts of a Slovene girl called Veronika. She appears as a character successful in life with no financial problems in the novel *Veronika Decides to Die*, by the Brazilian author Paulo Coelho (1998). She is recovered to a mental hospital after her suicide attempt due to her boredom of life. The novel is about her recovery process in this famous mental hospital in Slovenia. Agis analyzes the literary representations of ecological events from an ecolinguistic point of view. For instance, November alludes to darkness alongside sadness, whereas summer alludes to hope; the seaside, the sunshine, horizons, and a blue sky refer to hope, whereas the long nights and darkness in the hospital are associated with depression. The relationship between psychiatrists and patients is also educative, as mentioned. Veronika's escape from the hospital with a schizophrenic guy, who was mourning after his girlfriend's death, teaches why hopes are vital in life. Moreover, a contrast occurs between living crazily and living by obeying strict rules. To conclude, ecological metaphors leading to depression during the Cold War due to hard times and societal norms are mentioned. Accordingly, the ecological metaphors associated with hope, depression, and suicide in this novel are examined from a cognitive semiotic and linguistic perspective to make suicide and its correlated behaviors closer to the reader. Examples of such conceptual and mental metaphors include "the sea is the hope for a bright future," "darkness is hopelessness," "rain is hope," "sun is love," "cold weather is depression," "hot weather is joy," "sunbeams are angels," "night is evil," and "nature is relief."

Wouter Schrover (University of Amsterdam) returns to the debate in the Netherlands about the state's role in assisted suicide in which the renowned poet, essayist, and novelist Joost Zwagerman took part in 2001. In "Intertextuality and the Opposition to Suicide and Assisted Suicide in the Netherlands – The Case of Joost Zwagerman," Schrover considers the novel *Zes sterren* (*Six Stars*) (2002), in which the suicidal act committed by one of the main characters is morally evaluated in diverse ways by the other characters in the book. While some of them are ambivalent about it, others believe it is an act of cowardice and desertion—the novel thus hints at the notion of the *Dutch act*, which refers to suicide and has a strong negative connotation. This chapter compares the representation of suicide in *Zes sterren* to the position Zwagerman took as an essayist—most explicitly in *Door eigen hand. Zelfmoord en de nabestaanden* (*With One's Own Hand. Suicide and the Relatives*) (2005). To this end, it combines narratological and rhetorical analysis and traces interdiscursive and intertextual relations between Zwagerman's work and other writings on suicide (e.g., Alvarez' *The Savage God. A Study of Suicide*, 1971, and Jean Améry's *Hand an sich legen. Diskurs über den Freitod*, 1976). Moreover, the examination of Zwagerman's novelistic and essayistic work is deepened by a brief discussion of his suicide in 2015 and the media coverage it received.

Michelle Falkoff (Northwestern University, Illinois) details some books published in recent years that look at suicide from multiple perspectives; from those who are suicidal themselves—such as in Jasmine Warga's *My Heart and Other Black Holes* (2015) and Jennifer Niven's *All the Bright Places* (2015)—to those left behind in the wake of suicide—as in Cynthia Hand's *The Last Time We Say Goodbye* (2015) and Emily X.R. Pan's *The Astonishing Color of After* (2018). Her chapter, "Suicide in Contemporary Young Adult Novels," warns that even though many of these books provide valuable insight for teen readers who engage in suicidal ideation or who want to understand the motivations of those who contemplate suicide or have taken their own lives, some books may prove harmful for vulnerable readers, particularly given the age range of the readership. Falkoff examines the benefits and challenges of taking on this complex topic for a teen audience, and evaluates some existing literature to determine what makes some novels effective and others potentially damaging. Specifically, she looks at the strategies writers develop to communicate this complicated matter, including the evaluation of characters, structure, and language across multiple novels that address the topic in a variety of ways.

"'Our Precarious Selves': Suicide and Autoimmunity in Yiyun Li," by Andrew Bennett (University of Bristol, United Kingdom), aims to think about Yiyun Li's remarkable novel *Where Reasons End* (2019). Written in the months after the death by suicide of Li's 16-year-old son, the novel presents a series of conversations between a fictional mother, the narrator, and Nikolai, a fictional, suicided 16-year-old boy. The novel approaches questions of loss, trauma, anger, guilt, and sorrow obliquely, offering fragmentary, meditative, and often impatient, querulous conversations about language and time, music and books, memory and regret, knowing and not knowing, perfection and imperfection, writing and fiction. Generated out of a particular historical event, the novel explores the repercussions of a death that cannot be assimilated, accepted, ignored, accounted for, or forgotten. Immersed in the specificity of an individual, historical, familial death, and the contemporary American and Chinese-American contexts and cultures, the fictionality of Li's novel also perforce transcends the concrete actuality of the circumstances that engendered and necessitated its writing.

In an effort to examine the benefits and challenges of taking on this complex topic for a teen audience, from a pedagogical point of view, through literature—and to put a different end to this review—this book finishes with the special contribution "Leaving One's Comfort Zone to Write About Suicide: Arya's Story," by Jeffrey Berman (University at Albany, State University of New York). Berman presents in this book the results of an undergraduate course at the University of Albany that consists of having the students writing about love and loss and then sharing their writings with classmates to identify and prevent suicidal ideation. Writing and reading short literature and essays by students demonstrates the personal, educational, and therapeutic value of literature to engage them on the journey out of and back into their comfort zone. Moreover, both they and us can better understand the social and individual causes of suicide and how to dismiss from our minds and the spirit of others the idea to commit suicide.

A morbid phenomenon for some, a thorny issue for others; the appealing but serious topic of suicide leaves no one unmoved. It is always difficult to talk of suicide, but literature is undoubtedly a means to be closer to ourselves and others in moments of crisis and desperation. This is not a self-help book, but an academic one. But the authors in this title demonstrate that people can find understanding and reassurance in the fictional experiences and perspectives of others to be applied to real life. Whatever a social or personal issue/reasons—presumably both—hopefully this book is of some help in the task of highlighting literature potential to prevent suicide in the current society, and many might find in these pages the path towards the understanding of the causes and remedies of their suffering.

As the editor of *Suicide in Modern Literature*, I want to thank the contributors to this project and acknowledge their brave to engage in this thoughtful conversation. Some of us met in person on the occasion of the international workshop *Depression as Creative and Destructive Force in Contemporary Literature* I organized at Harvard University in May 2019, and are planning to meet again in 2022 online due to the COVID-19. It was the respect and commitment they demonstrated toward this socio-individual problem that I got the inspiration and strength to edit this book. I am truly grateful to Springer and my editor Lilith Dorko for making this collective work possible. My last words of gratitude are for the Department of Romance Languages and Literatures at Harvard University and the Department of Philosophy and Society at Complutense University of Madrid, and my respective supervisors there, Mariano Siskind and José Luis Villacañas Berlanga. This book has benefited from the research projects "Por una historia conceptual de la contemporaneidad" (PID2020-113413RB-C31), "Improvisation and emotional contagion" (PID2019-108988GB-I00), and "Institución y constitución de la individualidad" (PID2020-117413GA-I00), funded by the Spanish MICINN, and "Nuevas redes de solidaridad en la COVID-19: Comunidades emocionales, activismo de base y ayuda mutua," funded by the Fundación BBVA (Ayudas a Equipos de Investigación Científica sobre SARS-CoV-2 y COVID-19 en Humanidades).

> I was clear at the point where I was ready to give up, and it wasn't that I didn't have the motivation to... it was almost as if I couldn't bring myself to make a conclusion. I can look back on it now like it was a different person, and I refuse to ever get to that place again. There's a big difference, I discovered, between wanting to die and not wanting to live. When you want to die, you at least have a goal. When you don't want to live, you're really just empty. Brian Hugh Warner (Marilyn Manson), MTV News (2007).

Madrid, Spain
October 13, 2020

Josefa Ros Velasco

Contents

Psychology, Suicide, and Literature 1
David Lester
Testing Psychological Theories 2
Understanding Human Behavior in the Past 3
Psychological Analyses of Literature 3
Psychological Studies of the Author (and the Reader) 6
Other Points of Contact 7
Does Creative Writing Harm Suicidal People? 7
A Dissenting Voice 9
References 9

Part I Social Causes of Suicide in Modern Fictional Literature

Suicide and the Interpretation of Modernity: Edith Wharton's Early Fictions 15
Jared Stark
"A Moment of Unheard-of Audacity": "Only a Child" and the Paradox of Decriminalization 18
A New Normal: William James's "Is Life Worth Living?" and Wharton's "A Cup of Cold Water" 22
"A Vast System of Moral Sewage": *Sanctuary* at the Limits of Sociology. 25
Conclusion: Fiction as Witness 29
References 30

Suicide Across the Waves: On the Feminist Possibilities of Dramatic Suicide in Plays by Susan Glaspell, Marsha Norman, and Naomi Wallace 33
Noelia Hernando-Real
References 43

The Gendering of Suicidal Agency in Jeffrey Eugenides' *The Virgin Suicides* 47
Katrina Jaworski
Introduction 47
Karen Barad's Approach to Agency 50
The Virgin Suicides 52
The Cultural Context of Interpreting Gender 55
The Power of the Masculine Gaze 58
Feminine Bodies and Sexuality 61
Suburban Landscape and Mood 63
Conclusion 64
References 65

***Magic Friend, Beggar Maid* and *The Fair Princess, Method Actress* and *Loving Mother*: Fantasies of Love, Loss, and Desire in Joyce Carole Oates' Fictional Account of Norma Jeane's Reality** 73
Gail Shanley Corso
A Magic Friend in the Mirror 84
Beggar Maid into Fair Princess 86
Method Actress 88
Mother with Her Baby 89
Conclusion 90
References 92

Suicide Is Not for the Poor: Self-Death in Veristi Authors, Luigi Capuana and Giovanni Verga 95
Anita Virga
Suicide as a Downside of Modernity 97
Capuana and Verga's Elite Suicides 100
Capuana and Verga's Suicides Among the Poor 104
Conclusion 106
References 107

Irony, Suicide, and Social Criticism in Margarita Nelken's Short Novel: *Mi suicidio* (1924) 109
Juan A. Godoy Peñas
Introduction 109
Irony, Suicide, and Social Criticism 112
Conclusion 117
References 118

The True Life in the False One (*Das wahre Leben im falschen*): Suicide Attempts of Literary Heroes in Eastern German Literature 119
Angelika Potempa
References 130

***The Life of Others*: Marx and Durkheim on Suicide and Social Good(s)** 133
Ricardo Gutiérrez Aguilar
Introduction: *The Great Chain of Goods*—Sharing and the Economic Life of the Community 134
Life and the City: Advantages and Disadvantages of Modern Collective *Maladies* 139
Our Life for Others: Altruism, Real Socialism, and Suicide 145
References 151

Part II Existential and Psychological Reasons for Suicide in Modern Fictional Literature

Desire of Death, Suicide, and Salvation: Problems with Eternity in Miguel de Unamuno 155
Rodolfo Gutiérrez Simón
Suicides in Unamunian Narrative: A Selection 156
Premeditation: Regretful Agony 156
Death as an Escape from Hopeless Solitude 159
Hope, Hopelessness, and the Others: From the Desire for Immortality to the Difference Between the Hero and the Suicide 160
Life as a Novel 163
References 168

"The End of the World? Let Me Die": Guido Morselli's *Dissipatio H. G.* Between Suicide and Mankind's Dissolution 171
Roberto Risso
"An Event (Unimaginable)": Morselli's Movement Toward the Cave...... 171
In the Cave: Suicide in Morselli's *Dissipatio H. G.* 173
After the Cave: Dissipatio Humani Generis.......... 178
References 182

The Existential and Suicidal Crisis in the Work of Walker Percy......... 185
Barbara Hawellek
Introduction.......... 185
The Person of Walker Percy (1916–1990) 186
Percy's Phenomenology of Suicide.......... 187
Literary Works 187
The Existential Conflict: Loss and Transmission of Meaning.......... 188
Phenomena of the Existential Crisis in Selected Novels 188
Specific Coping Mechanisms for the Meaning Crisis.......... 195
Origin Models of the Existential Crisis 196
Connections to Modern Neuroscience 197
Relations to Philosophical Systems.......... 198
Summary.......... 200
References 201

What *Darkness* Reveals: A Look at Depression and Suicide in the Works of William Styron.......... 203
Robyn R. Gaier
Suicide and Moral Agency.......... 204
Styron and the Self as Other.......... 207
Compassion in Place of Judgment 211
Conclusion.......... 212
References 213

Part III Suicide Prevention Strategies of Modern Fictional Literature

Ecological Metaphors: Suicide Versus Life in Paulo Coelho's *Veronika Decides to Die*........... 217
Fazila Derya Agis

Introduction 217
Theoretical Framework and Analyses: Ecolinguistics and Cognitive Semiotics 219
Negative Nature Metaphors Related to Depression 220
Positive Nature Metaphors Related to Hope 226
Conclusion 232
References 235

Intertextuality and the Opposition to Suicide and Assisted Suicide in the Netherlands: The Case of Joost Zwagerman 239
Wouter Schrover
Introduction 239
Escape from Everyone and from Myself 241
Against Suicide Assistance 245
Concluding Remarks 248
References 249

Suicide in Contemporary Young Adult Novels 253
Michelle Falkoff
YA Literature as a Category 254
Suicide as a Popular Topic 255
Thirteen Reasons Why 256
  Suicide as a Revenge Fantasy 257
  Decentering Suicidal Characters 257
  Ignoring Mental Health Issues 258
  Escalating the Violence Onscreen 258
Suicide in YA Literature Post-*Thirteen Reasons Why* 259
  Gayle Forman, *I Was Here* 260
  Cindy Rodriguez, *When Reason Breaks* 260
  Cynthia Hand, *The Last Time We Say Goodbye* 260
  Jasmine Warga, *my Heart and Other Black Holes* 261
  Jennifer Niven, *All the Bright Places* 261
  Emily X.R. Pan, *The Astonishing Color of After* 261
  Karen McManus, *One of Us Is Lying* 262
Takeaways 262
References 263

"Our Precarious Selves": Suicide and Autoimmunity in Yiyun Li 267
Andrew Bennett
Suicidality: *Dear Friend, from My Life I Write to You in Your Life*............ 268
Surviving Suicide: *When Reasons End*.. 274
References 279

Epilogue: Leaving One's Comfort Zone to Write About Suicide: Arya's Story 281
Jeffrey Berman
Helping Students at Risk... 282
Arya 284
Avoiding Landmines 287
The Classroom as a Holding Environment 291
References 292

Index 293

Editor and Contributors

About the Editor

Josefa Ros Velasco is a postdoctoral researcher at Complutense University of Madrid, where she is the PI of the project "PRE-BORED. Well-being and prevention of boredom in Spanish nursing homes," funded by the UNA4CAREER program (Marie Sklodowska-Curie Actions/Una Europa/Horizon 2020/UCM). Prior to this, she was a postdoctoral researcher of the Postdoctoral Research Fellowships at Harvard University for Distinguished Junior Scholars program (2017/2021). She is a specialist in Boredom Studies from a multidisciplinary approach and is the founder and president of the International Society of Boredom Studies (www.boredomsociety.com / @BoredomSociety). She is the author of *La enfermedad del aburrimiento (The Disease of Boredom)* (Alianza Editorial, 2022) and the editor of books such as *The Faces of Depression in Literature* (Peter Lang, 2020), *The Culture of Boredom* (BRILL, 2020), and *Boredom Is in Your Mind* (Springer, 2019). Ros Velasco was awarded the Julián Marías Prize for excellent researchers in humanities and social sciences under 40 years (2020), and the UCM Alumni Researcher Prize (2021). Contact josros@ucm.es / @JosefaRosUCM.

Contributors

Fazila Derya Agis Independent Scholar, Ankara, Turkey

Ricardo Gutiérrez Aguilar University of Alcalá, Madrid, Spain

Andrew Bennett University of Bristol, Bristol, UK

Jeffrey Berman University at Albany, State University of New York, Albany, NY, USA

Gail Shanley Corso Neumann University, Aston, PA, USA

Michelle Falkoff Northwestern University, Evanston, IL, USA

Robin R. Gaier Youngstown State University, Youngstown, OH, USA

Juan A. Godoy Peñas University of Cincinnati, Cincinnati, OH, USA

Barbara Hawellek Beta Clinic Bonn, Bonn, Germany

Noelia Hernando-Real Autonomous University of Madrid, Madrid, Spain

Katrina Jaworski University of South Australia, Adelaide, SA, Australia

David Lester Stockton University, Galloway, NJ, USA

Angelika Potempa The University of Texas Rio Grande Valley, Edinburg, TX, USA

Roberto Risso Clemson UniversityClemson, SC, USA

Wouter Schrover University of Amsterdam, Amsterdam, The Netherlands

Rodolfo Gutiérrez Simón Complutense University of Madrid, Madrid, Spain

Jared Stark Eckerd College, St.Petersburg, FL, USA

Anita Virga University of the Witwatersrand, Johannesburg, South Africa

Abbreviations

ABC	American Born Chinese
CDC	Centers for Disease Control
DSM-5	Diagnostic and Statistical Manual of Mental Disorders, 5th Edition
EMS	European Modular System
fMRI	Functional Magnetic Resonance Imaging
FRG	Federal Republic of Germany
GDR	German Democratic Republic
NAMI	National Alliance on Mental Illness
NIMH	National Institute of Mental Health
PET	Positron Emission Tomographic
SED	Sozialistische Einheitspartei Deutschlands (Socialist Unity Party of Germany)
TAT	Thematic Apperception Test
YA	Young Adult Literature

Psychology, Suicide, and Literature

David Lester

Contents

Testing Psychological Theories 2
Understanding Human Behavior in the Past 3
Psychological Analyses of Literature 3
Psychological Studies of the Author (and the Reader) 6
Other Points of Contact 7
Does Creative Writing Harm Suicidal People? 7
A Dissenting Voice 9
References 9

Both psychology and literature focus on human behavior, and, as a result, there are several areas in which the interests of psychologists and writers converge. For example, Aldous Huxley was enamored by William Sheldon's theory that body type was associated with personality, and so Huxley ensured that the characters in his novels had the appropriate Sheldonian physique (Calcraft, 1980). Psychologists too have made use of literature in many ways. This relationship is useful when studying suicide.

D. Lester (✉)
Stockton University, Galloway, NJ, USA
e-mail: David.Lester@stockton.edu

J. Ros Velasco (ed.), *Suicide in Modern Literature*,
https://doi.org/10.1007/978-3-030-69392-3_1

Testing Psychological Theories

Literature can be used to test psychological theories. For example, theories of suicide can be tested using suicide notes, albeit an unusual form of literature. Thomas Joiner (2005) proposed that two factors were present in suicides—thwarted belongingness (disrupted social relationships) and perceived burdensomeness. Gunn et al. (2012) examined 261 suicide notes from Australia and found thwarted belongingness in the content of 30.7% of the notes and perceived burdensomeness in 10.3%. Only 4.2% had both themes, thereby disputing the generality of Joiner's theory.

Folk tales from primitive societies have been studied. For example, McClelland et al. (1966) looked for factors associated with heavy drinking in societies and found that those with heavy drinking had folk tales in which the characters had a feeling of weakness in the face of heavy demands, leading the men to dream of magical potency and to achieve this by drinking. Literature has also been used to study people's preference for different degrees of complexity. Kammann (1966) found that people prefer intermediate levels of complexity, but this level varies from person to person.

Suicides in literature have also been used to study a culture. Lester (1972) examined the suicides which occurred in the plays of the Norwegian Henrik Ibsen (1828–1906) to see if they conformed to the patterns described by Hendin (1964) for suicides in Norway, Sweden, or Denmark. Hendin used his clinical judgment to argue that suicide in Sweden was usually the result of failure to achieve a high level of performance, suicide in Denmark was the result of the loss of significant others, and suicide in Norway was the result either of loss of a significant other upon whom the suicide was dependent or of guilt over transgressions.

Apart from a brief mention in *Cataline* (2013) of the suicide of a woman after a rape, there are seven suicidal deaths in Ibsen's plays, five victim-precipitated homicides, and two equivocal deaths. In general, found that the suicides had suffered from dependency loss, whereas the victim-precipitated murders were experiencing guilt over transgressions. The suicides also appeared to be motivated by the desire to preserve or restore an ideal self-image.

For example, in *The Wild Duck* (2013), Hedvig is very attached to her parents, especially her father. Because of her poor eyesight, she does not go to school and has no friends her own age. Hedvig's suicide occurs after her father realizes that she is not his daughter, considers leaving home, and verbally rejects her. Hedvig shoots herself shortly after her father tells her to go away and not to come near him. Her suicide is clearly provoked by the rejection of her father. It would seem to be a dependency-loss suicide, which fits Hendin's description of Norwegian suicides.[1]

Understanding Human Behavior in the Past

The psychological study of historical figures, such as Erikson's (1962) of Martin Luther, was the basis of a new academic discipline—psychohistory. An example of a psychohistorical study is in my work (2004) on the suicide of Socrates (he drank hemlock rather than allowing the state to execute him). Whereas philosophers who have written about his death argue, on the whole, that his death was not suicide, I argued that his death was a form of suicide in which an individual forces others to kill him. This is often seen in modern times when an individual acts in such a way that police officers are forced to shoot him (a behavior known as suicide-by-cop).

McClelland (1958) used quantitative methods by scoring a selection of ancient Greek writings for the need to achieve. He found that this need declined steadily from 700 BC to 250 BC which was consistent with the historical events of that period. History and psychology can interact through literature in attempts to categorize historical epochs in psychological terms rather than in economic or social terms. Manuel (1965) examined utopian novels from the past 500 years and noted that they fall into three clear periods: utopias of calm felicity (pre-nineteenth century), the open-ended utopias of the nineteenth century, and contemporary utopias based either on the hypothesis of a growing spiritualization (a humanistic psychological influence) or on the fantasy of great sensate gratification (a psychoanalytic influence).

Psychological Analyses of Literature

The most common interaction of psychology and literature has been the use of psychological theories (especially psychoanalysis) to analyze literature. Niederland (1960) noted that the first example of this was an analysis by Freud of *Die Richterin* (*The Judge*) (1986) written by the Swiss writer, Conrad Ferdinand Meyer (1825–1898). Freud sent an essay to his friend, Wilhelm

[1] Interestingly, Ibsen considered moving to Denmark, but never did so. Furthermore, according to Meyer (1971), Ibsen did contemplate suicide during one stressful period in his life.

Fliess in 1898, in which he suggested that the novel was an unconscious defense against Meyer's memory of an affair with his sister.

Faber (1970) provided several examples of how an examination of suicide in literary characters can throw light on our understanding of suicide. In doing this, Faber explicitly stated that he viewed literary suicides as case studies (though he places the words in quotes) which may serve as archetypes of suicidal behavior and which may provide insights into suicidal behavior. He states that he is not interested in how the suicides further the literary aims or *esthetic contraptions* of the authors, their esthetic implications, or how they might throw light on the attitudes toward suicide of the society in which the play was written.

The suicide of Alcestis, Queen of Thessaly, illustrates some of the possible unconscious psychodynamics of voluntary altruistic suicide. Apollo learns that Alcestis' husband, Admetus, is to die prematurely and makes a deal with the Fates to spare his life. The Fates demand another death in Admetus' place, and only his wife, Alcestis, volunteers to die in his place.

The central theme in the play appears not to be that Alcestis has offered to die in place of her husband but that her husband has accepted her offer! After Alcestis realizes that her husband is going to accept her offer, she is filled with resentment toward him. She acts so as to induce guilt in him in order to punish him for accepting her offer. However, her aggression is expressed in part consciously and in part unconsciously.

On the day of her death, Alcestis does not emphasize the voluntary nature of her death. She speaks of herself as one who is about to be destroyed, implying that Admetus should have protected her from this destruction. She hints of betrayal and abandonment, focusing, for example, on her soon-to-be-motherless children. She expresses the hope that her daughter will marry a noble husband, implying that her own husband is not so noble.

In Admetus' presence, Alcestis breaks down and weeps, whereas with others she is more controlled. As soon as Admetus begins to experience the guilt and to suffer, Alcestis recovers her composure rapidly. She then extracts a promise from Admetus that he will not remarry, so that he will be less likely to forget Alcestis and her sacrifice.

Faber notes that Admetus is very dependent upon his wife, and it is this dependence that leads him in part to ask for and accept her sacrifice. However, his dependency on Alcestis makes her loss unbearable. He ends up begging her not to abandon him. We have, therefore, a relationship between a dependent person with few inner resources and a self-sacrificing person who resents being involved with a man who needs her in an infantile way and treats her as an object. Admetus uses Alcestis' sacrifice to stop living rather than anticipating the construction of a new life without her.

A clinical hypothesis generated by Faber's analysis is that voluntary altruistic suicides stress that they are victims; in contrast, obligatory altruistic suicides tend to protect their egos by transforming the will of others into their own will, that is, they see themselves as martyrs. I doubt that this hypothesis could have been formulated using cases of suicidal behavior found among the clinical material in the files of psychiatric hospitals or psychotherapists' offices. Faber, therefore, provided insights into altruistic suicide that had not been identified from case studies of real-world suicides.

Good examples of learning about suicide from literature come from the plays of Sophocles whom I (2002) called the first great suicidologist. In the play *Oedipus Rex* (*Oedipus the King*) (2005a), I noted that there are clues that Jocasta has known for a long time that Oedipus is her son and that the prophecy has been fulfilled. She is content with this, and she tries to prevent Oedipus from seeking the truth. When she fails, she dies by suicide, calling out to Laius, her first love and the father of Oedipus. She has lost her baby when they sent him to die, then her husband, and now her long-lost son and second husband, as well as a loss of status, losses that are too great for her to continue living. Oedipus, when he discovers the truth, goes to kill his mother but, when he finds her dead, turns his anger onto himself, a common psychoanalytic process.

In the play *Antigone*, Antigone, having lost her mother and father and her preferred brother—she sees her death as reuniting with Polynices in her "bridal bower" (2005b, p. 46, line 896)—goads Creon into executing her, a victim-precipitated homicide (Wolfgang, 1959). Haemon, rushing to save to Antigone, tries to kill his father, Creon, but fails and so turns the sword onto himself—another "murder in the 180th degree" (Shneidman, 1985, p. 34).

Literary styles have been studied. Skinner (1941) attempted to estimate whether the amount of alliteration in Shakespeare's sonnets exceed chance expectations. Rokeach et al. (1970) analyzed the values expressed in the *Federalist Papers* in order to ascertain the authorship of the disputed papers. A frequent approach has been to trace a theme through its many manifestations in literature. For example, McClelland (1964) traced the Harlequin theme (the association of sexuality and death in the same person) in past and current novels and plays. He then found that dying women gave more themes of illicit sexuality in their stories stimulated by the pictures in the Thematic Apperception Test (TAT) than did non-dying women, illustrating the Harlequin theme in real people.

I (1989) treated the poems of Sylvia Plath as if they were responses to the Rorschach inkblot test in order to see whether doing so throws light on her suicide. Piotrowski (1974) suggested that the use of shading in responses to the test (What do you see in this inkblot?) provides information as to whether the person will inhibit behavior under stress or act out. Light shading (using the variations in the gray parts of the inkblots) indicates inhibition, whereas dark shading (using the words, dark, black, night, etc.) indicates acting out.[2] I found that the use of dark shading increased dramatically as the day of Plath's suicide grew close, indicating the increased likelihood of acting out. For example, in her poem "Daddy" (1992), written a few months before her suicide, Plath used the word *dark* six times. In her first collection of poems, she used dark shading words an average of 0.65 times per poem.

Psychological Studies of the Author (and the Reader)

Another important area of study has been the psychological study of the author and the creative process. For example, Ghiselin (1963) argued that the unconscious and inspiration played a minimal role in the creative process, but rather a sense that the story was writing itself (compulsion) and flashes of self-consciousness. There have also been studies of the psychological state of authors. For example, Bellak (1964) treated the short stories of Somerset Maugham as if they were responses to the pictures of the TAT and scored the stories to measure Maugham's psychological needs. After an analysis of 10 of Maugham's 91 short stories, Bellak suggested that Maugham had a continuous struggle with his sexual and aggressive impulses. To control them, Maugham tried for emotional isolation and detachment, playing the role of an onlooker toward others.

Many writers base their novels and poems on their own experiences, and so their works can be considered autobiographical. This is true, for example, of the novelists Ernest Hemingway and Cesare Pavese and the poets Anne Sexton and Sylvia Plath, all of whom died by suicide, and some authors have also written diaries and letters which have been preserved. For example, I (2009) analyzed Pavese's suicide using his diary and novels.

The most notable study of the reaction of people to reading was stimulated by the Commission on Obscenity and Pornography (Anonymous, 1970) which sponsored research on the effects of pornography on people. In another

[2] Calling this *dark shading* is perhaps a poor choice of terms by Piotrowski (1974).

example of the study of the reaction of readers to literature, psychologists have speculated why children like fairy stories involving cannibalism (e.g., Bettelheim, 1977), but I (2020) have argued that a more relevant question is why parents choose to read stories involving cannibalism to children.

Other Points of Contact

Goodman (1963) has noted two areas in which psychology and literature relate. First, psychologizing can itself be viewed as a literary genre. A psychoanalytic case history in a scholarly journal is, for Goodman, a real novel or adventure. A second relationship that Goodman saw between psychology and literature is in the way that writers have been affected by psychological ideas. For example, contemporary writing takes into account the continuity of dream life, daydreams and waking life, the slips and errors we make in speech, fantasy, and wishful thinking.

Does Creative Writing Harm Suicidal People?

Is writing therapeutic for creative writers or is it a stressor that contributes to their psychological disturbance? Silverman and Will (1986) analyzed the life and suicide of Sylvia Plath and concluded that, although she tried to control her suicidal impulses by means of her poetry, she failed in this endeavor. Silverman and Will argued that poetry is successful when it bridges the inner worlds of the creative person and the audience—presumably they mean critically successful, for even poor poetry can serve a useful psychological function for the writer, even if it is merely cathartic. To be successful, poetry must first achieve a balance between the writer's use of the audience to serve his or her own narcissistic needs (a type of exhibitionism) and the desire to give others a way of structuring the terrors and anxieties that afflict us all.

When they apply their ideas to Sylvia Plath, Silverman and Will assert that the successful creative process is successful only when the unconscious forces in the writer operate silently and remain hidden from view. This assertion represents a rather traditional view of creative writing. It would seem to express a preference on the part of Silverman and Will for a particular type of literature rather than expressing a universal truth. The confessional style of poetry developed by W.D. Snodgrass and Robert Lowell and pursued by Anne Sexton is in direct opposition to Silverman and Will's view. In her later style, Plath revealed her deepest feelings in her poems, using her experiences to create the poem rather than to simply transform it. Silverman and Will note that she described her early poems as "proper in shape and number and every part" (1986, p. 142) but not alive. Her poems moved from being a reordering and reshaping of experience with a poetic purpose toward becoming expressions of herself. She identified with her poems, which made their rejection by publishers even more painful, and Silverman and Will label this change as a "narcissistic regression" (1986, p. 99).

The causal sequence which Silverman and Will propose for Plath has no evidence for or against it. It is simply one reading of Plath's life. Other, equally plausible, alternative paths can be proposed. For example, it is quite likely that Plath's participation, along with Anne Sexton with whom she became very close, in a poetry workshop run by Robert Lowell had a major impact on her writing style. Several members of his workshop adopted a more self-revealing content for their poems, and two received Pulitzer prizes for their work.

What is interesting is that, whereas in the early 1950s, her writing may not have helped her cope with the stressors, external and intrapsychic, with which she was confronted, in the later 1950s her switch to a more revealing and personalized style of writing may have helped her survive. Silverman and Will claimed that her writing failed to prevent her suicide. Perhaps it may have postponed her suicide?

Terry and I myself (1992) argued that writing poetry can be useful for suicidal individuals. Writing poems per se may not necessarily be helpful to the client (although they may be cathartic), but the revision of the initial drafts of poems may be therapeutically useful. Revising poems may serve a similar function for clients as the journal assignments devised by cognitive therapists by giving the clients intellectual control over their emotions and distance from the traumatic memories. Sexton revised her poems extensively and, in the process of revision, had to concentrate on form rather than content. This allows for both the action that therapists deem to be therapeutic and the distancing of the self from one's problems. Because Sexton ultimately chose the moment of her death, one should not discount the therapeutic help her writing afforded her.

Anne Sexton illustrates the dialectic in poetry as therapy, between expression and catharsis on the one hand and cognitive control on the other. Sexton, as long as she was able to stay psychiatrically stable, was able to apply the craft of poetry to her creative productions. Both Sexton and Martin Orne, her first therapist, believed that her poetry had helped her recover. Only toward the end of her life, as her ability to craft her poems declined, so did her mental stability dissipate.

Interestingly, both Plath and Sexton showed manic trends prior to their suicides, writing poems furiously, poems with more emotional expression and less poetic crafting. Rather than arguing that writing poetry contributed in part to their suicides, it makes as much sense to say that, in their final breakdowns, poetry was no longer able to help them deal with the intrapsychic forces driving them as it had in the past. As their inner turmoil increased, both wrote feverishly, almost like a safety valve letting out the steam under pressure in a boiler, but to no avail since the pressure was building up faster than they could release it.

But this final failure of the craft of poetry to keep Sylvia Plath and Anne Sexton alive does not, as Silverman and Will argue, signify total failure. Both were outstanding poets and functioned quite well given their probable affective disorders. I would argue that the craft of poetry kept both poets alive for many years after their self-destructive impulses first manifested themselves and so signifies success.[3]

A Dissenting Voice

Not everyone approves of this interaction between psychology and literature. Jaffe (1967) argued that a work of literature is contrived, serving only the writer's intent. The literary structure of the work (play, poem, or novel) forces the character into particular acts and mannerisms. Thus, we cannot learn about real people from a study of literary characters. We can learn only about unreal people. Furthermore, we must beware of discovering *facts* from literature when those writers incorporated that information into their works (see the use of Sheldon's ideas about physique and personality used by Huxley, noted above).

However, with care and forewarned, the psychologist can find a rich source of materials for study in the realm of literature.

References

Andreasen, N. C. (1987). Creativity and mental illness. *American Journal of Psychiatry, 144*(10), 1288–1292. https://doi.org/10.1176/ajp.144.10.1288

Anonymous. (1970). *Report of the commission on pornography and obscenity*. Bantam.

[3] It should be noted in passing that creative writing has been found to be strongly associated with affective disorder (Andreasen, 1987).

Bellak, L. (1964). Somerset Maugham. In R. H. White (Ed.), *The study of lives* (pp. 142–159). Atherton.
Bettelheim, B. (1977). *The uses of enchantment*. Alfred A. Knopf.
Calcraft, L. G. A. (1980). Aldous Huxley and the Sheldonian hypothesis. *Annals of Science, 37*, 657–671. https://doi.org/10.1080/00033798000200451
Erikson, E. (1962). *Young man Luther*. Norton.
Faber, M. (1970). *Suicide and Greek tragedy*. Sphinx Press.
Ghiselin, B. (1963). *The creative process*. Mentor Books.
Goodman, P. (1963). The psychological revolution and the writer's life view. *Daedalus, 92*, 297–311.
Gunn, J. F., Lester, D., Haines, J., & Williams, C. L. (2012). Thwarted belongingness and perceived burdensomeness in suicide notes. *Crisis, 33*(3), 178–181. https://doi.org/10.1027/0227-5910/a000123
Hendin, H. (1964). *Suicide in Scandinavia*. Grune & Stratton.
Ibsen, H. (2013). *Cataline*. Stagedoor.
Jaffe, A. (1967). *The process of Kafka's Trial*. Michigan State University Press.
Joiner, T. E. (2005). *Why people die by suicide*. Harvard University Press.
Kammann, R. (1966). Verbal complexity and preferences in poetry. *Journal of Verbal Learning and Verbal Behavior, 5*(6), 536–540. https://doi.org/10.1016/S0022-5371(66)80088-9
Lester, D. (1972). Suicide in Ibsen's plays. *Life-Threatening Behavior, 2*(1), 35–41. https://doi.org/10.1111/j.1943-278X.1972.tb00454.x
Lester, D. (1989). Application of Piotrowski's dark shading hypothesis to Sylvia Plath's poems written before her suicide. *Perceptual & Motor Skills, 68*(1), 122. https://doi.org/10.2466/pms.1989.68.1.122
Lester, D. (2002). Sophocles: The first great suicidologist. *Crisis, 23*(1), 34–37. https://doi.org/10.1027//0227-5910.23.1.34
Lester, D. (2004). Philosophy and suicide. In D. Lester (Ed.), *Thinking about suicide* (pp. 35–50). Nova.
Lester, D. (2009). Learning about suicide from the diary of Cesare Pavese. *Crisis, 30*(4), 222–224. https://doi.org/10.1027/0227-5910.30.4.222
Lester, D. (2020). *Easting people: Understanding cannibalism*. Nova.
Lester, D., & Terry, R. (1992). The use of poetry therapy. *The Arts in Psychotherapy, 19*, 47–52.
Lien, H., & Meyer, R. W. (2013). Hedvig (The Wild Duck). In *Memnon sound portraits of Ibsen characters*. Ozella.
Manuel, F. E. (1965). Toward a psychological history of utopias. *Daedalus, 94*(2), 293–332.
McClelland, D. C. (1958). The use of measures of human motivation in the study of society. In J. W. Atkinson (Ed.), *Motives in fantasy, action and society* (pp. 518–552). Van Nostrand.
McClelland, D. C. (1964). The Harlequin complex. In R. W. White (Ed.), *The study of lives* (pp. 94–119). Atherton.

McClelland, D. C., Davis, W., & Wanner, E. (1966). A cross-cultural study of folk tale content and drinking. *Sociometry, 29*(4), 308–333. https://doi.org/10.2307/2786291

Meyer, C. F. (1986). *Die Richterin*. Reclam.

Meyer, M. (1971). *Ibsen*. Doubleday.

Niederland, W. G. (1960). The first application of psychoanalysis to a literary work. *The Psychoanalytic Quarterly, 29*(2), 220–235. https://doi.org/10.1080/21674086.1960.11926171

Piotrowski, Z. A. (1974). *Perceptanalysis*. Privately Published.

Plath, S. (1992). *The collected poems*. Harper Perennial.

Rokeach, M., Homant, R., & Penner, L. (1970). A value analysis of the disputed federalist papers. *Journal of Personality and Social Psychology, 16*(2), 245–250. https://doi.org/10.1037/h0029857

Shneidman, E. S. (1985). *Definition of suicide*. Wiley.

Silverman, M. A., & Will, N. P. (1986). Sylvia Plath and the failure of emotional self-repair through poetry. *The Psychoanalytic Quarterly, 55*(1), 99–129. https://doi.org/10.1080/21674086.1986.11927132

Skinner, B. F. (1941). A quantitative estimate of certain types of sound patterning in poetry. *The American Journal of Psychology, 54*(1), 64–79. https://doi.org/10.2307/1417793

Sophocles. (2005a). *Oedipus the King*. Pocket Books.

Sophocles. (2005b). *Antigone*. Prestwick House.

Wolfgang, M. E. (1959). Suicide by means of victim-precipitated homicide. *Journal of Clinical and Experimental Psychopathology, 20*, 335–349.

David Lester has doctoral degrees from Cambridge University (UK) in social and political science and Brandeis University (USA) in psychology. He is an Emeritus Professor of Psychology at Stockton University in Galloway, New Jersey. He is a former President of the International Association for Suicide Prevention. He has published extensively on suicide, murder, and other issues in thanatology. His recent books include *Mass Murder* (Nova Science, 2004), *Katie's Diary: Unlocking the Mystery of a Suicide* (Routledge, 2004), *Suicide in Professional and Amateur Athletes* (Charles C. Thomas, 2012), *Suicide as a Dramatic Performance* (Transaction, 2015), *The End of Suicidology* (Nova Science, 2019), and *How Culture Shapes Suicidal Behavior* (Nova Science, 2019).

Part I

Social Causes of Suicide in Modern Fictional Literature

Suicide and the Interpretation of Modernity: Edith Wharton's Early Fictions

Jared Stark

Contents

"A Moment of Unheard-of Audacity": "Only a Child" and the Paradox of Decriminalization........ 18
A New Normal: William James' "Is Life Worth Living?" and Wharton's "A Cup of Cold Water"........ 22
"A Vast System of Moral Sewage": *Sanctuary* at the Limits of Sociology........ 25
Conclusion: Fiction as Witness........ 29
References........ 30

> Suicide is interpretation.
> Margaret Higonnet, "Speaking Silences: Women's Suicide"

On May 28, 1879, the front page of the *New York World* carried the story of the suicide of a 12-year-old boy, Harry Ackley, in a Philadelphia juvenile reformatory. After a week of solitary confinement imposed following a feeble attempt to escape the institution, Ackley had hung himself from the bars of his cell window, it was reported, "with a deliberateness of purpose appalling when it is considered that he was a mere child" (1879a, p. 1). The article also

J. Stark (✉)
Eckerd College, St. Petersburg, FL, USA
e-mail: starkjl@eckerd.edu

J. Ros Velasco (ed.), *Suicide in Modern Literature*,
https://doi.org/10.1007/978-3-030-69392-3_2

noted, however, that Ackley's act must have been "impelled" by the conditions of his incarceration. Indeed, a page-four editorial on the same day accused the boy's wardens of "homicide by official stupidity," while his mother charged that her son had died not by his own hands but of "mistreatment" (1879b, p. 4). The more detailed coverage in *The Philadelphia Press* expanded the scope of institutional responsibility. Only by chance and journalistic tenacity was the "mysterious secret" of the boy's death uncovered, raising questions about both the disciplinary methods and the public accountability of the House of Refuge—the name of which, the newspaper noted, had acquired ironic overtones (1879a, p. 1, 1879b, p. 6). Stories over the following days would report "other and worse cases of cruelty" and would bring debate over reformatory practices "to a white heat" (1879c, p. 6).

Among the flurry of reactions to this incident in the press was an 80-line poem printed in the *New York World* on May 30, 1879, over the pseudonym "Eadgyth." Edith Wharton would recall the circumstances surrounding her writing and publication of this poem some 40 years later:

> I had read an account of a little boy who had been put in the 'lock-up' for some childish offence, & had hanged himself in the night. This appealed to the morbid strain in my nature, & I wrote a poem on the subject, which I sent to the Editor of one of the New York papers—I think the World. (1990, p. 1091)

As her biographer Cynthia Griffin Wolff observes, the publication of "Only a Child" marks Wharton's "one youthful literary triumph" (1995, p. 47), launching a literary career that spanned the late nineteenth and early twentieth centuries, coming to a close on the eve of World War II. It also anticipates a lifelong preoccupation with stories of suicide. Perhaps most memorably, Lily Bart, in *The House of Mirth* (1905), takes her place along with Emma Bovary and Anna Karenina in a lineage of celebrated female heroines who take their own lives. But beyond *The House of Mirth*, Wharton's work establishes her as one of the great chroniclers of modern suicide. From her first published fiction, the short story collection *The Greater Inclination* (1899), to her final completed novel, *The Gods Arrive* (1932), suicide would appear in marginal or central roles in 9 of the 21 novels and novellas she published during her lifetime, as well as frequently in her short stories.[1]

[1]Among Wharton's novels that include stories of suicide, whether marginally or centrally, are: *Sanctuary* (1903 [1970]), *The House of Mirth* (1905), *The Fruit of the Tree* (1907), *Ethan Frome* (1911), *The Custom of the Country* (1913), *The Mother's Recompense* (1925), *The Children* (1928), and *Hudson River Bracketed* (1929). Short stories in which suicide plays a role include "A Cup of Cold Water," "The Portrait," "The Last Asset," and "The Day of the Funeral," as well as the unpublished fragment "Beatrice Palmatto" (according to the plot summary of which both Beatrice and her sister take their own lives). Hermann Sundermann's *The Joy of Living*, a play Wharton translated early in her career (1902), also has suicide as a central plot element.

This concern with suicide might be linked to certain biographical data—most directly the suicide of her father-in-law in 1891 and her own thoughts of suicide, confided at least once to Henry James (Lewis, 1975, p. 238). But considered in its full spectrum, Wharton's fiction is less preoccupied with her own possible suicide than with the question of how suicide might expose and illuminate the ethical, political, and cultural consequences of modernity. As is already the case in her juvenile poem, the central figure in Wharton's fictions of suicide is the figure of the witness rather than the suicide herself. To live the condition of modernity means for Wharton to live as the surviving witness to another's self-destruction.

In addition to the juvenile poem "Only a Child," the present essay discusses two of the first fictions of Wharton's adult writing career: one of her early stories "A Cup of Cold Water" (1899 [1968]) and the novella *Sanctuary* (1902 [1970]). In imagining the ethical and political dilemma of the witness, these texts respond to and participate in a notable turn-of-the-century shift in the ways suicide is conceptualized. By the end of the nineteenth century, industrialization, secularization, and political revolution had decisively unsettled traditional attitudes towards self-destruction and the institutions that enforced them, affecting both laws concerning suicide and its cultural meanings. With suicide no longer officially marked as inhuman, sinful, or criminal, with the corpses of suicides no longer subject to desecration nor their estates to forfeiture, with the decline of political structures organized around the sovereign's right to kill, it became possible, and necessary, to reconsider what suicide meant and how it could be defined and interpreted. As such, suicide becomes a privileged object of analysis in emerging medical, psychological, and sociological discourse and even a test of their validity. Debates over the meaning of suicide thus track late-nineteenth- and early-twentieth-century efforts to discover, invent, or limn the conditions of modern selfhood and society.[2] Wharton's writing both explicitly and implicitly participates in these new explanatory frameworks, generating new ways of plotting and interpreting suicide. But it does not simply ratify modern explanations of suicide. Her writing, I argue, also critically exposes the ways in which these frameworks, despite their claims to give the meaning and legitimacy of suicide its due, work to limit or vitiate the radical uncertainties to which any interpretation of suicide is subject.

[2] Minois (1999) provides a fascinating and synthetic account of cultural attitudes toward self-destruction in Europe from the middle ages to the early twentieth century. Other crucial works in the cultural history of suicide include Bayet (1922), Gates (1988), and MacDonald and Murphy (1990). A partial history of suicide in the USA is provided in Kushner (1989).

"A Moment of Unheard-of Audacity": "Only a Child" and the Paradox of Decriminalization

The newspaper coverage of the Ackley death registers a paradigm shift in the interpretation of suicide in Europe and the USA that takes place largely over the course of the nineteenth century. Criminal and moral discourses are increasingly supplanted in this period by medical, psychological, and sociological understandings. These new disciplinary approaches sought to identify the underlying causes of suicide, treating it as a symptom of physical, psychological, and environmental factors. As A. Alvarez succinctly puts it in his classic study, *The Savage God*: "'To be or not to be' had given way to 'the reason why'" (1971, p. 99).

While some reports of the boy's death seem to cling to the earlier paradigm, effectively blaming or criminalizing his act—his appalling deliberateness of purpose—a more vocal chorus saw his death as the symptom of social ills and as one of the many symptomatic suicides that were reported almost daily, often on the front pages, and which fueled concerns over a possible suicide epidemic.[3] Wharton's poem joins this chorus. Like the newspaper items to which it responds, "Only a Child" indicts the boy's wardens of criminal negligence and laments a more general climate of indifference. In contrast to an imagined jury that misguidedly "found— he came to / His death by his own hands!" (1879, p. 4, lines 15–16), thus treating the boy as a convicted criminal, the poem insists instead on the boy's victimization. Against the judgment that Ackley died "by his own hands," the poem thus focuses on the innocence of those hands:

> Poor little hands! that should have known
> No subtler arts than these—
> To seek for violets newly blown
> Beneath the April breeze,
> Or gaily bind unchidden

[3] For instance, in May, 1879, *The New York Times* reported 23 suicides, 4 on its front pages. Supplementing these news reports were frequent editorials on suicide, its causes, and its meanings. Apparent increases in suicide rates in the USA during the second part of the nineteenth century led to frequent reports of a possible "suicide epidemic," for which media coverage was also often held responsible (Kushner, 1989). The most comprehensive study of the rhetoric of suicide epidemic in the nineteenth century is Lieberman ("Une Maladie Épidemique," 1987 and *Leaving You*, 2003). A striking manifestation of the anxiety over a suicide epidemic in England is found in Hardy's *Jude the Obscure* (1896 [1978]), in which the suicide of Little Father Time is immediately recognized as a symptom of a threat to the social fabric, "the beginning of the coming universal wish not to live" (p. 411).

The daisies into sheaves,
Or reach the bird's nest hidden
Among the budding leaves.
(1879, p. 4, lines 17–24)

As these lines show, the poem might be justly accused of adopting a moralizing tone (Benstock, 1994, p. 37). Yet alongside its sentimentality, it also registers a more profound anxiety and a more profound insight concerning the implications of casting the suicide as a victim rather than a criminal. If, on the one hand, the decriminalized and symptomatic interpretation of suicide illuminates and potentially indicts the conditions—medical, psychological, political, and social—that are said to cause suicide, on the other hand, the symptomatic interpretation also potentially deprives suicide of its transgressive intentionality. Rather than commit suicide, one is impelled or driven to it. Suicide becomes homicide ("homicide by official stupidity," to recall the wording of the *New York World*). Even as the discourses of suicide that succeed its decriminalization seem to recognize the noncriminal, legitimate intentionality of the one who claims the right to die, they paradoxically suppress that intentionality by attributing the suicide to external causes.

For the young "Eadgyth," this paradox appears less as a consciously-analyzed problem than as the hinge that joins the writer's plight to that of the incarcerated boy. The critical role of the poem in the writer's life becomes clear in her 1934 autobiography, *A Backward Glance* (1934 [1964]), published at the age of 72. In this book, Wharton gives the poem unexpected importance by counterfactually dating its publication prior to the private publication of her *Verses* in 1878. Consequently, "Only a Child" appears as "a more significant starting-point for the new writer," as Millicent Bell observes (1955, p. 64). As significantly, *A Backward Glance* places the publication of the poem immediately after a famously chilling moment when an "icy comment" from her mother, Wharton recalls, "shook me crudely out of my dream of writing fiction" (1964, p. 73). In defiance of this "icy comment," in defiance of the familial, social, and gender norms that militate against her writing, Wharton characterizes the publication of "Only a Child" as "a moment of unheard-of audacity" (1964, p. 73). This audacity inheres not only in submitting the poem for publication but in the poem's very form. For when she submitted the poem—to no less a figure than one she calls the "Editor of the World" (1990, p. 1092)—the young writer prefaced it with a letter "apologizing for the fact that my metre was 'irregular,' but adding firmly that, though I was only a little girl, I wished this irregularity to be respected as it was 'intentional'" (1964, p. 74).

According to this autobiographical account of the publication of "Only a Child," Wharton's preoccupation with stories of suicide thus begins with a moment that links suicide to her first experiment in authorship, her first challenge to the silencing regime of family and society. More specifically, the plight of the young writer and the plight of the boy converge around two related questions. What does it mean to discover intention in an act that might otherwise appear as an error? And how can one bear witness to an act of audacity in something that is otherwise silent, otherwise 'unheard-of'?

The title of the poem captures the tensions that characterize both the boy's death and the young Eadgyth's act of writing. On the one hand, echoing the prevailing sentiment of the press coverage, the poem's title bemoans the isolation, silencing, and discipline to which the child is subjected. He was only a *child*: How could he have deserved such harsh treatment? And how could a "mere child" be accused of deliberately taking his own life? Yet the title also hints at the potential of the child's agency, of his exceptional ability ("*Only* a Child") to find a way to subvert the carceral regime, to act in defiance of his imposed silence and isolation, to perform a definitive escape, perhaps even to make himself heard through the walls of his solitary confinement. Not simply an event dictated by external forces, the boy's suicide constituted for the young Wharton an active *appeal*.

Yet how might one respond to an appeal that is silent and that is also self-silencing? This silence is at the heart of the first stanza, which recounts the discovery of the boy's hanging corpse. "The little hands were numb, / And the piteous voice entreating / In death at last was dumb" (1879, p. 4, lines 6–8). This silence returns in the later reimagining of the scene of death:

His little hands had nought to do
But beat against the wall,
Until at last too tired they grew—
Poor little hands, so small!
And so he lay there voiceless,
Alone upon the ground;
If he wept, his tears were noiseless,
For he feared to hear their sound.
At last perhaps the silence grew
Too deep—it dazed his head—
And his little hands had naught to do;
And so—they found him dead!
(1879, p. 4, lines 57–68)

In depicting the boy's death as the result of inactivity and silence, and not as a form of active resistance, the poem casts doubt on its own expressive capacity. For at the moment it recounts the boy's death, the poem itself falls silent. The hiatus that marks this death ("And so—") draws the limit of both identification and interpretation and consequently calls into question the poet's ability to ground her own act of writing on the site of the boy's suicide. Indeed, when read together with the newspaper article that depicted Ackley in his cell with "nothing to read, nothing to do; only the floor upon which to sit, and only his thoughts to keep him company" (*New York World,* 1879a, p. 1), it becomes unclear whether the poem says anything in its own voice about the scene or instead merely reproduces the newspaper's language.

The only place where the poem may maintain the possibility of the child's agency—that is, the possibility that the child's suicide is a meaningful appeal in itself and not simply a futile symptom of madness or resignation—would be in the almost imperceptible orthographic shift from "nought" (1879, p. 4, line 57) to "naught" (p. 4, line 67), where the latter includes in its semantic field the sense of something destructive ("naughty") not included in its partial synonym "nought."[4] The "noiseless" and "voiceless" child takes his own life, as it were, in the unvoiced alteration of *o* into *a*. Is this orthographic shift simply an oversight on the part of the young writer or merely an artifact of negligent copyediting on the part of the newspaper? Or does it constitute another "intentional irregularity"? With no way to resolve this question, the agency of the text, like that of the child, remains irrecuperably mediated by the institutions that regulate and produce it (as juvenile delinquent, as published poem). By the same token, agency is not entirely erased by this mediation, since for each there remains the possibility of *intentional error*, of something that might *seem to be* a mistake or lapse, the symptom of something external to the boy or to the poet, but that nonetheless may be "intentional."[5] Binary categories of intended and unintended action, which in turn dictate attributions of guilt and innocence, become insufficient for grasping the significance of the boy's death. For the poem situates the boy's death at a moment where both the boy's and the poem's intentions become radically uncertain. In providing a model or pretext for the writer's "moment of unheard-of audacity," the boy's "appalling act" thus exposes the poem and its readers to the limits of interpretation.

---

[4] According to the *Oxford English Dictionary*. In "Life and I" (1990), Wharton describes several crucial childhood episodes when she was found "naughty." See also, for instance, Ophelia's admonition of Hamlet: "You are naught, you are naught" (Shakespeare 1603 [1973], III.ii.173).

[5] Underlining this possibility is the fact that while "Only a Child" displays numerous metrical irregularities, none is as evident as one produced at the very site of the inscrutable shift from "nought" to "naught." By repeating the one line—"His little hands had nought to do" (p. 4, line 57)—ten lines later but with an extra syllable appended—"*And* his little hands had naught to do" (p. 4, line 67)—the poem displays an *internal* metrical inconsistency discernible without reference to any external standard.

The poem, consequently, allows the unintelligibility of the boy's suicide by risking its own intelligibility.

A New Normal: William James' "Is Life Worth Living?" and Wharton's "A Cup of Cold Water"

The radical undecidability and unintelligibility that inhabit the act of suicide—and the act of writing—in "Only a Child" continue to inform Wharton's mature engagements with modern frameworks for interpreting suicide. Among these, I suggest, is an engagement with a position embodied in the philosophical modernism of William James. Although her writings do not give explicit evidence of her readings of James until several years later, and although her early story, "A Cup of Cold Water," published in the 1899 collection, *The Greater Inclination*, does not explicitly mention James, it is not unlikely that Wharton would have been familiar, directly or indirectly, with the ideas developed in his 1895 lecture, "Is Life Worth Living?," published two years later in his *The Will to Believe* (1895 [1979]).[6] Whether or not Wharton specifically had James' lecture in mind, "A Cup of Cold Water" dramatizes and challenges the same modern dilemma puzzled over by James—how to justify suicide prevention when suicide is no longer considered a priori as a moral, legal, or religious transgression.

In "Is Life Worth Living?," James seeks to develop an argument against suicide. Rather than adhere to traditional metaphysical or theological preconceptions or to the suicide taboo, however, he adopts a fundamentally modern position according to which suicide is taken to be a priori both conceivable and legitimate:

> That life is *not* worth living the whole army of suicides declare [...] We, too, as we sit here in our comfort, must 'ponder these things' also, for we are of one substance with these suicides, and their life is the life we share. (1979, p. 38)

This solidarity means that the argument against self-killing must find a new basis and form: "What I propose is to imagine ourselves reasoning with a fellow-mortal who is on such terms with life that the only comfort left him is

[6] In a letter from September 7, 1902, Wharton mentions reading, and not finishing, James' *The Varieties of Religious Experience* (1902) (Menon, 2003). Later letters also give evidence of her familiarity with James' philosophy. From the start of her friendship with Henry James in 1900, William would also be part of Wharton's extended social circle. For a sustained consideration of intersections between James' philosophy and Wharton's writing, see Kress (2002).

to brood on the assurance, 'You may end it when you will'" (1979, p. 39). The imagined scenario of an empathetic dialogue presages some of the cultural and institutional changes that would take place at the beginning of the twentieth century, when, for instance, the first suicide prevention organizations were formed—a short-lived "anti-suicide commission" in Cleveland in 1905 (*The New York Times,* 1905), the National Save-A-Life League in New York City in 1906, and the Anti-Suicide Bureaus of the Salvation Army, the first of which opened in London the same year (Colt, 1991, pp. 287–289). These organizations, like James' lecture, signal a transfer of responsibility from the suicide, or potential suicide, to the community.

Yet to assume responsibility for another's possible suicide, James' argument suggests, means to admit the possibility of one's own. The affirmation of the right to die thus affects a change in the very nature and meaning of suicide:

> The certainty that you now *may* step out of life whenever you please, and that to do so is not blasphemous or monstrous, is itself an immense relief. The thought of suicide is no longer a guilty challenge and an obsession. (1979, p. 45)

Whereas the traditional prohibition of suicide posits it as an exceptional act—whether monstrously exceptional as a crime, sin, or act of madness, or heroically exceptional as an act of martyrdom or rebellion—the modern legitimation of the right to die vitiates its exceptionality. The reason for refraining from suicide, in this light, is no longer that it severs one from the community, but rather that it would fail to demonstrate or effect such a division. Life is worth living because I can—but refuse to—commit suicide. In an argument that anticipates, despite vast differences, Albert Camus' *The Myth of Sisyphus* (1942 [1991]), James writes: "It is only by risking our persons from one hour to the next that we live at all" (1979, p. 53). Suicide becomes the sign and promise of self-determination precisely at the moment it is rejected.

Wharton's "A Cup of Cold Water" stages and assesses the consequences of the modern attitude toward suicide I associate here with James. The decline of metaphysical truths that structures James' inquiry is mirrored in Wharton's story by the loss of ethical absolutes:

> Was not the staunchest code of ethics but a trunk with a series of false bottoms? Now and then one had the illusion of getting to absolute right or wrong, but it was only a false bottom—a removable hypothesis—with another false bottom underneath. There was no getting beyond the relative. (1968, p. 158)

Based on this pointed assessment of modernity, Wharton's protagonist, a bank clerk named Woburn, decides to flee the country to evade embezzlement charges after a series of failed financial speculations. The critical scene in the story takes place in that eminently modern setting, a hotel, the night before his planned flight.[7] Upon hearing sobs from the adjoining room, Woburn peers through the keyhole to witness a woman holding a revolver and preparing her suicide note. As she lifts the gun to her head, he breaks down the door:

> "I saw what you were going to do and I had to stop you"
> She looked at him for a moment in silence, and he saw the terrified flutter of her breast; then she said, "No one can stop me for long. And besides, what right have you—"
> "Everyone has the right to prevent a crime," he returned, the sound of the last word sending the blood to his forehead.
> "I deny it," she said passionately. "Everyone who has tried to live and has failed has the right to die."
> (1968, p. 162)

Woburn's flushed reaction to his own utterance signals both his identification with Ruby Lee—he realizes that from the perspective of his employers he too is a criminal—and a recognition that in labeling her act a crime he reproduces the false-bottomed ethics of which he sought and seeks to disburden himself. Ruby Lee's affirmation of the right to die forces this realization and leads him to attempt another mode of intervention, consonant with James' imagined dialogue: "Tell me what has gone wrong, and let's see if there's no other way out of it" (1968, p. 162).

Ruby Lee's difficulties, like Woburn's, are financial; having left her husband for another man only to be in turn abandoned, she is penniless and without means to afford her hotel bill and train fare back to the Midwest.[8] As the title of the story predicts, Woburn successfully cools Ruby Lee's suicidal passion. This is achieved, however, not by rekindling her will to live nor by creating a better or different future, but simply, in a gesture that seems to encapsulate James' reasoning, by extinguishing the urgency of her determination to die: "It was curious how her passion was spending itself in words; he saw that she would never kill herself while she had anyone to talk to" (1968, p. 164). Ruby Lee is saved, not (as romantic convention would have it) through a

---

[7] On the significance of the hotel as a characteristically modern space in Wharton's writing, see Klimasmith (2002).

[8] It is interesting to note that a similar situation—the attempted suicide of a jilted woman in a New York hotel—prompted Baptist minister Henry Marsh Warren to found the National Save-A-Life League in 1906 (Colt, 1991).

revitalizing affirmation of a passionate attachment to the world or to another, but rather through an encounter with a stranger whose disinterested and dispassionate listening seems to allow her to attain a certain distance from her own situation. Similarly, Woburn's own "thought of flight" is canceled by his encounter with Ruby Lee. Though he is left alone with her revolver and seems on the verge of using it, he too decides against suicide. Instead, he returns to the bank the next day to "face the future which the last hours had prepared for him" (1968, p. 171).

But whether Woburn and Ruby Lee enter the future capable of resisting the forces that first led to their suicidal gestures remains unresolved. For although both relinquish their thoughts of suicide in order to live, as James would put it, "from day to day," they remain no less isolated than before. They are again subject to conditions identical to those they initially sought to escape. In their last moment together, as Woburn installs Ruby on a train returning to the Midwest, the narrative registers the alienating effects of their return to social space: "he felt that the people in the other seats were staring at them" (1968, p. 170). A few hours later, Woburn will think of Ruby Lee on her homebound train with a touch of self-satisfaction. But his refusal to give her his address or full name has also permanently severed their relationship. The story thus evinces a deep suspicion of the ethics of suicide prevention. For if ethics demand Woburn's intervention at Ruby Lee's moment of crisis, it is far from certain that survival constitutes an unqualified good. Indeed, the story asks whether a chance to defy convention and to transform the future has been missed or even whether such defiance and transformation are possible. In the end, Woburn and Ruby Lee's return to social anonymity casts a shadow on Jamesian pragmatic optimism, pointing instead to the wings where forces beyond Woburn's and Ruby Lee's control—the forces of desire and of economic and social structures—remain untouched.

"A Vast System of Moral Sewage": *Sanctuary* at the Limits of Sociology

In immersing both the would-be suicide and the witness or Samaritan in an inescapable social field, "A Cup of Cold Water" moves toward the sociological interpretation of suicide developed over the course of the nineteenth century and consolidated by Durkheim in his 1897 *Suicide: A Study in Sociology* (1951). For Durkheim, as for James, there is no difference in principle between the suicide and the non-suicide, no intrinsic monstrosity or madness, heroism or genius, in the one who takes her own life. Consequently, suicide must be recognized as a potentially meaningful, relevant act. But where suicide for James sheds light on individual, internal meaning, for Durkheim its significance pertains to "realities external to the individual" (1951, pp. 37–38). Whereas, for James, the other's suicide challenges me to consider (and reject) my own possible suicide, and therefore allows me to perceive myself as a self-determining individual, for Durkheim, the other's suicide supplies evidence of the determining power of social conditions. Suicides are significant for Durkheim to the extent that they generate the statistics that tell the story and diagnose the present conditions of a given society. Rather than signs of personal or private meaning or difference, these statistics become transparent signifiers granting the sociologist access to the "real" social dynamics that determine individual behavior. Sociology thus manages to acknowledge the potentially communicative dimension of suicide while also disallowing the suicide's heroism or radical alterity.

Kate Orme's efforts to grasp the social and ethical meanings of suicide in Wharton's second novella, *Sanctuary*, published in 1903, can be set against the background of the sociological interpretation of suicide. It addresses what are also the fundamental questions of sociological inquiry: What impact does suicide have on society? How is society implicated in the suicides of its members? And what ethical consequences does this complicity entail?

In the first part of *Sanctuary*, Kate learns that a woman has drowned herself and her child in a nearby lake. Prior to her death, the woman's failed lawsuit—in which she claimed to be married to the late brother of Kate's fiancé, Denis Peyton—had produced a passing scandal in Kate's social world, "a darkness [that] had crossed her sky and left it as unclouded as before" (1970, p. 109). The discovery of the suicide, however, divides the world of *Sanctuary* in two. The Peyton family, falling back on conventional attitudes and anxious to "hush up" any scandal, attributes the woman's actions to her "fallen" nature. "Why, I suppose it was her last throw, and she was desperate; we don't know how many times she may have been through the same thing before" (1970, p. 113), contends Denis—a claim that anticipates one prominent reading of Lily Bart in *The House of Mirth*.[9] Denis' mother shores up the case:

[9] In this reading, Lily's death appears as entirely unexceptional, a symptom of larger realities that produce, contain, and explain it. Spangler (1979), for instance, sees *The House of Mirth* as one of several turn-of-the-century American novels, along with Dreiser's *Sister Carrie* (1900) and London's *Martin Eden* (1909) that exemplify Durkheim's analysis of suicide, according to which "modern society is a killer, the suicide its victim" (1951, p. 296).

> Surely religion teaches us that suicide is a sin? And to murder her child! [...] Of course one is shocked at the woman's crime—but, if one looks a little deeper, how can one help seeing that it may have been designed as a means of rescuing that poor child from a life of vice and misery? (1970, p. 129)

Against these self-serving recriminations, the deaths of the woman and her child generate in Kate a critical perspective on society:

> But hitherto she had been like some young captive brought up in a windowless palace whose painted walls she takes for the actual world. Now the palace had been shaken to the base, and through the cleft in the walls she looked out upon life. (1970, p. 115)

Through this breach, Kate understands the suicide as a proclamation of outrage and innocence, as proof that the woman's claims were in fact legitimate. When Denis concedes this fact, as well as his own complicity in covering it up, Kate is transformed into a sort of skeptical sociologist:

> She had begun to see that the fair surface of life was honeycombed by a vast system of moral sewage. Every respectable household had its arrangements for the private disposal of family scandals [...] Who was she to pass judgment on the merits of such a system? The social health must be preserved: the means devised were the result of long experience and the collective instinct of self-preservation. (1970, p. 136)

Far from exceptional, the woman's suicide and the efforts to dismiss its implications are revealed as part of a larger social pattern, a "vast system." Indeed, the very sphere of the "private" appears here as the effect of collective interests.

But even as she learns to read the other's suicide as a symptom of underlying social realities, Kate remains constantly aware, and in the grip of, the event that affords her this perspective. Her identification with the suicide thus precludes the presumed distance or neutrality of the sociologist:

> I found myself exulting that you and I were so far from it—above it—safe in ourselves and each other—and then the other feeling came—the sense of selfishness, of going by on the other side; and I tried to realize that it might have been you and I who—who were down there in the night and the flood— (1970, pp. 116–117)

Rather than appear as a symptom of deeper social dynamics, the other's suicide issues an ethical imperative, calling on her to relinquish the distanced position of spectator.

Denis' reply, however, reasserts the limits of Kate's position:

> "Upon my soul," he said with a laugh, "you must have a nice opinion of us both."
>
> The words fell chillingly on the blaze of her self-immolation. Would she never learn that Denis was incapable of mounting such hypothetical pyres? He might be as alive as herself to the direct demands of duty, but of its imaginative claims he was robustly unconscious. The thought brought a wholesome reaction of thankfulness.
>
> "Ah, well," she said, the sunset dilating through her tears, "don't you see that I can bear to think such things only because they're impossibilities? It's easy to look over into the depths if one has a rampart to lean on." (1970, p. 117)

Denis' failure of imagination shows that Kate can only relate to the other's suicide by transforming it into a hypothesis or fiction. This fiction seems to allow Kate to grasp her own reality, but only belatedly. She can imagine her own ethical "self-immolation" only from a position of safety that necessarily misses the significance of the very experience it seeks to fathom.

Suicide in *Sanctuary*, then, rather than provide a stable ground for the apprehension of social reality, reveals the epistemological error on which Kate's ethical and social views are based.[10] But this error, the novella suggests, is a necessary one, resulting from the structural limits or "impossibilities" that preclude knowledge of the experience of death. What separates Kate from her society, in other words, is also what separates her from herself. For as she attempts to pursue the consequences of the actuality unveiled by the other's suicide, she increasingly finds herself divided between a set of outward behaviors that conform to social norms—she marries Peyton, raises a son, and watches in passive silence as he negotiates his own ethical relation to society—and a set of covert motivations, justifications, and actions that generate an internal story for her about her own resistance to and impact on her world, that is, about her ability to respond to the "imaginative claims" issued by the suicide. Thus, she imagines that by marrying Peyton, she does not endorse the system he represents but rather "might expiate and redeem his fault by becoming a refuge from its consequences" (1970, p. 139). When her son, like his father before him, faces "his hour, his one irrecoverable moment" (1970,

[10] Kate's acute sense of shame as analyzed by Raphael would therefore be the affective equivalent or consequence of this error (1991).

p. 190), she pictures her own silence as a form of action. At the end of *Sanctuary*, her son seems to validate this fiction:

> If you'd said a word—if you'd tried to influence me—the spell would have been broken. But just because the actual *you* kept apart and didn't meddle or pry, the other, the you in my heart, seemed to get a tighter hold on me. (1970, p. 201)

As this "happy" ending realizes Kate's ethical vision, however, it also exposes the limits of her agency, which can be exercised only through another form of what she earlier called her "self-immolation." If bearing witness to suicide allows her to perceive her social world as a "vast system of moral sewage," and if it seems to represent for her a way of resisting that world, it does so only as she repeats that suicide in metaphorical form. She acts only by withdrawing.

Conclusion: Fiction as Witness

From "Only a Child" to *Sanctuary*—and extending through all her writing, up to her final novel, *The Gods Arrive*—Wharton's fictions of suicide address not only the personal or psychological implications of self-destruction, but, more generally, the decisive role figures of suicide play in modern visions of the ethical subject and ethical society. For characters like Woburn and Kate Orme, as for thinkers like William James and Durkheim, suicide or the thought of suicide seems to grant an otherwise unobtainable purchase on reality, one that cuts through the mystifications of theology or ideology in order to expose a more authentic ground for individual or social life. And yet Wharton's fictions also insist on the limits of the witness' or interpreter's grasp of suicide, limits that undermine the effort to find in suicide a stable point of orientation. Wharton's fictions of suicide are thus not simply mimetic attempts to document the reality of suicide in literary form. Instead, they expose the ways that modern frameworks for determining the reality, truth, or cause of suicide are themselves inherently fictions that bear witness to—without being able to account for—what remains, insistently, an act of unheard-of audacity.[11]

---

[11] This essay is substantially revised from an earlier version that appeared in *The Edith Wharton Review* (Stark, 2002). I am grateful to Elaine Golin, Anupama Rao, Johannah Rodgers, and Augusta Rohrbach for their astute comments.

References

Alvarez, A. (1971). *The savage god*. W.W. Norton.
Bayet, A. (1922). *Le suicide et la morale*. Felix Alcan.
Bell, M. (1955). 'Eadgyth' Wharton in the *New York World*, 1879. *The Yale University Library Gazette, 30*(2), 64–69.
Benstock, S. (1994). *No gifts from chance*. Charles Scribner's Sons.
Camus, A. (1991). *The myth of Sisyphus*. Vintage International Editions.
Colt, G. H. (1991). *The enigma of suicide*. Touchstone.
Dreiser, T. (1900). *Sister Carrie*. Doubleday.
Durkheim, É. (1951). *Suicide: A study in sociology*. The Free Press.
Gates, B. (1988). *Victorian suicide: Mad crimes and sad histories*. Princeton University Press.
Hardy, T. (1978). *Jude the obscure*. Penguin.
Higonnet, M. (1986). Speaking silences: Women's suicide. In S. Suleiman (Ed.), *The female body in western culture* (pp. 68–83). Harvard University Press.
James, W. (1902). *The varieties of religious experience*. Longmans Green and Co.
James, W. (1979). Is life worth living? In W. James (Ed.), *The will to believe and other essays in popular philosophy* (pp. 34–56). Harvard University Press.
Klimasmith, B. (2002). The 'hotel spirit': Modernity and the urban home in Edith Wharton's *The Custom of the Country* and Charlotte Perkins Gilman's short fiction. *Edith Wharton Review, 18*(2), 25–35.
Kress, J. M. (2002). *The figure of consciousness: William James, Henry James, and Edith Wharton*. Routledge.
Kushner, H. (1989). *Self-destruction in the promised land: A psychocultural biology of American suicide*. Rutgers University Press.
Lewis, R. W. B. (1975). *Edith Wharton: A biography*. Harper and Row.
Lieberman, L. (1987). Une maladie epidémique: Suicide and its implications in nineteenth-century France. Doctoral Dissertation, Yale University.
Lieberman, L. (2003). *Leaving you: The cultural meaning of suicide*. Ivan R. Dee.
London, J. (1909). *Martin Eden*. Macmillan.
MacDonald, M., & Murphy, T. R. (1990). *Sleepless souls: Suicide in early modern England*. Oxford University Press.
Menon, P. (2003). 'Beings of different language': Pragmatist meets idealist in Edith Wharton's *The Reef*. *The New Compass: A Critical Review, 2*. http://people.auc.ca/disanto/dec2003/menon.html. Accessed 5 Oct 2020.
Minois, G. (1999). *History of suicide: voluntary death in Western Culture*. Johns Hopkins University Press.
New York World. (1879a, May 28). Suicide of a little boy. *New York World*, p. 1.
New York World. (1879b, May 28). The Ackley suicide. *New York World*, p. 4.
Raphael, L. (1991). *Edith Wharton's prisoners of shame*. St. Martin's Press.
Shakespeare, W. (1973). Hamlet. In G. Blakemore Evans (Ed.), *The Riverside Shakespeare* (pp. 1141–1186). Houghton Mifflin.

Spangler, G. M. (1979). Suicide and social criticism: Durkheim, Dreiser, Wharton, and London. *American Quarterly, 31*(4), 496–516. https://doi.org/10.2307/2712269
Stark, J. (2002). Wharton's suicides. *The Edith Wharton Review, 18*(2), 12–25.
Sundermann, H. (1902). *The joy of living*. Charles Scribner's Sons.
The New York Times. (1905, November 13). Mr. Johnson's latest experiment. *The New York Times*, p. 8.
The Philadelphia Press. (1879a, May 27). Driven to death. *The Philadelphia Press*, p. 1.
The Philadelphia Press. (1879b, May 28). The Ackley atrocity. *The Philadelphia Press*, p. 6.
The Philadelphia Press. (1879c, May 29). The latest horror. *The Philadelphia Press*, p. 6.
Wharton, E. (1878). *Verses*. C. E. Hammett, Jr.
Wharton, E., [Eadgyth]. (1879, May 30). Only a child. *New York World*, p. 4.
Wharton, E. (1899). *The greater inclination*. Charles Scribner's Sons.
Wharton, E. (1905). *The house of mirth*. Charles Scribner's Sons.
Wharton, E. (1907). *The fruit of the tree*. Charles Scribner's Sons.
Wharton, E. (1911). *Ethan Frome*. Charles Scribner's Sons.
Wharton, E. (1913). *The custom of the country*. Charles Scribner's Sons.
Wharton, E. (1925). *The mother's recompense*. D. Appleton and Co.
Wharton, E. (1928). *The children*. D. Appleton and Co.
Wharton, E. (1929). *Hudson River bracketed*. D. Appleton and Co.
Wharton, E. (1932). *The gods arrive*. D. Appleton and Co.
Wharton, E. (1964). *A backward glance*. Charles Scribner's Sons.
Wharton, E. (1968). A cup of cold water. In R. W. B. Lewis (Ed.), *The collected short stories of Edith Wharton* (Vol. 1, pp. 151–172). Scribner's Sons.
Wharton, E. (1970). Sanctuary. In E. Wharton (Ed.), *Madame de Treymes and three novellas* (pp. 105–202). Collier.
Wharton, E. (1990). Life and I. In E. Wharton (Ed.), *Novellas and other writings* (pp. 1069–1096). Library of America.
Wolff, C. G. (1995). *A feast of words: The triumph of Edith Wharton*. Addison-Wesley.

Jared Stark is Professor of Comparative Literature at Eckerd College in St. Petersburg, Florida. He is the author of *A Death of One's Own: Literature, Law, and the Right to Die* (Northwestern UP, 2018). Other essays on suicide and literature have appeared in *Modernism/Modernity*, *The Yale Journal of Criticism*, and *Connect*. He has also published, with Alina Bacall-Zwirn, *No Common Place: The Holocaust Testimony of Alina Bacall-Zwirn* (Nebraska UP, 1999), along with numerous essays on Holocaust literature and testimony.

Suicide Across the Waves: On the Feminist Possibilities of Dramatic Suicide in Plays by Susan Glaspell, Marsha Norman, and Naomi Wallace

Noelia Hernando-Real

Contents

References.......... 43

Gender has been identified as a key category that can facilitate a comprehensive approach to the study of suicide, for decades now understood as an epidemiological growing concern worldwide (Barroso, 2019). Statistics have proved the existence of such a gender divide. While it is estimated that men are more often performers of lethal suicides (77.97% male performers vs. 22.03% female performers), it is also registered that for every man who attempts suicide, three women do so as well (American Association of Suicidology, 2019). Necessarily, any earnest approach to understanding why women commit suicide starts by questioning the influence of gender concerns in leading more women to consider self-slaughter. Theater, this literary genre known for holding a mirror up to nature, has always been aware of suicide as both a personal and political choice and as a powerful dramatic tool. Indeed, suicide has been integral to theater from its early days. Classical drama, such as Sophocles' *Ajax* (ca. 450 BC [1979]) and *Antigone* (441 BC [2005]), Renaissance plays loved by audiences now and then, such as Shakespeare's

N. Hernando-Real (✉)
Autonomous University of Madrid, Madrid, Spain
e-mail: noelia.hernando@uam.es

J. Ros Velasco (ed.), *Suicide in Modern Literature*,
https://doi.org/10.1007/978-3-030-69392-3_3

Romeo and Juliet (ca. 1596 [1839]) or *Hamlet* (ca. 1600 [1860]), and modern drama, such as Miller's also canonical *Death of a Salesman* (1949 [2007]), have taught us that self-sought death can be preferable to a life of grief or shame or even to accusations of lack of patriotism. But in the same way that in suicide research, gender has recently been incorporated as an analytical tool, very significantly, a closer look at plays that deal with suicide and their reception reveals a consistent gender bias as to the ways and reasons male and female protagonists commit suicide. This essay undertakes the analysis of an apparently paradoxical theatrical choice: US women playwrights' use of their female protagonists' self-sought death as part of a feminist agenda. To do so, three plays by three different authors are used as case studies: Susan Glaspell's *Bernice* (1919 [2010]), Marsha Norman's *'night, Mother* (1983), and Naomi Wallace's *And I and Silence* (2011). This chronological perspective allows for the necessary placement of these playwrights and their works within their own Feminist Waves. By discussing the reasons that lead the female protagonists to commit suicide in their time and the social implication of their suicides, conclusions will be drawn as regards wider political claims that women were/are making at the time. At the same time, the analysis of the varied theatrical and dramatic techniques these playwrights employ in their depiction of suicide will illustrate these women's understanding of the means to make their audiences empathize with the suicidal protagonists and then how necessary it is to keep theater looking into new ways of presenting suicide.

Through the works presented in this essay, it can be said that Susan Glaspell (1876–1948), Marsha Norman (1947), and Naomi Wallace (1960) are representative of women writers' feminist concerns within the three Feminist Waves. Susan Glaspell, a New Woman herself, endorsed any movement that meant the amelioration of women's lives in the days prior to the passage of the 19th Amendment to the US Constitution. Her most well-known play, *Trifles* (1916 [2010]), in fact, advocates for women's right to sit in juries and, in sum, to have the right to vote; this was one of the main concerns of First Wave feminists, together with access to higher education, changes regarding marriage and divorce laws, and access to the professions, among other demands. As Glaspell said in a 1921 interview: "I am interested in all progressive movements, whether feminist, social, or economic" and she took active part through her writing (qtd. in Rohe, 1921, p. 18). Marsha Norman's early career places her within a reinvigorated Second Feminist Wave, rooted in the Civil Rights movement and making strong demands for changes in women's objectification in the media, women's rule over their own (sexual) bodies, and women's opportunities in the workplace. Naomi Wallace's works seem to respond to the growing feminist awareness of essentialist definitions of womanhood by earlier feminists, claiming the vital need to reconsider the importance that class or ethnicity, for instance, have always played in the subjugation of women. Third Wave feminists, on the whole, have sought to emphasize the significance of the particular at the expense of the general.

A bond that brings together these women playwrights widely separated in time—in fact by three waves of the feminist movement—is their understanding of the dramatic power of suicide to make feminist demands. Glaspell's *Bernice*, a play written just one year before women were granted the right to vote in the USA, opens with the death of the protagonist, an absent character. Although Bernice, an average white upper-middle-class housewife, has died of natural reasons, the audience soon learns that on her deathbed she made her maid promise she would tell her husband she had killed herself. From the structural point of view, Glaspell uses suicide as the conflict that makes the plot unfold, guiding the audience in this Ibsenite psychological drama into understanding why this woman had this shocking last wish. The play is a psychological approach to suicide, with characters, on the one hand, elucidating the reasons Bernice could have had to commit suicide and, on the other hand, the reasons other characters find to understand why Bernice has lied. All in all, Glaspell's approach shares with suicidology one important premise: "In the aftermath of a suicide, those who knew the deceased always dwell on the question 'why?'" (Fincham et al., 2011, p. 1). While Glaspell uses the concept of suicide as the starting point of *Bernice*, in contrast, both Marsha Norman and Naomi Wallace use suicide to build up to the climax of their plays. Nevertheless, each playwright approaches this climax in diametrically opposed ways. Norman's two-character play *'night, Mother*, written in the early 1980s, almost starts with Jessie's terrible confession: "I'm going to kill myself, Mama" (1983, p. 13). Consequently, similar to Glaspell's strategy, throughout the course of the play, the audience is explicitly and implicitly invited to understand the many reasons Jessie, an undiagnosed depressed white woman in her late 30s or early 40s, has to end her life. Her final death is but the logical conclusion of her initial statement. In *And I and Silence*, on the other hand, Wallace allows the audience to bear witness to Dee and Jamie's bright dreams for the future. In contrast with the two other plays, where time is used in a traditional way, *And I and Silence* alternates scenes in the past, set in 1950, when Jamie, an African American girl of 17, and Dee, a white girl of 16, meet in prison, with scenes from the present, set in 1959, now with Dee and Jamie living together outside prison. The 1950s setting, symbolically laden with the connotations of the early days and struggles of the Civil Rights movement in the USA (Herrera Medalle, 2015), serves Wallace to remind contemporary audiences of the ordeals Jamie and Dee go through in their attempt to sustain a mixed-race relation. Furthermore, the alternation of scenes from the past and the present leads spectators to "interpret the hopes and then the anguish and the distress of Jamie and Dee" and thus to "understand their final decision" (Ozieblo, 2018, p. 164).

Significantly, although perhaps unsurprisingly, the three plays have met mixed reviews as regards the use of the strategy of dramatic suicide, too often aligning it with a support of patriarchal views of womanhood. For instance, the case of Bernice, who masks her natural death as suicide, is apparently meant to make her husband feel loved. That is, Bernice wants her husband to believe she has committed suicide because she could not stand his infidelities any longer. After her fake suicide, Craig is reassured at last, as he says, "Bernice *killed* herself because she loved me so" (2010, p. 99). Scholars such as Cheryl Black believe that "Bernice's bizarre, post-mortem sacrifice seems a compensatory gesture, a sign that she had little to give [her husband] in life" (2005, p. 56). Critics of Norman's *'night, Mother* have been more direct. For example, for William Demastes, Jessie's suicide is a "defeatist resolution" to escape her entrapment (1993, p. 109). Feminist critics Jill Dolan, Jeanine Forte, and Linda Ginter Brown have gone even further suggesting that with Jessie's suicide, Norman was pleasing a male audience and then reasserting patriarchal ideology (Dolan, 1988; Forte, 1989; Brown, 1996a). Wallace's *And I and Silence* has also received similar reviews. Charles Isherwood, writing for *The New York Times*, notes that "the sensational conclusion still feels strained and, yes, even melodramatic, more appropriate to one of the purplish women-behind-bars movies than Ms. Wallace's high-toned, low-energy drama" (2014). And for Rovie Herrera Medalle, the play's end offers no glimpse of hope, and it is tragic and defeatist in the sense that for Dee and Jamie there is no other escape (2015). However, it is my contention that the male gaze misinterprets these dramatic suicides, favoring a reading of female characters' suicide as the weak solution of powerless characters. In contrast, I believe Glaspell, Norman, and Wallace dismantle the male gaze and invite their audiences to share a female gaze, an understanding of why these women claim suicide as empowerment and not as defeat.

To start with, it must be noted that the three plays share the traditional home setting, a setting that holds some of the reasons for the protagonists' suicide and that, consequently, rather than reassert questions patriarchal values. As Linda McDowell and Joanne P. Sharp have noted, in the West the social construction of home has erected this figure "as a place of familial pleasures, a place of leisure and rest – for men a sylvan and tranquil respite from the rigours of the city or the workplace and for women a supposedly safe haven" (1997, p. 263). And at the same time, as Rosemary George says, "The word 'home' immediately connotes the private sphere of patriarchal hierarchy, gendered self-identity, shelter, comfort, nurture and protection" (1999, p. 1). As has been affirmed, home has usually been associated with "family, child-bearing, and hence emotional and physical sustenance" (Valentine, 1997, p. 288). Home, in short, is woman's place, the source of stability, reliability, and authenticity. D.A. Leslie denounces that:

> feminine identity has tended to be more spatially confined than that of men. Whereas male subjectivity is defined in terms of control over space, female subjectivity becomes that which must be controlled by being bounded: the house itself may be seen as a system of control and surveillance. (1997, p. 304)

Bernice, Jessie, Dee, and Jamie all dwell in houses that look like prisons and that represent women's incarceration in social roles that prompt their suicides. As Patrizia Velotti and Giulio Cesare Zavattini have stated, there are substantial reports that show a consistent link between demographic and contextual factors (age, gender, socioeconomic status) and/or behavioral and psychological factors, which may co-occur and thus lead to conditions for suicide (2018). Glaspell and Norman opt for realistic representations of homes to represent such co-occurrences. The house in *'night, Mother* is "way out on a country road" (1983, p. 3), and as Mama says, Jessie "doesn't go to the front steps" (1983, p. 54). Similarly, the house setting in *Bernice* is also apart from civilization. It is "up on a hill," out "in the country" (2010, p. 94), and very difficult to reach; no one could come on time for Bernice's last breath, not even the doctor. Glaspell and Norman use the physical isolation of their protagonists' houses to subtly suggest reasons for their suicides: They felt isolated and detached and thus unable to reach out for help. In *And I and Silence*, Wallace opts for a minimalist representation of Dee and Jamie's dwelling: "The Present takes place on the outside, in a city, in a small, mostly bare room" (2011, p. 3), "Their room is made up of a minimum of furniture" (2011, p. 7), and indeed they only have one bed, which they alternate with sleeping on the floor. Dee and Jamie's room in the present is symbolic of their extreme poverty; the setting is minimalist pretty much because Dee and Jamie cannot own anything. Significantly, Wallace denotes this setting with a conscious geographical indeterminacy to suggest the universality of her protagonists, forcing her audience to realize that there are many other Dees and Jamies out there. Dee and Jamie's isolation, like Bernice's and Jessie's, is evident as they cannot leave this room together. If they do, they fall prey to verbal and physical abuse:

Dee	Here we can't get out together. We can't sit together. We can't walk together anymore.
Jamie	We can walk together.
Dee	Then why don't we?
Jamie	You know why.
Dee	Sure. 'Cause folks on the street see us together, everyone thinks you're my maid. Me, have a maid? [...so we tell] the truth: that we're both servants. That we are friends. What do we get then?
Jamie	Be quiet.
Dee	What do we get? An orange crush bottle flying through the air. Then another 'cross my back. Guts from the butcher in your hair. Doors slamming behind us. (2011, p. 43)

This repeated abuse, as Barbara Ozieblo has noted, "derive[s] from the hatred and fear inspired by those who are different" and "it is augmented by the fact that this is a friendship among women" (2018, p. 165), a friendship that indeed seems to develop into lesbian love as the play advances. Nevertheless, instead of considering their room a haven or a shelter, this enclosing space reminds Dee and Jamie of their isolation and lack of opportunities.

As advanced earlier, the protagonists' prison-like houses, besides suggesting suicidal drives based on isolation and detachment, also signal these women's incarceration in social roles. In this regard, it is necessary to reconsider the way in which gender has been spatialized, as also the traditional binary between public and private spaces. Traditionally, the public arena was obviously the male place, while women could rejoice in the sanctity of their private homes. But given that the private is controlled by the same social definitions working in the public arena (including women's roles, socializing practices, and power relations), the long-held opposition between public and private spheres reveals itself as an artificial and deceiving trick. As Michael Keith and Steve Pile affirm, "all spatialities are political because they are the (covert) medium and (disguised) expression of asymmetrical relations of power" (1993, p. 220).

The close examination of the geographies of *Bernice*, *'night, Mother*, and *And I and Silence* reveals how there is no such difference between the public and the private, since the same organizing principles of the outside, patriarchal, world govern these houses and act as triggers for the protagonists' suicidal ideas. In Glaspell's play, Craig does not arrive on time to see his wife on her deathbed because he was away, on one of his very common trips, to be with his present flame. Paradoxically, the one who is seen departing from their given social role is Bernice and not Craig, the unfaithful husband. As Laura, Craig's sister and patriarchy's spokesperson in the play, very directly says, "[Bernice] should have wanted to [hold Craig.] It's what a wife should want to do" (2010, p. 101). And not only was Bernice considered a failed wife for not being able to hold her husband but also a failed mother and woman, as, after a miscarriage, she never bore a child. Appallingly, no one seems to consider the traumatizing event this miscarriage must have been for Bernice, who then perhaps chose to live in seclusion in this house playing the attentive nurse to her traumatized veteran father. Furthermore, most Glaspell scholars have underlined Bernice's choice to live in seclusion, detached from society (Friedman, 1995), but frequently visited by her friend Margaret, a very modern woman who lives in New York City and is an open advocate of women's rights. I agree with Black that, "barring heterocentric assumptions, there is as much evidence in the play to suggest a sexual relationship between Margaret and Bernice as there is between Craig and Bernice" (2005, p. 56). One wonders if Bernice's lie about her natural death and fake suicide does not hold dreams she had in the past, an idea Bernice entertained for having failed in her prescribed social roles and the impossibility of living her love for Margaret openly. As has been noted, completed suicide promoted by trauma is very often preceded by suicidal thoughts (Maltsberger et al., 2018).

Marsha Norman has been firm in her definition of how prescribed social roles for women have been determinant in her portrait of female characters who depart from such roles. In her own words:

> I'm saying that the things that we've been taught will make us happy don't always end up making us happy. We, as women, I think, have been sold a real bill of goods about what a good life is. I think this version of the good life is based upon what the species needs us to do and what society needs us to do. [...] Yet, we *are* used by society – to calm the men down and take care of the children – you know, breed the children and take care of the children we breed. (qtd. in Brown, 1996b, p. 203, emphasis in original)

Jessie in *'night, Mother* is representative of women used by society, women who have been sold this bill of goods about what a good life is. In fact, it is because of the many things that Jessie has been forced to do that she finds her way out in suicide. When she tells her mother about her plans for that night, Mama, wavering between incredulity and despair, asks her daughter, "What's the matter with you?" Jessie's revealing answer is simply "I'm tired. I'm hurt. I'm sad. I feel used" (1983, p. 28). This answer encapsulates many of the signals specialists highlight as indicative of potential suicides, including behavioral, emotional, social, and family scenarios (Velotti & Zabatini, 2018). Jessie is described as "pale and vaguely unsteady physically" (1983, p. 2), and she confesses she feels people reject her because she is not attractive. That her husband abandoned her and obliged her to move in with her mother ratifies both her thwarting self-esteem and the difficult economic situation in which she has been left. Moreover, she has a difficult relationship with her son, a criminal who only visits her to rob her. Significantly, Jessie also suffers from epilepsy, and seizures have determined her to live in seclusion: She felt people were afraid of her when this happened, and this illness also forced her to stop working, sending her home and making her feel useless. Jessie, when she puts what defines her at the moment against what her life should be, considers herself a failure as a productive worker, as a wife, as a mother, and, in sum, as a woman. When Jessie found herself failing according to her social definition, she came home to Mama, only to be reminded of all her failures and to be imprisoned in this house as the housewife to her mother. Jessie is tired of being used: Of cooking, of doing Mama's nails, of cleaning, and of filling all kinds of containers with sweets—the activities she is performing tonight in front of the audience for the last time before committing suicide. Nevertheless, tonight, this routine is fundamentally different because of Jessie's choice, her suicide provides these common activities with a different meaning. As Eric Brantley has put it, "In setting her mother's house in order one last time […] Jessie is defining the suffocating, sterile existence of the years she has lived there since her marriage ended" (2004).

Naomi Wallace's technique of alternate chronologies in her play allows for the interplay between public and private in obvious ways. To start with, the private and the public are fused in the settings to embody a physical and metaphysical prison. Dee and Jamie's 1959 room setting has been discussed earlier as representative of poverty. Moreover, as Ozieblo has noted, Wallace goes one step further, since this room resembles a prison cell "in its lack of comfort and decoration" and also "in their inability to leave it" (2018, p. 169). The cell in the scenes from the past is simply described as "a bare prison cell" (2011, p. 12), a bare room with "a small window" (2011, p. 15). Dee's cell's window gives onto a brick wall, while Jamie's, more luckily as she ironically remarks, offers her a piece of tree. This lack of view, representative of the dehumanizing spatialities of federal prisons, symbolically enhances these girls' lack of opportunities; the colorful horizon they imagine outside prison will just be the same brick wall, now that of their 1959 room. In prison, Dee and Jamie have to stand the abuse of prison guards, who hit them, steal their juice, and put worms in their food, who disapprove of mixed-race relationships, and who punish them by putting them in *the hole*. In the present, Dee and Jamie suffer almost identical mistreatment: Male bosses who abuse them, boyfriends who use them, female bosses who hit them, they suffer the scarcity of food, and they must be confined in their own hole, the bare room they share. As Josephine Machon has affirmed, "these dreams to rise above poverty and racial inequality are violently dashed when life outside of prison proves to be harsher, more confining, and ultimately more destructive than their earlier incarceration" (2013, p. 92). That Dee and Jamie's dreams involve finding a husband and working as servants, being fed on leftovers, painfully reflects how these two young women have internalized what is to be expected from women of their circumstances. And it is even more painful to discover that even this "dream" is denied to them. Wallace has Dee and Jamie rehearse endlessly how to achieve their dream. That is, they are so aware that there is a social role they must perform, that they want to be excellent at it. In prison and in their room, they practice how to be "a happy servant" (2011, p. 18), how to clean, how to polish, how to sing, how to be graceful, but also how to accept being beaten and insulted and how to put limits to the sexual advances of bosses. Dee and Jamie's naivety is crushed by reality no matter how earnestly they have rehearsed and results in their one-time performance, that of their suicide.

Paradoxically, suicide in *Bernice*, *'night, Mother*, and *And I and Silence* is the whirling force that brings the plays to life and eventually empowers Bernice, Jessie, and Dee and Jamie. As has been noted, "Disconcerting for a feminist reading of the play, however, is the fact that Bernice's power lies in her death" (Ozieblo, 2008, p. 43). But it is exactly in death where Bernice's power lies, specifically in her fake suicide. On the one hand, because her husband, the unfaithful husband, will live all his life thinking his wife killed herself because of his actions. And on the other hand, because those who loved her in earnest, such as her friend Margaret, have been forced to put themselves in Bernice's position and understand why she could have wished her own death. *'night, Mother* and *And I and Silence*, where Norman and Wallace force their audiences to either hear or see the suicides, allow for symbolic readings of the ways suicides are committed, readings that support theatrical female empowerment. As suicidology scholars have noted, women usually attempt suicide by poison, while men most often choose weapons, most commonly firearms (SAVE, 2020). Jessie shoots herself with her father's gun, which she cleans in front of her mother as part of the routine she is doing tonight. Jessie locks herself in her bedroom and while her mother pounds again and again and screams "Jessie! Please!" "we hear the shot, and it sounds like an answer, it sounds like No" (1983, p. 89). Jessie's dramatic suicide denotes agency, that she has chosen an answer and this is No to life. As she had said earlier in the play:

> I can't do anything either, about my life to change it, make it better, make me feel better about it. Like it better, make it work. But I can stop it. Shut it down [...] It's all I really have that belongs to me and I'm going to say what happens to it. And it's going to stop. And I'm going to stop it. (1983, p. 36)

Dee and Jamie's deaths in *And I and Silence* replicate some of the same agency clues Norman employed in her play but, significantly, they kill themselves in front of the audience. The reasons and definitions of suicide Wallace makes her characters utter toward the end of the play constitute the climax, while their very deaths enact the resolution to the conflict. As Jessie in *'night, Mother*, Dee and Jamie also want it to "stop," they want to "go away," to "quit" this place, and they also present it as empowerment: So they feel "That world is ours," that they are not "givin' up"; they are "givin' in, to a world where [they] almost are. Almost. Are." They see suicide as "a kind of travel" to a "quiet place" they can go together and prove they are the owners of their lives (2011, pp. 55–56). The end of the play brings together two scenes, one from the past, when Young Dee and Young Jamie are saying goodbye in prison, promising to one another they will meet again and be always together, and the scene in the present, in which Dee and Jamie commit suicide. Here, as Machon has said, "Past and present are fused in a visceral present where time coils, helix-like, to communicate the power of hope amidst the destruction of dreams" (2013, p. 95). As Jessie, they die in what can be considered an unwomanly way; they use "an elegant knife" (2011, p. 64). This knife is indeed the only thing they have ever stolen, therefore making it obvious that they choose death as an answer to a classist and capitalist world that has denied them of any opportunity to fulfill their dreams. The same happiness young Dee and Jamie show when saying goodbye in prison echoes in how happy they feel while dying, as they explicitly say so. They die together and by putting their hands together as Jamie pushes the knife first into Dee's stomach and then into hers. The last seconds of the play describe how the two women "are both calm, as though at the centre of a storm" meeting eternal silence as the characters say "Hush" (2011, p. 68). Ozieblo has read this end as a direct reference to the title of the play and the lines from Emily Dickinson's "I Felt a Funeral, in my Brain" (2018, p. 170) that inspired it. For Ozieblo, the play shows that there "is no other escape into anything other than silence," since "they have always been the wrecks of humanity" (2018, p. 170). While this intertextual reading is convincing, I favor a more positive reading of the end in which, as Machon above, the power of hope can overcome the destruction of dreams and the destruction of lives. Hopefully, the audience will feel shocked by their suicide onstage, and rather than disregarding them as "melodramatic" (Isherwood, 2014) or not completely "convincing" (Hempstead, 2014) will understand its dramatic power as a Brechtian *gestus* meant to move the audience to action.

To conclude, the three plays discussed here show how powerful dramatic suicide has been across the three Feminist Waves. Such feminist readings require a departure from a male gaze perspective that obliges the audience to see female characters who kill themselves as simply the victims of a patriarchal world where they do not fit. By looking at Bernice's, Jessie's, and Dee and Jamie's conception of suicide from their own perspectives, the audience is able to recognize in these women empowered heroines who give up their lives so that we, who are the real people outside the auditorium, can see their suicides as a personal phenomenon with enormous political implications. Their suicides reveal social ills that the audience is left to ponder about and, hopefully, react and amend.

References

American Association of Suicidology. (2019). Facts and statistics 2018 [Updated 2020]. *American Association of Suicidology*. https://suicidology.org/facts-and-statistics/. Accessed 11 Mar 2020.

Barroso Martínez, A. A. (2019). A critical literature review of the research on suicide from a gender perspective. *Social Medicine, 12*(2), 118–124.

Black, C. (2005). Making queer new things: Queer identities in the life and dramaturgy of Susan Glaspell. *Journal of Dramatic Theory and Criticism, 20*(1), 49–69.

Brantley, E. (2004, November 15). Theater review; mother-daughter angst, with death in the wings. *The New York Times*. https://www.nytimes.com/2004/11/15/theater/reviews/motherdaughter-angst-with-death-in-the-wings.html. Accessed 9 Apr 2020.

Brown, L. G. (1996a). A place at the table. Hunger as metaphor in Lillian Hellman's *Days to Come* and Marsha Norman's *'night, Mother*. In L. G. Brown (Ed.), *Marsha Norman: A casebook* (pp. 63–85). Garland.

Brown, L. G. (1996b). More with Marsha Norman. In L. G. Brown (Ed.), *Marsha Norman: A Casebook* (pp. 197–220). Garland.

Demastes, W. (1993). Jessie and Thelma revisited: Marsha Norman's conceptual challenge in *'night, Mother*. *Modern Drama, 36*(1), 109–119. https://doi.org/10.1353/mdr.1993.0039

Dolan, J. (1988). *The feminist spectator as critic*. University of Michigan Press.

Fincham, B., Shiner, M., Scourfield, J., & Langer, S. (2011). *Understanding suicide. A sociological autopsy*. Palgrave Macmillan.

Forte, J. (1989). Realism, narrative, and the feminist playwright: A problem of reception. *Modern Drama, 32*(1), 115–128. https://doi.org/10.3138/md.32.1.10

Friedman, S. (1995). Bernice's strange deceit: The avenging angel in the house. In L. Ben-Zvi (Ed.), *Susan Glaspell: Essays on her theater and fiction* (pp. 155–163). University of Michigan Press.

George, R. M. (1999). *The politics of home. Postcolonial relocations and twentieth-century fiction*. University of California Press.

Glaspell, S. (2010). *The complete plays of Susan Glaspell*. McFarland.

Hempstead, P. (2014, August 25). Review of *And I and Silence*. *Theatermania*. https://www.theatermania.com/off-broadway/reviews/and-i-and-silence_69659.html. Accessed 5 Mar 2020.

Herrera Medalle, R. (2015). Race on trial. The battle against segregation in Naomi Wallace's *And I and Silence*. In A. Howe Kritzer & M. Lopez-Rodriguez (Eds.), *Woman on trial. Gender and the accused woman in plays from Ancient Greece to the contemporary stage* (pp. 277–289). Teneo Press.

Isherwood, C. (2014, August 25). Bonding behind bars. *The New York Times*. https://www.nytimes.com/2014/08/26/theater/and-i-and-silence-a-prison-drama-by-naomi-wallace.html. Accessed 5 Mar 2020.

Keith, M., & Pile, S. (1993). Conclusion: Towards new radical geographies. In M. Keith & S. Pile (Eds.), *Place and the politics of identity* (pp. 220–226). Routledge.

Leslie, D. A. (1997). Femininity, post-fordism, and the 'new traditionalism'. In L. McDowell & J. P. Sharp (Eds.), *Space, gender, knowledge. Feminist readings* (pp. 300–317). Arnold.

Machon, J. (2013). Naomi Wallace and the politics of desire. In S. T. Cummings & E. S. Abbitt (Eds.), *The theatre of Naomi Wallace* (pp. 89–102). Palgrave Macmillan.

Maltsberger, J. T., Goldblatt, M., Ronningstam, E., Weinberg, I., & Schechter, M. (2018). Traumatic subjective experiences invite suicide. In M. Pompili (Ed.), *Phenomenology of suicide. Unlocking the suicidal mind* (pp. 147–165). Springer.

McDowell, L., & Sharp, J. P. (1997). *Space, gender, knowledge. Feminist Readings*. Arnold.

Miller, A. (2007). *Death of a salesman*. Methuen Drama.

Norman, M. (1983). *'night, Mother*. Noonday Press.

Ozieblo, B. (2008). Susan Glaspell. In B. Ozieblo & J. Dickey, *Susan Glaspell and Sophie Treadwell* (pp. 11–90). Routledge.

Ozieblo, B. (2018). Embodied agency: A cognitive approach to Naomi Wallace's *And I and Silence*. In I. Duran, R. Gualberto, E. De Lorenzo, C. M. Mendez-Garcia, & E. Valls (Eds.), *A critical gaze form the Old World. Transatlantic perspectives on American studies* (pp. 159–176). Peter Lang.

Rohe, A. (1921, December 18). The story of Susan Glaspell. *New York Morning Telegraph*, p. 18.

SAVE. (2020). *Suicide facts 2020*. Suicide Awareness Voice Education. https://save.org/about-suicide/suicide-facts/. Accessed 12 Mar 2020.

Shakespeare, W. (1839). *Romeo and Juliet*. J. Pattie.

Shakespeare, W. (1860). *Hamlet*. Sampson Low.

Sophocles. (1979). *Ajax*. Arno Press.

Sophocles. (2005). *Antigone*. Prestwick House.

Valentine, G. (1997). (Hetero)sexing space: Lesbian perceptions and experiences of everyday spaces. In L. McDowell & J. P. Sharp (Eds.), *Space, gender, knowledge. Feminist readings* (pp. 284–300). Arnold.

Velotti, P., & Zavattini, G. C. (2018). Emotional dysregulation and suicide risk: If you'll leave me, I'll kill myself! In M. Pompili (Ed.), *Phenomenology of suicide. Unlocking the suicidal mind* (pp. 131–145). Springer.

Wallace, N. (2011). *And I and silence*. Faber and Faber.

Noelia Hernando-Real is an Associate Professor of English and American Literature at the Autonomous University of Madrid (Spain). She has authored *Self and Space in the Theater of Susan Glaspell* (McFarland, 2011) and *Voces contra la mediocridad: la vanguardia teatral de los Provincetown Players, 1915–1922* (Publicaciones Universidad de Valencia, 2014). She has co-edited several volumes, such as *Performing GenderViolence. Plays by Contemporary American Women Dramatists* (Palgrave Macmillan, 2012), a special issue of the Spanish feminist journal *Asparkía*, devoted exclusively to North American women playwrights (2012); the special issue of the *Complutense Journal of English Studies* "Staging the Sounds of a Nation;" and the bilingual collections *En torno a espacios y género – Negotiating Gendered Spaces* (Fundamentos, 2013), and *Estudios de Género: Visiones Transatlánticas - Gender Studies: Transatlantic Visions* (Fundamentos, 2016). Noelia Hernando-Real is the President of the International Susan Glaspell Society.

The Gendering of Suicidal Agency in Jeffrey Eugenides' *The Virgin Suicides*

Katrina Jaworski

Contents

Introduction ... 47
Karen Barad's Approach to Agency ... 50
The Virgin Suicides ... 52
The Cultural Context of Interpreting Gender ... 55
The Power of the Masculine Gaze ... 58
Feminine Bodies and Sexuality ... 61
Suburban Landscape and Mood ... 63
Conclusion ... 64
References ... 65

Introduction

While researchers across academic disciplines are yet to agree on a common definition of suicide—albeit for very good reasons—on the surface, suicide is commonly understood as an explicitly individual and private act (Andriessen, 2006; De Leo et al., 2006; Silverman, 2016). Or, as Michael Kral (2019, p. 19) outlines, "suicide is the voluntary taking of one's own life." In this way,

K. Jaworski (✉)
University of South Australia, Adelaide, Australia
e-mail: Katrina.Jaworski@unisa.edu.au

J. Ros Velasco (ed.), *Suicide in Modern Literature*,
https://doi.org/10.1007/978-3-030-69392-3_4

as Kral (2019, p. 20) notes, "calling suicide a death produced by a willful act of the self implies consciousness and choice, yet suicide is usually seen as an irrational behavior by a clouded mind." Regardless of whether suicide is a product of rational or irrational choices, it is clear that suicide is understood in anthropocentric terms. That is, there is an assumption that agency is entirely human, because of the individual desire and intention to die, made manifest through the content of the body and mind. The problem with this anthropocentric viewpoint is with how agency is interpreted.[1] Agency is framed as something a person possesses or is meant to possess, as if agency is something human beings possess by virtue of being human.

Things become more complicated when the agency of suicide is read through the cultural lens of gender. Statistical differences regularly tell us that more men than women die by suicide, whereas more women than men attempt suicide (Callanan & Davis, 2011; Choo et al., 2017). Based on outcome, largely determined by mortality rates, suicide is interpreted as a male phenomenon, where men are seen as completers and women as attempters (Canetto, 1992–1993, 1995, 1997; Canetto & Lester, 1998; Coleman & Casey, 2011; Dahlen & Canetto, 2002; Range & Leach, 1998). A range of actions, or self-destructive behaviors, also informs the interpretation of men as completers and women as attempters (Andriessen, 2006; Jaworski, 2014). As I have argued elsewhere, this interpretation is important because it contributes to the interpretation of two important facets of suicide: suicide methods and motivation or reasons for suicide (Jaworski, 2010a, 2014).

Traditionally, men prefer to use more lethal methods such as firearms, whereas women prefer to use methods considered less violent such as drug overdoses. Methods such as firearms are considered not only more visually and physically violent but also male, masculine, and active. Methods such as drug overdoses are viewed as less visually and physically violent and lethal and more feminine. Where the former is viewed as serious and willful, the latter is viewed as passive, reactive, and attention-seeking, configured by a fear of bodily disfigurement (Brockington, 2001; Callanan & Davis, 2011; Canetto & Sakinofsky, 1998; Galligan et al., 2010; Rich et al., 1992; Stack & Wasserman, 2009). Specifically, overdoses are said to imply dependence,

[1] I too have adopted an anthropocentric view of suicide in my earlier work (see Jaworski, 1999, 2002, 2003, 2005, 2008, 2010a, b, c, d, 2012, 2014, 2015, 2020, as some examples). Although I am not the first scholar to theorize suicide and agency through the lens of new materialism, this chapter departs from my earlier work on the performativity of suicide even though it is clear, at least to me in retrospect, that I would eventually arrive at the point of rethinking agency. I guess I needed time to arrive at this point in ways which make sense to me as a thinker and writer.

ambivalence, weakness, failure, foolishness, impulsivity, helplessness, and manipulation (Brockington, 2001; Cato & Canetto, 2003a, b; Dahlen & Canetto, 2002; Lewis et al., 1994). Such binary differences—male/active versus female/passive—are the reason for interpreting completed suicides as masculine and attempts as feminine (Callanan & Davis, 2011; Canetto, 1992–1993, 2008; Canetto & Sakinofsky, 1998; Coleman & Casey, 2011; Galligan et al., 2010). This is despite the fact that some women choose hanging and others do not survive drug overdoses (Jaworski, 2014; Range & Leach, 1998).

The interpretation of reasons for suicide suffers the same analytical fate when it comes to gender differences. One of the most enduring myths in western culture is that women die for love, whereas men die for glory (assuming they are heterosexual) (Canetto, 1992–1993). Women's suicides are often interpreted through the lens of relationship breakdown as a result of emotional turmoil. In contrast, men's suicides are read as signals of courage, pride, and resistance against external circumstances such as economic hardship, severe physical illness, and social isolation (Canetto, 1992–1993; 1997; Lieberman, 2003; Range & Leach, 1998). It is assumed that men assert their independence and physical prowess in crisis, whereas women internalize crisis by becoming depressed, dependent, and passive (Canetto & Lester, 1998; Coleman & Casey, 2011; Galligan et al., 2010; Langhinrichsen-Rohling et al., 1998, 2009). This is despite the fact that some studies demonstrate that male and female completed and attempted suicides are often motivated by reasons outside traditional explanations (Jaworski, 2014). Women engage with suicide due to sexual and emotional abuse, neglect, and economic hardship. Likewise, men engage with suicide as a result of emotional breakdowns and social isolation (Dahlen & Canetto, 2002; River, 2014). Through the combined focus on means of and reasons for suicide, male suicide is read as *publicly resisting* loss, whereas female suicide as *privately reacting* to it (Canetto & Lester, 1998; Jaworski, 2014). Importantly, whether resisting or reacting, both agentic responses are framed as an entirely human affair.

In response to the problem of agency and gender in suicide, this chapter analyzes the gendering of suicide in *The Virgin Suicides* (1993), written by Jeffrey Eugenides. Drawing on the new materialist feminist scholarship of Karen Barad, I will argue that agency in suicide is more than human, because that which is human depends on nonhuman materiality. I will also argue that the feminine, traditionally interpreted as reactive and passive in suicide, is in fact agentic. The chapter will begin by discussing the cultural context interpreting gender, and the way this context influences the interpretation of the suicides of the teenage Lisbon sisters—Cecilia, Bonnie, Therese, Lux, and Mary. I will then analyze the power of the masculine gaze and the way it frames and reframes the five suicides. I will also analyze the gendering of feminine bodies and sexuality. Finally, I will consider the significance of the suburban landscape and mood as key to understanding suicidal agency.

Karen Barad's Approach to Agency

Throughout the chapter I will draw heavily on the scholarship of the particle physicist and feminist theorist, Karen Barad (2007) and her work on agential realism. Critically deploying the work of Michel Foucault, Judith Butler and Niels Bohr, Donna Haraway, Vicki Kirby, Joseph Rouse, and others, Barad (2003, 2007) argues that we need a posthumanist performative account of agency, where agency is both human and nonhuman, best understood through its influence on the material and discursive world.[2] For Barad, agentic realism offers such an account because it:

> challenges the positioning of materiality as either a given or a mere effect of human agency [...] materiality is an active factor in the process of materialization. Nature is neither a passive surface awaiting the mark of culture nor the end product of cultural performances. (2007, p. 183)

In this sense, agency is not "aligned with human intentionality and subjectivity" but rather "is 'doing' and 'being' in its intra-activity" (Barad, 2007, pp. 177–178). Barad's (2003, 2007) account of agency is significant not only because agency is not always human but also because she reframes the biology or materiality of bodies as dynamic and active instead of mute and passive.

It is clear that Barad's (2003, 2007) account of agentic realism shares similarities with Judith Butler's (1990, 1993) theorization of performativity, which I have deployed extensively in earlier work to theorize the performativity of suicide (Jaworski, 2010a, 2014). Briefly, in her earlier work, Butler (1990) reworks Nietzsche's claim that there is no doer behind expressed deeds as both the doer and the deeds are constituted expression themselves, rather than the

[2] By posthumanist, Barad is referring to the "crucial recognition that non-humans play an important role in natural cultural practices, including everyday social practices, scientific practices, and practices that do not include humans" (2007, p. 32). As Barad states, "my use of 'posthumanism' marks a refusal to take the distinction between 'human' and 'nonhuman' for granted, and to found analyses on this presumably fixed and inherent set of categories" (2007, p. 32).

doer being the origin of the deeds. Thus, gender as performative is constituted by repeated acts over time within the regulatory framework of heteronormativity, which make the body look like the source of expressing gender rather than being a discursive effect like gender (Butler, 1990, pp. 33, 136). Later on, Butler reformulates her initial contention to argue that gender as performative is a "reiterative and citational practice by which discourse produces the effects it names" (Butler, 1993, p. 2). As such, norms precede, constrain, and exceed what we can and cannot do through our bodies and the bodies of others (Butler, 1993, 1997). In light of this, gendering, as Butler (1993) argues, and as I will show later, refers to the process of materializing or invoking meaning. In this sense, agency is possible because what we do and how we do things with and through our bodies draws "upon and reengage[s] conventions which have gained their power precisely through a *sedimented iterability*" (Butler, 1995, p. 134). Agency is present, but its presence is located at the very moment of a practice brought into being through performative actions (Butler, 1992, 1993, 1995).

Barad (2003, 2007) finds Butler's account of performativity useful yet problematic. On the one hand, Butler's account questions normative conditions and practices of representing. On the other hand, Butler's conception of materiality focuses on human bodies alone. While Butler (2004, p. 87) argues that the body is "irreducibly cultural and material at once," Barad questions this irreducibility because, as she interprets, Butler privileges the discursive over the material and "fails to recognize matter's dynamism" (2007, p. 64). For Barad (2007), bodies are not passive matter or mute surfaces upon which culture and history make their mark nor is discourse and language privileged over the material. Among other things, Barad (2007) turns to the notion of intra-action instead of the more common term, interaction, to develop her account of agentic realism. Unlike interaction, which assumes that "there are separate individual agencies that precede their interaction," the notion of intra-action "recognizes that distinct agencies do not precede, but rather *emerge through*, their inter-action" (Barad, 2007, p. 33, my emphasis). If agencies of different kind appear distinct, this distinctiveness exists because of their "*mutual entanglement*" (Barad, 2007, p. 3), or the way different materials, people, ideas, and contexts constantly change, blend, mutate, influence, and work inseparably in the course of bringing objects and subjects into being (Alaimo, 2008; Hickey-Moody, 2020; Tuana, 2008).[3]

[3] Barad's (2003, 2007) work, as innovative as it is, has been subject to critique. Unfortunately, I do not have the room in this chapter to consider this critique. For insightful and thought-provoking critiques, see Ahmed (2008), Braunmühl (2018), Norris (2016), Sullivan (2012), and Van der Tuin (2008).

In light of the above, what is so important about Barad's (2003, 2007) reconceptualization of agency to the analysis of suicide in this chapter? As Anu Salmela (2018, p. 3) argues in the context of female suicides in late-nineteenth-century Finland, Barad's new materialism is important because "it brings out the material dimension of suicides that scholars have hitherto largely neglected because of their focus has been on discourses." Furthermore, as Salmela (2018, p. 3) also argues, Barad's work "helps to question whether suicide [i]s a thoroughly human phenomenon," which "departs from the idea of things having a fixed essence" and therefore helps to analyze suicide "as a non-deterministic and ever-varying phenomenon." This is especially useful in the analysis of Jeffrey Eugenides' *The Virgin Suicides* because, as I will demonstrate, the novel offers an opportunity to think through the degree to which human and nonhuman agents influence the way the gender of suicide is interpreted in the context of the suicides of the five Lisbon sisters.

The Virgin Suicides

The Virgin Suicides is a novel narrated by ten middle-aged men who have come together during the 1990s to recall and explain the dramatic event of their teenage years, namely, the suicides of the mysterious five adolescent Lisbon sisters—Cecilia (13), Lux (14), Bonnie (15), Mary (16), and Therese (17)—which took place during the 1970s in their upper-middle-class neighborhood of Grosse Point, Michigan. As Cline (2018) and Iler (2017) pinpoint, the book retroactively constructs 13 months between the first and last suicide—approximately between June 1973 and July 1974. Thus, *The Virgin Suicides* is about loss, trauma, memory, and longing, as much as it is about obsession and voyeurism. Importantly, as Hoskin (2007) notes, the literary gothic form underpins the novel, where the suburb, pristine, and placid as it may appear hides horrors just below its surface. In an attempt to recount the past, the novel "operates like a weather system, with its own distinct logic" (Cline, 2018). Rooms, streets, neighborhoods, and landscapes are described in elaborate detail, demonstrating the degree to which the neighborhood boys were, and still are, obsessed with the five sisters.

The novel is not character or plot driven. What could be classified as an ending to the story, namely, the deaths of the five Lisbon sisters, is revealed in the first few pages.[4] This kind of structuring of the novel, as Shostak (2009, p. 813) writes, turns death into "the premise, not the endpoint, of

[4] As Eugenides remarks in an interview: "In that book, the first paragraph was the first thing I wrote, and it was a blueprint for the entire novel […]. The way I did it in *The Virgin Suicides* was to say: five sisters commit suicide; the first one does in chapter one, and then almost the entire book proceeds without anyone else killing herself, at least until the end […]. So suspense has been created about something that

storytelling," which means "the secrets of the narratives lie in the girls' mysterious motivation for suicide—the why, not the what." In this sense, the novel is driven by a desire to find an explanation only to realize that there will never be an explanation, or at least not one that makes sense to the narrators.[5] As Hoskin explains:

> [...] the deaths of the Lisbon girls constitutes their entrapment in the stagnated world of nostalgia, their memory forever trapped in objects, repetitive dreams, and rows of pleasant houses on suburban streets. These boys will always be outsiders looking in and looking back at the Lisbon house, and the girls will always be inside, illuminating a lack of not only temporal, but also physical proximity. (2007, p. 219)

For Shostak (2009), this turns the narrators into readers of their own memories and testimonies. Perhaps, this is one of the many reasons why *The Virgin Suicides* is a novel constituted by contradictions, which are "at once lyrically macabre, comically elegiac and, tenderly violent, and improbably realistic" (Shostak, 2009, p. 828).

Unsurprisingly, *The Virgin Suicides* has attracted scholarly attention in the literary and filmic circles.[6] From a literary studies perspective, Millard (2017) argues that *The Virgin Suicides* is a coming-of-age novel, whereas Kelly (2010) see it as an observer-hero tragedy. Shostak (2009, 2013), Dines (2012), and Iler (2017) focus on the narrative voice in the novel. Initially identifying it as an unusual first-person plural narrative voice, and later as impossible narrative voices, Shostak (2009, 2013) argues that this collective yet singular "we" offers the reader the chance to see the events according to different points of view. From a more humanities-based perspective, Wilhite (2015), Womack & Mallory-Kani (2007), and Dines (2012) focus on the sociopolitical context of the novel, examining the political upheavals during

has already been revealed. That was the trick of that book in terms of plot" (Schiff & Eugenides, 2006, p. 113).

[5] Interestingly, as Eugenides explains, "It's really not a book about suicide – it's a book about surviving suicide, or knowing someone who has committed suicide. The book never answers definitively why the girls do it, but it's about the feeling you're left with if someone you know and love does commit suicide" (Schiff & Eugenides, 2006, p. 114).

[6] *The Virgin Suicides* was made into a film by the director Sofia Coppola, who also wrote the screenplay in consultation with Jeffrey Eugenides. In drawing on extant literature, I mainly refer to scholarship focused on the novel rather than the film for obvious reasons, even though as some researchers have rightly pointed out, the film is a very faithful adaptation of the novel (Backman Rogers, 2018; Cline, 2018; Hoskin, 2007; Monden, 2013). Therefore, it makes sense to refer to some of the research on the filmic adaptation in so far as it visually captures the written content very well. In its readability, the novel is very visual and speaks to how something presents or appears rather than the content itself.

the 1970s in the USA, including the Watergate scandal and the resignation of the then US President Richard Nixon; the racial riots of the 1960s and the racism of whiteness; discourses of isolation and privatism; and the false nature of the American Dream. Hoskin (2007) and Dines (2012) focus on the role of nature and landscape in the novel, whereas Cline (2018), Collado-Rodríguez (2005), and Kostova (2013a, b) focus on trauma and death. Examining what is cultural and visual, Monden (2013) and Backman Rogers (2018) unpack analytically the significance of the body and gender in relation to feminine aesthetics of embodiment, girlhood, voyeurism, misogyny, and eroticism.

While existing scholarship addresses the context of the five suicides, very few pay attention to suicide itself. Monden's (2013) deft analysis considers suicide in the context of adolescent crisis. In so doing, Monden (2013) argues that the suicides represent a challenge to, and criticism of, the culturally and socially forced dependency and passivity on women. Thus, the five sisters exercised agency in the context of gender. Such agency, however, is interpreted through the anthropocentric terms only. Kostova (2013a) and Wilhite (2015) explicitly evoke a Durkheimian reading of the suicides by recognizing a relationship between individual deaths and collective suicidal outcomes, with suicide functioning as a barometer of social ills, described in the novel as "a symbol of what was wrong with the country" (Eugenides, 2011, p. 231). This is despite the fact that Durkheim has been extensively critiqued in the last 100 years, especially in regard to the degree to which his account of suicide and agency is masculine and masculinist (Lehmann, 1994; Jaworski, 1999, 2014; Witz & Marshall, 2003). Finally, Jafari et al. (2017) analyze gender through Thomas Joiner's (2005) interpersonal-psychological theory of suicide behavior. The authors argue that Cecilia and Lux were driven to suicide because of love: Cecilia because of an unrequited love interest and Lux because she was abandoned by Trip Fontaine. While Jafari et al. (2017) acknowledge the impact of isolation imposed by Mrs. Lisbon, their interpretation deprives the five sisters of mastery over their final destiny as if being female and feminine stands in the way of exercising agency *properly*.[7] Like previous analyses, no attention is given to considering whether human and nonhuman aspects contribute to the exercise of suicidal agency.

[7] For a brilliant critique of Joiner's theory from a perspective of gender, see Hjelmeland and Knizek (2020).

The Cultural Context of Interpreting Gender

I want to begin the task of analyzing the gendering of suicidal agency by considering the cultural context of interpreting suicide in *The Virgin Suicides*. While very important, this context is not only the sociocultural backdrop against which the story is set. Instead, the context I have in mind is embodied in the material practices each sister uses to kill herself, made evident in the collective yet singular "we" and the way this "we" refracts how different people interpret gender. In this way, the suicides of the five sisters are performative in so far as the use of various methods of suicide, and the interpretation of motives reiterate and cite what it means to kill oneself through the lens of gender. In Baradian terms, context is the apparatus, which co-constitutes some meanings at the expense of others. Context embodies *conditions of possibility*, enabled through a web of people that tell the story of the five suicides.

The performative character of suicide is made evident almost immediately in the novel. As the youngest of the five Lisbon sisters, Cecilia is the first to attempt suicide by "slitting her wrists like a Stoic while taking a bath, and when they found her, afloat in the pink pool, with the yellow eyes of someone possessed and her small body giving off the odor of a mature woman" (Eugenides, 2011, p. 3). Cecilia's agency is possible not only because she chose a particular method, but also because the materiality of the bath, razor, blood, and water co-constitutes the act, together with corporeal characteristics of her body, accentuated by a cultural and religious ideal found in western philosophy. The "blood on the bath mat; Mr. Lisbon's razor sunk in the toilet bowl, marbling the water" also co-constitutes the materiality of Cecilia's suicidality (Eugenides, 2011, p. 4). While Cecilia survives her attempt, she later jumps from the second story bedroom window during a party, impaling herself on the spike of the nearby fence. Eugenides evoked this moment as follows: "the wind sounded huffed, once, and then the moist thud jolted us, the sound of a watermelon breaking open" (2011, p. 30). The finality of Cecilia's death emerges through the entanglement with the natural world, sound, physical objects, and a metaphor used to explain the corporeal violence. It also emerges through Mr. Lisbon "trying to lift her off the spike that had punctured her left breast, travelled through her inexplicable heart, separated two vertebrae without shattering either, and come out her back, ripping the dress and finding the air again" (Eugenides, 2011, pp. 30–31). This, I think, shows the degree to which agency is rendered visible through movement as much as the specific features that mark the body as suicided.

The rest of the Lisbon sisters kill themselves on, or shortly after, the first-year anniversary of Cecilia's death. Bonnie hangs herself in the basement. Bonnie's pink dress and white confirmation stockings embody the suicide, as do the shoes and balloons left over from Cecilia's party. The narrators go on to say that: "She spun slowly, and at one point her face broke out of the seaweed of balloons, showing us the reality of the death she'd chosen. It was a world of blackening eye sockets, blood pooling in lower extremities, stiffening joints" (Eugenides, 2011, pp. 215–216). Unlike Bonnie, Mary gasses herself in the oven, described as having: "put her head in the oven shortly thereafter, on hearing Bonnie kick the trunk from under herself" (Eugenides, 2011, p. 216). Therese is next, who overdoses on "sleeping pills washed down with gin" (Eugenides, 2011, p. 216). Lux dies by carbon monoxide poisoning after sealing herself inside the garage with the car running and is found "in the front seat, gray-faced and serene, holding a cigarette lighter that had burned its coils into her palm" (Eugenides, 2011, p. 216). Mary survives, but only for another month. In the end, she kills herself "in a sleeping bag, and full of sleeping pills," described as wearing too much smudged make-up, a black dress and veil (Eugenides, 2011, p. 237).

Whether it is the use of the rope to hang, gassing in the oven, swallowing of sleeping pills or poisoning oneself with carbon monoxide, these material practices and their objects work together in proximity to materialize death. That is, you cannot separate the means of suicide from the inscriptions on the bodies, because bodies, objects, the immediate material environment and ideas of what it takes to kill oneself work in a dynamic performative relationship through which suicidal agency emerges. Indeed, the five sisters exercise their human agency, but their agency is simultaneously entangled with nonhuman agencies. While we may be able to tell a difference between such agencies, my contention is that you cannot separate them to make sense of the suicides. Importantly, physical bodies are not passive as if waiting for intent to materialize before making its corporeal mark visible. Rather, female bodies actively co-constitute the intent to die through the act of killing oneself. Regardless of whether the outcome is survival or death, it is clear that the female bodies of the Lisbon sisters were agentic instead of passive. Importantly, nonhuman agency does not undermine human agency: What is human and nonhuman works together to enable one another.

If gender has not been evoked explicitly so far in the analysis, it is because gender has been part of the picture all along. This is not simply because the five sisters possess female bodies. Instead, gender is hailed performatively through the way the neighbors try to explain the motives behind the five suicides. In relation to Cecilia, two local mothers blame the parents, suggesting that Cecilia did not want to die, but rather: "wanted out of that house," because "she wanted out of that decorating scheme" (Eugenides, 2011, p. 17). Others wonder whether "it was true that the girl had only fallen and cut herself" (Eugenides, 2011, p. 18). Some neighborhood kids think Cecilia was copying Seneca given her religiosity, whereas others thought an unreciprocated teenage crush is the reason for her death. The hospital psychiatrist, Dr. Hornicker, notes that Cecilia's attempt is "an act of aggression inspired by the repression of adolescent libidinal urges" (Eugenides, 2011, p. 21). Despite the visceral violence, Cecilia did not mean "to end her life. Her act was a cry for help" (Eugenides, 2011, p. 21). The local parish priest listed Cecilia's death as an accident (as were the other sisters), because it was difficult to tell what the sisters "were really trying to do" (Eugenides, 2011, p. 38). Initially, Cecilia's death is not reported in the newspapers because of its "sheer prosaicness," in contrast to the murder suicides committed by fathers who were fired at the automotive plants due to the economic recession (Eugenides, 2011, pp. 93–94).

Regardless of whether it is the interior design of the house, a teenage crush (which turns out to be an incorrect judgment), the psychiatric assessment, religious interpretations, or media representations, Cecilia's suicidal agency is continually questioned and erased by those around her because she was a girl. She is engendered as girlish not simply because she was 13 but because her femininity is perceived as passive and as lacking any sense of autonomy (Driscoll, 2002; Monden, 2013). Despite the fact that her death is so violent, it is as if Cecilia's female and feminine body renders her incapable of deciding properly or exercising suicidal agency fully. Ultimately, she is read as pathological, attention-seeking, and desiring rescue instead of death. This diffracting demonstrates the degree to which gendered discourses operate in the gendering of Cecilia's death.

Of course, Cecilia's suicide is not the only one interpreted through gender. As the narrators tell us, many are convinced that Cecilia's death caused other deaths. That is:

> In the bathtub, cooking the broth of her own blood, Cecilia had released an airborne virus [...]. The other girls, safe in their own rooms, had smelled something strange, sniffed the air, but ignored it. Black tendrils of smoke had crept under their doors, rising up behind their studious backs to form the evil shapes of smoke or shadow take on in cartoons: a black-hatted assassin brandishing a dagger; an anvil about to drop. (Eugenides, 2011, p. 158)

What is interesting about this explanation is that it renders the other four sisters as passive and reactive as well. Here, the world of biology vis-à-vis contagion and infection precludes the Lisbon sisters from being agentic, meaning they could not possibly do this of their own volition. But this is not the only explanation for what is framed as a "suicide pack" toward the end of the novel (Eugenides, 2011, p. 223). Instead, the suicides are interpreted as "reasoned refusal to accept the world as it was handed down to them, so full of flaws" (Eugenides, 2011, p. 245). For me, this is perhaps the truest explanation, given Mrs. Lisbon's complete isolation of her daughters from the rest of the world. In so doing, it offers a different reading of the five suicides: A challenge and critique of the "culturally and socially imposed passivity and dependency, and those who impose such burdens" (Monden, 2013, p. 153). Thus, the suicides of the five sisters are willful and deliberate, demonstrating that what is rendered as female and feminine is agentic.

The Power of the Masculine Gaze

In her germinal essay first published in 1975, the feminist critic and film scholar Laura Mulvey (1990) first introduced the concept of the male gaze or the sexual pleasure associated with looking in traditional Hollywood cinema's use of scopophilia. This involves the camera directing and encouraging the viewer to stare at the female body, thus creating a mode of looking associated with the male protagonist's point of view. Traditionally, as Mulvey (1990, p. 62) explains, the displayed woman has two functions: "as erotic object for the characters within the screen story, and as erotic object for the spectator within the auditorium, with a shifting tension between the looks on either side of the screen." However, as E. Ann Kaplan (2010) notes, the gaze is not literally male, but rather a masculine position activated through the act of looking. While this concept is nowadays more accurately described as a heterosexual masculine gaze, it still frames the man as a bearer of the look, or the subject in control of the looking, whereas the woman is a spectacle through which her place is to be the bearer of meaning instead of a meaning-maker (Bloom, 2017; Chandhuri, 2006; Mulvey, 1990; White, 2017). In other words, what is male is active, whereas what is female is passive.

Given its context, the concept of the masculine gaze is often applied to analyze films, television shows, visual arts, advertisements, and any other visual content. Yet, as Elizabeth Skomp (2003) shows, this concept can be applied to the analysis of literature. Skomp (2003) re-adapts the three aspects of Mulvey (1990) notion of the male gaze: The gaze of the author; the gaze of men within a narrative; and the gaze of readers. For the purpose of the analysis here, I focus on the gaze of the boys/men in the novel. This gaze is important not only because it permeates the novel but also because it frames the intelligibility of the five suicides. The storytelling of the collective "we" directs the gaze of the male subjects at the female body. In this sense, the neighborhood boys are the subjects, the active bearers of the look in control of the direction of the story. The five Lisbon sisters are the passive objects of the obsessive, youthful male heterosexual desire, which records every detail of their feminine, eroticized bodies.

The masculine gaze objectifies the bodies of the five sisters in a number of ways. First, we, as readers, know what they look like:

> They were short, round-buttocked in denim, with roundish cheeks that recalled the same dorsal softness. Whenever we got a glimpse, their faces looked indecently revealed, as though we were used to seeing women in veils. No one could understand how Mr. and Mrs. Lisbon had produced such beautiful children. (Eugenides, 2011, pp. 7–8)

Specifically, Bonnie is described as being a foot taller than her sisters, with a "sallow complexion and sharp nose of a nun"; Therese has "a heavier a face, the cheeks and eyes of a cow," a "big girl" with a high forehead and cupid lips; Mary has darker hair and "a widow's peak and fuzz above her upper lip"; Lux "radiates health and mischief" with a tight fitting dress; and Cecilia always wears a vintage "wedding dress with the shorn hem" (Eugenides, 2011, pp. 26, 59, 102). Secondly, we know certain details about the content of the Lisbon house such as "crumpled panties," "stuffed animals," "a crucifix draped with a brassiere," or the "gauzy chambers of canopied beds" (Eugenides, 2011, p. 9). Third, we know some of their thoughts when the neighborhood boys read Cecilia's diary, claiming that they "felt the imprisonment of being a girl, the way it made your mind active and dreamy, and how you ended up knowing which colors went together" (Eugenides, 2011, p. 43). Finally, we know what the five sisters did, whether it is: "the pink heel of a hand flattening against the glass, then rubbing back and forth to uncover the bright mosaic of an eye, looking out at us," or watching Lux's sexual trysts on the roof of her house (Eugenides, 2011, pp. 145, 160).

Powerful and far-reaching as it might seem, the masculine gaze does not always work. During the night of Cecilia's party, the boys are surprised to discover that "instead of five replicas with the same blond hair and puffy cheeks we saw that they were distinct beings, their personalities beginning to transform their faces and reroute their expressions" (Eugenides, 2011, p. 26).

Furthermore, those boys who take the Lisbon sisters to the homecoming dance discover that:

> At home, each boy had pictured the Lisbon girls amid the stock scenery of our impoverished imaginations – cavorting in the surf or playfully feeling at the ice-skating rink, dangling ski-hat pom-poms like ripe fruit before our faces. In the car, however, beside the actual living girls, the boys realized the paltriness of these images. Inverse properties were also discarded: notions of the girls as damaged or demented [...] they had something to say about the families in each one, which meant *they had been looking out at us as intensely as we had been looking in.* (Eugenides, 2011, pp. 123–124, my emphasis)

In fact, as the novel draws to an end, the narrators realize "the girls had been trying to talk to us all along, to elicit our help, but we'd been too infatuated to listen. Our surveillance had been so focused we missed nothing but a simple returned gaze" (Eugenides, 2011, p. 199). This, as Shostak (2009, p. 817) argues, reveals that "the narrators' vision of the girls is just that, a vision determined by their subject position as innocent males and shaped by the narcissism of their youth."

The failure of the masculine gaze reveals the degree to which the gaze functions as an "agential cut," which "cut 'things' together and apart" (2007, p. 178). The gaze divides different agencies, framing what is to be included and excluded (Barad, 2014; Warefield, 2016). Therefore, if something appears as distinct, it means it has been "cut." With this in mind, I want to suggest that the masculine gaze of the narrators cuts into what we can and cannot know about the Lisbon sisters, and the way we come to know of them through a girlish white *form* of femininity. This form, I want to suggest, depends on not simply *what* is described in such detail, but rather on *how* what is described engenders the five sisters. Interestingly, the sisters are almost always represented as passive even though the playing of records, the use of Virgin cards to communicate, and the flashing lights portray the sisters as anything but passive. In this way, the material world in the shape of objects renders the sisters as agentic even though the masculine gaze attempts to frame out their agency. Perhaps it is the narrators themselves who are reactive and passive, unable to see past their masculine heterosexual desires.

Feminine Bodies and Sexuality

While the sisters are responding to bad circumstances, the narrators do not perceive them as having agency, not only because they are unaware of being watched but also because of the urge to help them to escape their confinement. In their passivity, the sisters come across as beautiful, smiling, playful, mysterious, mature, and all-knowing despite their fragility and vulnerability. As the narrators describe: "Added to their loveliness was a new mysterious suffering, perfectly silent, visible in the blue puffiness beneath their eyes or the way they would sometimes stop in mid-stride, look down, and shake their heads as though disagreeing with life" (Eugenides, 2011, p. 52). In contrast, the neighborhood boys appear to be free, active, naïve, and immature, busy with trying to solve the mystery of the Lisbon sisters and, toward the end, busy with trying to rescue them. In this sense, the gendering of the five sisters as much as the neighborhood boys abides by the traditional ideas of heterosexual masculinity and femininity, where the former embodies instrumentality and activity and the latter embodies passivity and emotions. Unlike the neighborhood boys, the five sisters are bound to the material conditions of their feminine bodies, made evident in descriptions such as: "five glittering daughters in their home-made dresses, all lace and ruffle, *bursting with their fructifying flesh*" (Eugenides, 2011, p. 8, my emphasis).[8] The bodies of the neighborhood boys are never of any importance throughout the novel. Their masculinity is somehow disembodied.

Unlike her sisters, Lux, the second youngest of the five sisters, is framed as promiscuous, with a talent for evading her mother's strict Catholic watchful eye. In the first half of the novel, the narrators recall Lux's countless trysts with faceless teenage boys from her school, which they see as a sign of "her disequilibrium" (Eugenides, 2011, p. 68). This includes Lux's date with Trip Fontaine, which culminates in them having sex on the football field during the homecoming dance. This framing of heterosexual teenage promiscuity continues in the second half of the novel when Lux sneaks boys and men onto the roof of the Lisbon house: "It was crazy to make love on the roof at any time," the narrators tell us, "but to make love on the roof in winter suggested derangement, desperation and self-destructiveness far in excess of any pleasure snatched beneath the dripping trees" (Eugenides, 2011, pp. 149–150). Dr. Hornicker sees Lux's promiscuity as a sign of confusing sex with love, whereby "sex

[8] It is important to note that the five sisters are aware of the way their agency was interpreted. In response to who was going to take whom to the homecoming dance, Mary said: "They're just going to raffle us off" (Eugenides, 2011, p. 116).

became a substitute for the comfort she needed as a result of her sister's suicide" (Eugenides, 2011, p. 86). Although Lux can be read momentarily as being in possession of her sexuality, she is predominantly framed as fragile, unstable, and out of control.

In contrast, I am going to suggest that things are different once we take a bird's eye view of the function of Lux's feminine body and sexuality. That is, feminine bodies and sexuality play a key role in regaining a sense of autonomy and self-assertion even if the consequences are deadly. This is most evident when the neighborhood boys finally make their way to the Lisbon house in an attempt to help the four sisters escape their confinement in the evening of June 14. Upon entering the house, the boys encounter Lux, who appears to be waiting for them:

> She looked down at herself, adjusted the halter, tucked with one thumb the exposed plumpness on her right side. Then she looked up again as thought into each of our eyes at once, and began walking forward [...]. She took one more step and her face reappeared. For a second it didn't seem alive: it was too white, the cheeks too perfectly carved, and the arched eyebrows painted on, the lips made of wax. But then she came closer and we saw the light in her eyes we have been looking for ever since [...]. She came up to Chase Buell. She came so close her breath stirred his hair. And then, in front of us all, Lux unbuckled the belt [...]. All the while she stared into his eyes, rising on the balls of her feet, and in the quiet house we heard the pants unsnap [...]. Lux's eyes, burning and velvet, glowed in the dim room [...]. Even though she was doing it to Chase Buell, we could all feel Lux undoing us, reaching out for us and taking us as she knew we could be taken. Just at the last second, another soft thud came from downstairs. (Eugenides, 2011, pp. 210–211)

Lengthy as it is, this excerpt demonstrates the degree to which Lux is not only in control of her sexuality but also utilizes her position as an object of sexual desire to enable the suicides of her other sisters. My point, then, is this: Just because someone embodies a form in the shape of a female body, which is interpreted as pretty and girlish, does not mean this form is passive and incapable of embodying intentional action. While the suicides of the four sisters do not lead to livable outcomes, nonetheless they escape a living death. They are adolescent girls in crisis who do not need adult intervention, because they orchestrate an intervention themselves, making the boys realize they "were pawns in this strategy, useful for a time" (Eugenides, 2011, p. 212). In a nutshell, all five sisters demonstrate that you can be agentic *because* of femininity, not *despite* it. Such agency, however, is not individual, but rather enabled by the content of the material world, be it their clothes, the house they lived in, the EMS trucks that came to collect their bodies, the school they went to, or the neighborhood they lived in.

Suburban Landscape and Mood

The suburban landscape is inescapably part of the gendering of suicide in *The Virgin Suicides*. As Dines (2012) writes, death and decay occur in synchrony with the five deaths in the Lisbon household. So, what can we make of this landscape and what does it evoke? For me, the landscape co-constitutes the meaning of loss of beauty, youth, and life, as much as it co-constitutes emptiness and absence made evident in the way of the five deaths. This begins within the first few pages of the novel, when we find out that Cecilia attempted suicide during June's fish-flying season:

> when each year our town is covered by the flotsam of those ephemeral insects. Rising in the clouds from the algae in the polluted lake, they blacken windows, coat cars and street-lamps, plaster the municipal docks and festoon the rigging of sailboats, always tin the same brown ubiquity of flying scum. (Eugenides, 2011, p. 4)

The synchrony with nonhuman agencies does not stop with the world of insects, algae, and polluted water. The landscape is dotted with dying trees, marked ready for removal because of the Dutch elm disease. As more trees disappear so do the sisters. The elm in front of the Lisbon house is the last tree to be removed, which "stood blighted, trying to raise its stunted arms, a creature clubbed mute, only its sudden voicelessness making us realize it had been speaking all along" (Eugenides, 2011, pp. 178–179). In this sense, nonhuman agencies vis-à-vis suburban landscape embrace the suicidal agency of the Lisbon sisters through death.

The synchrony of human and nonhuman agencies within the suburban landscape, I want to suggest, creates a mood of decay. Mood, as Saige Walton (2018) argues in the context of film, "does not belong to single entity or body, least of all human." Instead, mood is a mode of feeling (Highmore, 2013) that emerges through the suburban landscape as it resonates with feelings of loss, grief, and longing in the novel. This is evident not only through the decaying natural world but also through the materiality of the Lisbon house. Initially, the house is portrayed as a "comfortable suburban house," "full of stark colonial furniture," and "orange carpeting and a brown vinyl sofa," among other things (Eugenides, 2011, pp. 8, 25). During the year of the suicides, desolation begins to creep in: "the blue slate roof, which in certain lights had resembled a pond suspended in the air, visibly darkened. The yellow bricks turned brown. Bats flew out of the chimney in the evening" (Eugenides, 2011, p. 88). This desolation is as material as it is metaphorical, for once Mrs. Lisbon institutes total isolation, the house is described as receding "behind its mists of youth being choked off" and as having "truly died" once Mr. Lisbon loses his teaching job at the local high school (Eugenides, 2011, pp. 145, 162). In this sense, then, we can read suicidal agency as a movement and process via human and nonhuman entities, rather than only a specific outcome of intent. As the house unravels, so do the four sisters as they draw closer to their final days.

Conclusion

In concluding this chapter, I want to re-emphasize that *The Virgin Suicides* offers us an opportunity to think through the degree to which human and nonhuman agents influence the way the gender of suicide is interpreted and can be interpreted. Unlike earlier interpretations, this novel is not misogynistic despite the clear presence of sexism and patriarchy during a tumultuous period of the American history and politics in which the story of the five Lisbon sisters is set. If anything, the narrating voice Eugenides (2011) develops offers us opportunities to see not only the cracks in the patriarchal system, but also the degree to which sexism has violent implications in the context of suicide.

By arguing that human and nonhuman agencies engender suicidal agency, this chapter demonstrated that the gendering of suicide depends on a number of aspects, which, as I examined, include the context of interpretation; the power of the masculine gaze; significance of feminine bodies and sexuality; and finally, suburban landscape and mood. Importantly, the chapter has demonstrated that bodies are not passive nor are they mere surfaces upon which culture is inscribed. Read through the analytical lens of posthumanist agency, the five bodies of the Lisbon sisters embody agency, made evident through movement, co-constituted through objects, things, people, ideas, and the natural biological world. Without these agents, as it were, it is impossible to make sense of what *The Virgin Suicides* offers to its readers.

By interpreting the suicides of the Lisbon sisters, this chapter argued that young women are not necessarily passive or uncertain in their suicidal intentions just because they embody a girlish aesthetic of femininity or are pervasively seen as objects of masculine heterosexual desire. If they are interpreted as passive, it is because they are framed as such. Once we challenge this framing, it is possible to re-read passivity outside the active/passive binary and see it as a form of agency. Young women do not have to exhibit characteristics of masculine violence nor does this mean they do not want to die. On the contrary, young women like the Lisbon sisters do die, and society does them a disservice by not taking their struggles seriously by considering them less important than the significantly higher rates of male suicide. Furthermore, society does them a disservice by assuming that what is vulnerable and fragile is voiceless and lacks determination. In this sense, the living or those left behind to make sense of suicide are just as much part of the gendering of suicide as are those who choose suicide. In this sense, then, Dr. Armstrong, who stitched up Cecilia's wrist wounds should have listened more carefully when she said: "Obviously, Doctor [...] you've never been a thirteen-year-old-girl" (Eugenides, 2011, p. 7).

References

Ahmed, S. (2008). Imaginary prohibitions. Some preliminary remarks on the founding gestures of the 'new materialism'. *European Journal of Women's Studies, 15*(1), 23–39. https://doi.org/10.1177/1350506807084854

Alaimo, S. (2008). Trans-corporeal feminisms and the ethical space of nature. In S. Alaimo & S. Hekman (Eds.), *Material Feminisms* (pp. 237–264). Indiana University Press.

Andriessen, K. (2006). On "intention" in the definition of suicide. *Suicide & Life-Threatening Behavior, 36*(5), 533–538. https://doi.org/10.1521/suli.2006.36.5.533

Backman Rogers, A. (2018). Imagining absence as abjection: The female body in Sofia Coppola's *The Virgin Suicides*. *Screening the Past*, 43. http://www.screeningthepast.com/2018/02/imaging-absence-as-abjection-the-female-body-in-sofia-coppolas-the-virgin-suicides. Accessed 5 Oct 2020.

Barad, K. (2003). Posthumanist performativity: Toward an understanding of how matter comes to matter. *Signs, 28*(3), 801–831. https://doi.org/10.1086/345321

Barad, K. (2007). *Meeting the universe halfway: Quantum physics and the entanglement of matter and meaning*. Duke University Press.

Barad, K. (2014). Diffracting diffraction: Cutting together-apart. *Parallax, 20*(3), 168–187. https://doi.org/10.1080/13535645.2014.927623

Bloom, J. D. (2017). *Reading the male gaze in literature and culture: Studies in erotic epistemology*. Plagrave Macmillan.

Braunmühl, C. (2018). Beyond hierarchical oppositions: A feminist critique of Karen Barad's agential realism. *Feminist Theory, 19*(2), 223–240. https://doi.org/10.1177/1464700117741243

Brockington, I. (2001). Suicide in women. *International Clinical Psychopharmacology, 16*(2), S7–S19. https://doi.org/10.1097/00004850-200103002-00003
Butler, J. (1990). *Gender trouble: Feminism and the subversion of identity.* Routledge.
Butler, J. (1992). Contingent foundations: Feminism and the question of "postmodernism". In J. Butler & J. W. Scott (Eds.), *Feminists theorize the political* (pp. 3–21). Routledge.
Butler, J. (1993). *Bodies that matter: On the discursive limits of "sex".* Routledge.
Butler, J. (1995). For a careful reading. In S. Benhabib, J. Butler, D. Cornell, & N. Fraser (Eds.), *Feminist contentions: A philosophical exchange* (pp. 127–144). Routledge.
Butler, J. (1997). *Excitable speech.* Routledge.
Butler, J. (2004). *Undoing gender.* Routledge.
Callanan, V. J., & Davis, M. S. (2011). Gender differences in suicide method: Do women avoid facial disfiguration? *Sex Roles, 65,* 867–879. https://doi.org/10.1007/s11199-011-0043-0
Canetto, S. S. (1992–1993). She died for love and he for glory: Gender myths of suicidal behavior. *Omega, 26*(1), 1–17. https://doi.org/10.2190/74YQ-YNB8-R43R-7X4A
Canetto, S. S. (1995). Men who survive a suicidal act: Successful coping or failed masculinity? In D. Sabo & D. F. Gordon (Eds.), *Men's health and illness: gender, power and the body* (pp. 292–304). Sage Publications.
Canetto, S. S. (1997). Gender and suicidal behavior: Theories and evidence. In R. W. Maris, M. M. Silverman, & S. S. Canetto (Eds.), *Review of suicidology* (pp. 138–167). Guildford Press.
Canetto, S. S. (2008). Women and suicidal behavior. *The American Journal of Orthopsychiatry, 78*(2), 259–266. https://doi.org/10.1037/a0013973
Canetto, S. S., & Lester, D. (1998). Gender, culture, and suicidal behavior. *Transcultural Psychiatry, 35*(2), 163–190. https://doi.org/10.1177/136346159803500201
Canetto, S. S., & Sakinofsky, I. (1998). The gender paradox in suicide. *Suicide & Life-Threatening Behavior, 28*(1), 1–23. https://doi.org/10.1111/j.1943-278X.1998.tb00622.x
Cato, J. E., & Canetto, S. S. (2003a). Young adults' reactions to gay and lesbian peers who became suicidal following "coming out" to their parents. *Suicide & Life-Threatening Behavior, 33*(2), 201–210. https://doi.org/10.1521/suli.33.2.201.22774
Cato, J. E., & Canetto, S. S. (2003b). Attitudes and beliefs about suicidal behavior when coming out is the precipitant of the suicidal behavior. *Sex Roles, 49*(9–10), 497–505. https://doi.org/10.1023/A:1025880622932
Chandhuri, S. (2006). *Feminist film theorists: Laura Mulvey, Kaja Silverman, Teresa de Lauretis, Barbara Creed.* Routledge.

Choo, C. C., Harris, K. M., & Ho, R. C. (2017). Prediction of lethality in suicide attempts: Gender matters. *Omega, 80*(1), 87–103. https://doi.org/10.1177/0030222817725182

Cline, E. (2018, October 2). "The virgin suicides" still holds the mysteries of adolescence. *The New Yorker*. https://www.newyorker.com/books/second-read/the-virgin-suicides-still-holds-the-mysteries-of-adolescence. Accessed 5 Oct 2020.

Coleman, D., & Casey, J. T. (2011). The social nature of male suicide: A new analytic model. *International Journal of Men's Health, 10*(3), 240–252. https://doi.org/10.3149/JMH.1003.240

Collado-Rodríguez, F. (2005). Back to myth and ethical compromise: García Márquez's traces on Jeffrey Eugenides's "The Virgin Suicides". *Atlantis, 27*(2), 27–40.

Dahlen, E. R., & Canetto, S. S. (2002). The role of gender and suicide precipitant in attitudes towards nonfatal suicidal behavior. *Death Studies, 26*, 99–116. https://doi.org/10.1080/074811802753455235

De Leo, D., Burgis, S., Bertolote, J. M., Kerkhof, A. J. F. M., & Bille-Brahe, U. (2006). Definitions of suicidal behavior. Lessons learned from the WHO/EURO Multicentre Study. *Crisis, 27*(1), 4–15. https://doi.org/10.1027/0227-5910.27.1.4

Dines, M. (2012). Suburban gothic and the ethnic uncanny in Jeffrey Eugenides's *The Virgin Suicides*. *Journal of American Studies, 46*(4), 959–975. https://doi.org/10.1017/S0021875812000722

Driscoll, C. (2002). *Girls: Feminine adolescence in popular culture and cultural theory*. Colombia University Press.

Eugenides, J. (2011). *The virgin suicides*. Bloomsbury.

Galligan, S. B., Barnett, R. V., Brennan, M. A., & Israel, G. D. (2010). Understanding the link between gender role conflict, resilience and propensity for suicide in adolescent and emerging adult males. *International Journal of Men's Health, 9*(3), 201–210. https://doi.org/10.3149/jmh.0903.201

Hickey-Moody, A. (2020). New materialism, ethnography, and social engaged practice: Space-time folds and the matter of agency. *Qualitative Inquiry, 26*(7), 724–732. https://doi.org/10.1177/1077800418810728

Highmore, B. (2013). Feeling our way: Mood and cultural studies. *Communication and Critical/ Cultural Studies, 10*(4), 427–438. https://doi.org/10.1080/14791420.2013.840387

Hjelmeland, H., & Knizek, B. L. (2020). The emperor's new clothes? A critical look at the interpersonal theory of suicide. *Death Studies, 44*(3), 168–178. https://doi.org/10.1080/07481187.2018.1527796

Hoskin, B. (2007). Playground love: Landscape and longing in Sofia Coppola's *The Virgin Suicides*. *Literature/Film Quarterly, 35*(3), 214–221.

Iler, D. R. (2017). Suicide and the afterlife of the cold war: Accident, intentionality, and periodicity in Paul Auster's *Leviathan* and Jeffrey Eugenides's *The Virgin*

Suicides. Modern Fiction Studies, 63(4), 737–758. https://doi.org/10.1353/mfs.2017.0055
Jafari, S., Jafari, S., & Astar, R. K. (2017). The acquired capability for lethal self-injury: Case studies of Plath's *The Bell Jar* and Eugenides' *The Virgin Suicides*. *International Journal of Applied Linguistics and English, 6*(5), 21–26. https://doi.org/10.7575/aiac.ijalel.v.6n.5p.21
Jaworski, K. (1999). Challenging a classic: Gendered dilemmas in Durkheim's *Suicide*. In M. Collis, L. Munro, & S. Russell (Eds.), *Proceedings of challenges and prospects: Sociology for a New Millennium, the Australian Sociological Association Annual Conference* (pp. 231–238). Monash University.
Jaworski, K. (2002). Bodily inscriptions and gender in legal discourses of suicide. *Sister in Law, 6*, 168–184.
Jaworski, K. (2003). Suicide and gender: Reading suicide through Butler's notion of performativity. *Journal of Australian Studies, 76*, 137–146. https://doi.org/10.1080/14443050309387832
Jaworski, K. (2005). (Un)desirable acts of death: Gendered truths in the cultural production of suicide. In E. Lorek-Jezinska & K. Wieckowska (Eds.), *Corporeal inscriptions: Representations of the body in cultural and literary texts and practices* (pp. 2019–2220). The Nicolaus Copernicus University Press.
Jaworski, K. (2008). 'Elegantly wasted': The celebrity deaths of Michael Hutchence and Paula Yates. *Continuum Journal of Media & Cultural Studies, 22*(6), 777–791. https://doi.org/10.1080/10304310802452446
Jaworski, K. (2010a). The gender-ing of suicide. *Australian Feminist Studies, 25*(63), 47–61. https://doi.org/10.1080/08164640903499752
Jaworski, K. (2010b). The male preserve of martyrdom': Palestinian female suicide bombers in Australian newsprint media. *Feminist Media Studies, 10*(2), 119–132. https://doi.org/10.1080/14680771003672247
Jaworski, K. (2010c). What it means to see: Reading gender in medical examinations of suicide. In T. Rudge & D. Holmes (Eds.), *Abjectly boundless: Boundaries, bodies and health work* (pp. 49–65). Ashgate.
Jaworski, K. (2010d). The author, agency and suicide. *Social Identities, 16*(5), 675–687. https://doi.org/10.1080/13504630.2010.509572
Jaworski, K. (2012). The visibility of difference: Gender and suicide in psy-knowledge. In G. Araoz (Ed.), *Mad/Sad/Bad: philosophical, political, poetic and artistic reflections on the history of madness* (pp. 105–116). Inter-Disciplinary Press.
Jaworski, K. (2014). *The gender of suicide: Knowledge production, theory and suicidology*. Ashgate.
Jaworski, K. (2015). Suicide, agency and the limits of power. In L. Broz & D. Munster (Eds.), *Suicide and agency: Anthropological perspectives on self-destruction, personhood and power* (pp. 183–201). Ashgate.
Jaworski, K. (2020). Towards ethics of wonder and generosity in critical suicidology. *Social Epistemology, 34*(6), 589–600. https://doi.org/10.1080/02691728.2020.1725923

Joiner, T. E. (2005). *Why people die by suicide*. Harvard University Press.

Kaplan, E. A. (2010). Is the gaze male? In M. Furstenau (Ed.), *The film theory reader: Debates and arguments* (pp. 209–221). Routledge.

Kelly, A. (2010). Moments of decision in contemporary American fiction: Roth, Auster, Eugenides. *Critique, 51*(4), 313–332. https://doi.org/10.1080/00111611003643905

Kostova, B. V. (2013a). Collective suffering, uncertainty and trauma in Jeffrey Eugenides's *The Virgin Suicides*: Of bystanders, perpetrators and victims. *Atlantis, 35*(2), 47–63.

Kostova, B. V. (2013b). Working through collective trauma: Metafiction, intertextuality, and the need for externalization and relativisation of trauma in *The Virgin Suicides*. *Estudios Ingleses de la Universidad Complutense, 21*, 66–85. https://doi.org/10.5209/rev_EIUC.2013.v21.43274

Kral, M. J. (2019). *The idea of suicide: Contagion, imitation, and cultural diffusion*. Routledge.

Langhinrichsen-Rohling, J., Lewinsohn, P., Rohde, P., Seeley, J., Monson, C. C., Meyer, K. A., & Langford, R. (1998). Gender differences in the suicide-related behaviors of adolescent and young adults. *Sex Roles, 39*(11–12), 839–849. https://doi.org/10.1023/A:1018824621193

Langhinrichsen-Rohling, J., Friend, J., & Powell, A. (2009). Adolescent suicide, gender, and culture: A rate and risk factor analysis. *Aggression and Violent Behavior, 14*, 402–414. https://doi.org/10.1016/j.avb.2009.06.010

Lehmann, J. M. (1994). *Durkheim and women*. University of Nebraska Press.

Lewis, J. R., Atkinson, J., & Shovlin, J. (1994). Gender differences in attributions about suicide and alcohol use. *Omega, 28*(2), 139–149. https://doi.org/10.2190/NBWG-HPP6-AR8N-RUPT

Lieberman, L. (2003). *Leaving you: The cultural meaning of suicide*. Ivan R. Dee.

Millard, K. (2017). *Coming of age in contemporary American fiction*. Edinburgh University Press.

Monden, M. (2013). Contemplating in a dream-like room: *The Virgin Suicides* and the aesthetic imagination of girlhood. *Film, Fashion & Consumption, 2*(2), 139–158. https://doi.org/10.1386/ffc.2020139_1

Mulvey, L. (1990). Visual pleasure and narrative cinema. In P. Erens (Ed.), *Issues in Feminist Film Criticism* (pp. 28–57). Indiana University Press.

Norris, M. (2016). Ecocriticism and moral responsibility: The question of agency in Karen Barad's performativity theory. *The Journal of the Midwest Modern Language Association, 49*(1), 157–184. https://doi.org/10.1353/mml.2016.0026

Range, L. M., & Leach, M. M. (1998). Gender, culture, and suicidal behavior: A feminist critique of theories and research. *Suicide & Life-Threatening Behavior, 28*(1), 24–36. https://doi.org/10.1111/j.1943-278X.1998.tb00623.x

Rich, A. R., Kirkpatrick-Smith, J., Bonner, R. L., & Jans, F. (1992). Gender differences in the psychosocial correlates of suicidal ideation among adolescents. *Suicide*

& Life-Threatening Behavior, 22(3), 364–373. https://doi.org/10.1111/J.1943-278X.1992.TB00741.X

River, J. (2014). Suicide and hegemonic masculinity in Australian men. In D. Lester, J. Gunn, & P. Quinnett (Eds.), *Suicide in men: How men differ from women in expressing their distress* (pp. 248–261). Charles C. Thomas Publisher.

Salmela, A. (2018). Fleshy stories. New materialism and female suicides in late nineteenth-century Finland. *International Journal of History and Cultural Modern, 6*(1), 1–27. https://doi.org/10.18352/hcm.545

Schiff, J. A., & Eugenides, J. (2006). A conversation with Jeffrey Eugenides. *The Missouri Review, 29*(3), 100–119. https://doi.org/10.1353/mis.2007.0007

Shostak, D. (2009). "A story we could live with": Narrative voice, the reader, and Jeffrey Eugenides's *The Virgin Suicides. Modern. Fiction Studies, 55*(4), 808–832. https://doi.org/10.1353/mfs.0.1642

Shostak, D. (2013). "Impossible narrative voices": Sofia Coppola's adaptation of Jeffrey Eugdenides's *The Virgin Suicides. Interdisciplinary Literary Studies, 15*(2), 180–202. https://doi.org/10.5325/intelitestud.15.2.0180

Silverman, M. M. (2016). Challenges to defining and classifying suicide and suicidal behaviors. In R. C. O'Connor & J. Pirkis (Eds.), *The international handbook of suicide prevention* (pp. 11–35). Wiley Blackwell.

Skomp, E. (2003). Misogyny, the male gaze, and fantasies of female death: *Eto Ia, Edichka* and *Russkaia Krasovitsa. New Zealand Slavonic Journal*, 137–142.

Stack, S., & Wasserman, I. (2009). Gender and suicide risk: The role of wound site. *Suicide & Life-Threatening Behavior, 39*(1), 13–20. https://doi.org/10.1521/suli.2009.39.1.13

Sullivan, N. (2012). The somatechnics of perception and the matter of the non/human: A critical response to new materialism. *European Journal of Women's Studies, 19*(3), 299–313. https://doi.org/10.1177/1350506812443477

Tuana, N. (2008). Viscous porosity: Witnessing Katrina. In S. Alaimo & S. Hekman (Eds.), *Material feminisms* (pp. 188–213). Indiana University Press.

Van der Tuin, I. (2008). Deflationary logic. Response to Sara Ahmed's 'imaginary prohibitions: Some preliminary remarks on the founding gestures of the "new materialism"'. *European Journal of Women Studies, 15*(4), 411–416. https://doi.org/10.1177/1350506808095297

Walton, S. Air, atmosphere, environment: film mood, folk horror and *The VVitch*. (Screening the Past, 43, 2018). http://www.screeningthepast.com/2018/02/air-atmosphere-environment-film-mood-folk-horror-and-the-vvitch. Accessed 5 Oct 2020.

Warefield, K. (2016). Making the cut: An agential realist examination of selfies and touch. *Social Media + Society*, April–June, 1–10. https://doi.org/10.1177/2056305116641706

White, M. (2017). Gaze. In L. Ouellette & J. Gray (Eds.), *Keywords for media studies* (pp. 75–77). New York University Press.

Wilhite, K. (2015). Face the house: Suburban domesticity and nation as home in *The Virgin Suicides*. *Mod. Fiction Stud., 61*(1), 1–23. https://doi.org/10.1353/mfs.2015.0008

Witz, A., & Marshall, B. L. (2003). The quality of manhood: Masculinity and embodiment in the sociological tradition. *The Sociological Review, 51*(3), 339–356. https://doi.org/10.1111/1467-954X.00424

Womack, K., & Mallory-Kani, A. (2007). "Why don't you just leave it up to nature?": An adaptationist reading of the novels by Jeffrey Eugenides. *Mosaic, 40*(3), 157–173.

Dr. Katrina Jaworski is a Senior Lecturer in Cultural Studies at the Justice and Society Academic Unit, University of South Australia. Having published on the topic of suicide for 20 years, her research focuses on the agency of suicide, with attention to gender, body, sexuality, ethics, and poetry. She also works on the Rwandan genocide, the philosophy of dying bodies, trauma, and the cultural politics of thinking. To date, she has authored/co-edited the following books: *The Gender of Suicide: Knowledge Production, Theory and Suicidology* (Routledge, 2014); *Women Supervising and Writing Doctoral Dissertations: Walking on the Grass* (Lexington, 2015); and *Rethinking Madness: Interdisciplinary and Multicultural Reflections* (Brill, 2013).

Magic Friend, Beggar Maid and *The Fair Princess, Method Actress* and *Loving Mother*: Fantasies of Love, Loss, and Desire in Joyce Carole Oates' Fictional Account of Norma Jeane's Reality

Gail Shanley Corso

Contents

A Magic Friend in the Mirror 84
Beggar Maid into Fair Princess 86
Method Actress 88
Mother with Her Baby 89
Conclusion 90
References 92

While many books, articles, films, and songs[1] have been written about the iconic star and sensual beauty, Marilyn Monroe, aka Norma Jeane Baker or Mortensen, her identity as an emotionally sensitive woman aspiring to achieve depth as a dramatic actress and to secure unconditional love and acceptance, has been buried in a mass of information about her life and conflicting narratives by biographers about her death at age 36 by overdose, further qualified

[1] "Candle in the Wind" lyrics by Elton John and Bernie Taupin, *Goodbye Yellow Brick Road*, MCA Records (1973).

G. S. Corso (✉)
Neumann University, Aston, PA, USA
e-mail: gcorso@neumann.edu

J. Ros Velasco (ed.), *Suicide in Modern Literature*,
https://doi.org/10.1007/978-3-030-69392-3_5

on the Coroner's Report (August 17, 1962) as a "probable suicide" (qtd. in Smith, 2004, p. 55). Claims about her diva behavior on location for films, her numerous sexual alliances, and false claims about her inability to deliver her lines obscure her triumphs and mute her interiority. Nonfiction representations about Marilyn persist about her constant need for painkillers, sedatives, and amphetamines. Biographers speculate about her unhappy, even lost childhood, caused by her not knowing the identity of her biological father and her forced separation from her mother (Gladys) whose need to be institutionalized for most of Norma Jeane's life prevented the child from having any semblance of a stable home environment during her formative years. In *Life* magazine's commemorative issue, *Remembering Marilyn*, the authors explain how Gladys and Norma Jeane "would remain virtual strangers, but Monroe, as soon as she was able, always saw to it – even in her will – that money was set aside for her mother's care" (Sullivan & Daspin, 2017, p. 26). Marilyn provided for the mother whose mental illness (paranoid schizophrenia) prevented a healthy mother-and-daughter relationship. Surrogate mothers attempted to fill this nurturing role, but lack of continuity of any one person for several years in this capacity pervades narratives about Marilyn. More modern understandings of what is understood as a healthy relationship between a mother and daughter or the ongoing presence of a single caregiver upon the development of a young woman have been made explicit (Gilligan, 1982).

The absence of such a long-term nurturing relationship contributes to psychological problems for a child, such as Marilyn. Carol Gilligan describes cases of women whose identity development and growth in moral judgment seem arrested, and she identifies possible contributing factors: "[…] in the absence of care from others, they are unable to care for a child or themselves. The issue is one of responsibility and life is seen as dependent on relationships" (1982, pp. 125–126). Gilligan emphasizes the importance of a nurturing relationship between a girl and her mother or a trusted guardian. For Gilligan, "the path that leads to maturity for woman is one that emphasizes 'relationships of care' and 'ongoing attachment' to others as opposed to 'individual achievement'" (1982, p. 170). In the absence of such a relationship in Norma Jeane's formative years, she aspires to the model of stardom. Her identity transforms into that of a pure white, blonde beauty, that follows as Lotta Kähkönen describes this desirable image of 1950s Hollywood with its requirement for chalky white makeup, shockingly-stark-platinum-blonde-white hair, and "skin painted exceptionally pale" in certain films and when in front of the camera (2009, p. 294). Famous images of Marilyn in skin-tight sparkling white dresses or in low-cut white dresses that sensuously move with the air draw attention to her image in strong contrast to the darkness around her. With this image, almost a blend of those constructed for other Hollywood icons of sexuality, Jean Harlow also known as "Baby," Bridget Bardot, and Jayne Mansfield, Norma Jeane's look, as analyzed by Kähkönen (2009), exemplifies the Hollywood ideal of the beautiful woman as a vamp. This image works toward erasing her identity as a living and breathing woman, stripped of her ethnicity and roots to poverty or lower-middle-class origins. All of her whiteness and compulsion to conjure that desirable image of the fantasy goddess obscures the needs of the real woman and transports her fans into the Hollywood-scripted image of her.

Storytellers, even 59 years after her death, still attempt to understand this woman as a complex enigma. Various theories have been claimed about circumstances leading to her death, and even disagreement about the nature of her death-suicide whether intentional or accidental by overdose, possible homicide victim caught in the crossfire of schemes by the Mafia, or by Jimmy Hoffa, or by disgruntled individuals from the CIA who felt betrayed by the Kennedys during the crisis in Cuba.[2] For these conspiracy theories, it is claimed that Marilyn became the bait used to entrap and publicly humiliate the Kennedy brothers, President of the United States, John F. Kennedy, and Robert F. Kennedy, then Attorney General, who were alleged to have had affairs with Marilyn.

In the John F. Kennedy Presidential Library, many have written about accomplishments of Robert F. Kennedy. In two areas nationally he became instrumental in effecting equity and social justice:

> Attorney General Kennedy launched a successful drive against organized crime, and convictions against organized crime figures rose by 800% during his tenure. He also became increasingly committed to helping African Americans win the right to vote, attend integrated schools and use public accommodations. (n.d., para. 6)

Aside from these accomplishments that angered those who held onto racist beliefs and others who led the infrastructure of the underworld, the Kennedy archive chronicles how the Kennedys also disturbed those in favor of military action in relation to the Cuban Missile Crisis:

> During the 1962 Cuban Missile Crisis, for instance, he helped develop the Kennedy administration's strategy to blockade Cuba instead of taking military

[2] Matthew Smith (2004) in *Marilyn's Last Words* identifies groups that might have held grudges against the Kennedys.

> action that could have led to nuclear war. He then negotiated with the Soviet Union on removal of the weapons. (n.d., para. 8)

Marilyn is alleged to have had relationships with both men, as explained by many biographers; her adoration for each man in power was well known. It is alleged that her house was under technological surveillance by various groups passionate about undoing the Kennedys.

Gloria Steinem though identifies several stories about Marilyn and her childhood that seem to reveal more about her true identity and her emotional pain throughout her entire life. The first story relates to her telling at least two biographers about a childhood experience with a male who was a trusted caretaker in one of the six foster homes in which she had lived:

> [...] the account of rape by an elderly boarder when she was eight was most disbelieved [...]. Whatever its facts, her memory of being sexually humiliated as a child, and then of being humiliated again by disbelief, seemed too full of pain to be artificial. Certainly, the stammering she attributed to that trauma was real. (Steinem, 1986, p. 51)

Steinem writes with sympathy about Marilyn and explains how her having to leave her mother's friends as her caretaker and her subsequent move to an orphanage added to her challenges and doubts about those ties of unconditional love that bind. Steinem also adds how through this iconic woman, all women can empathize with her struggles at that time to be taken seriously in the professional role, to break through stereotypes of ineptitude and powerlessness. Marilyn's struggles persisted as she resisted the stereotypes of being a dumb blonde, of being an unresourceful person who was compelled to sleep her way to stardom. She was believed from her earliest beginnings to have an erotic but illusory power over men:

> Marilyn's career began when she was discovered by an Army photographer assigned 'to take morale-building shots of pretty girls' in a defense plant for *Yankee* and *Stars and Stripes* magazines and Marilyn was a pretty eighteen-year old worker on the assembly line. That photographer's commanding officer, a young captain who spent World War II supervising this kind of morale-building work from his desk in a movie studio, was Ronald Reagan [future President of the United States]. (Steinem, 1986, p. 97)

While Marilyn's images were published in numerous magazines, on calendars, and as posters, she seems to have struggled considerably to survive as a professional and to sustain relationships. Steinem chronicles how Marilyn self-reported to various biographers her attempts throughout her life to commit suicide:

> she had attempted suicide twice before she was nineteen. When she was twenty-four, Natasha Lytess saved her a third time. There were three near-deaths during her marriage to Arthur Miller, and at least two more close calls before the final act. (1986, p. 154)

Aside from these close calls with death, Steinem identifies how Marilyn had "a dozen or so illegal abortions" (1986, p. 142). These risky, life-threatening experiences Steinem connects to Marilyn's awareness of intergenerational mental illness in her family, some unresolved trauma that she experienced as a child and young woman, and her ongoing displacements from her home with her mother, Gladys, to foster homes, and then to the orphanage. Several of her caretakers from her childhood, too, experienced mental health issues:

> Of the women whom Marilyn knew as a very young child, her mother's mother died in a mental hospital; her own mother has spent most of her life institutionalized as well; Ana Lower died of a stroke (although Marilyn apparently believed she died of malnutrition); and Grace McKee died of suicide. The teachers of her earliest lessons on femaleness offered life examples that were sad or tragic. (1986, p. 94)

Whether or not Marilyn commit suicide intentionally or unintentionally or whether she became a victim of homicide as revenge toward the Kennedys by any of the brothers' detractors remains a mystery. Through drama in two plays by her last husband, Arthur Miller, the *intellectual playwright* as Joyce Carol Oates labels him in *Blonde* (2009), we recognize his emotional paralysis and inability to connect to his wife Marilyn. More interestingly, through the novel *Blonde*, Joyce Carol Oates portrays what seems to be the real Marilyn—Norma Jeane's complex interior life, her fears, and her struggle to survive.

Marilyn seems to have had four husbands—James Dougherty from June 1942–1946, Robert Slatzer for three days in 1952, Joe DiMaggio from January 14, 1954, to September 1954, and Arthur Miller, June 29, 1956, to January 20, 1961, ironically, the same day as John F. Kennedy's inauguration as President of the United States. Her last ex-husband, playwright, Arthur Miller, in two of his plays creates a tragedy about unfulfilled love in a relationship between with a female character who seems to reflect his former wife's energy and torments and with a male character who reflects his own inability to cope with creative aspirations and needs of a woman. In Act II of *After the*

Fall, produced in 1964, soon after Marilyn's death by "probable suicide" on August 5, 1962, Maggie, the singer, explains to Quentin how she likes to identify as "Sarah None" or "Miss None" (2015, p. 560). This anonymity indicates issues that Maggie has with her own identity. Marilyn, like Maggie, was forced to change her name as she began to construct her identity in films. Quentin in the following lines like Arthur Miller also identifies for Maggie how she allows others to exploit her: "QUENTIN. It's not the money they take, it's the dignity they destroy. You're not a piece of meat; you seem to think you owe people whatever they demand!" (2015, p. 564).

As Maggie continues her career, her relationship with Quentin suffers. When they are around other people, she feels especially estranged from him. She perceives that he makes her feel lonely and ashamed. She even questions her sanity. At one point, when arguing with him, she says, "What are you trying to make me think, I'm crazy?" (2015, p. 574). For Maggie, Quentin becomes a projection of all the men who have used or abused her. When Quentin tells Maggie that he has spoken to her doctor, he admits his concerns about being in such an unstable relationship with her:

> QUENTIN. Do you know any more who I am? Aside from my name? I'm all the evil in the world, aren't I? All the betrayal, the broken hopes, the murderous revenge? *She pours pills into her hand, and he stands. Now fear is in his voice.* A suicide kills two people, Maggie, that's what it's for! So I'm removing myself, and perhaps it will lose its point. *He resolutely starts out. She falls back on the bed….* (2015, p. 580)

In this drama, Maggie indeed kills herself, but Quentin survives by turning to Holga, for yet another attempt at love in a relationship with a woman who is a survivor of a globally-recognized traumatic experience, the Holocaust. Maggie though has succumbed to her personal sense of worthlessness, an effect of her experiences with gaslighting. Critics have perceived this play as paralleling too closely Miller's own troubled relationship with Marilyn. John Stinson interprets Miller's inclusion of Maggie as a way for the playwright to show a character as victim:

> a victim who did not die in vain, but one who prompted the agonizing guilt, and as the vision of Quentin/Miller […]. [Miller] does not want Marilyn Monroe's death to be a meaningless piece of pathos […] but really an example, and thus a *felix culpa* [a happy guilt]. (1967, p. 240)

Maggie/Marilyn becomes for Quentin/Miller a sacrificial lamb. Perhaps this rendition of a struggling relationship between Maggie and Quentin becomes for Miller his justification for withdrawing from his relationship with Marilyn before the impending suicide or death which he may have felt that he could not prevent. Stephen Marino identifies how Quentin, while he attempted to save Maggie, did it for all the wrong reasons—"not out of pure love, but for power" which makes him complicit with her fall (2005, p. 52).

Arthur Miller later in his life returns to his inspiration, Marilyn, in yet another play. In *Finishing the Picture* (2009) that premiered on September 21, 2004, at the Goodman Theatre in Chicago, Illinois, Kitty, who ironically remains silent throughout the three acts, is portrayed as the temperamental actress whose marriage to Paul, the scriptwriter for the film in which she stars, mirrors considerably what biographers have written about Marilyn Monroe and Arthur Miller during the production of *The Misfits* (1961), the film which Miller also had scripted. In *Finishing the Picture*, the producer like the producer and studio for *The Misfits* considers abandoning the project due to its delays and cost overruns attributed partially to Kitty's troubling absence or presence in a less-than-timely way on sets. In *Finishing*, several characters attempt to understand Kitty's erratic behavior. Paul, Kitty's husband, identifies Kitty's inability to accept love as the cause for her deep depression that precludes her from functioning well with commitments to others and with time management:

> PAUL. What I think? Her life has her by the throat, there is no way to reach into her that I know of. We're all a little bit angry at her, that's inevitable- but the key to this lock is probably love. Which she can't accept. (Miller, 2009, p. 224, Act. I)

Paul sees his wife, Kitty, that beautiful goddess, as "a mockery, phantom, a curl of smoke…" in relation to her image of flawless beauty and erotic allure (2009, p. 229, Act. I). When other characters in the play see Kitty's meltdowns as she wanders through the halls of the trailer nude, dazed, and lost, they consider how and why she continues to enrapture, even enthrall, them despite their frustrations with her. The director, Derek, comments to the producer, Ochsner, on why Kitty behaves as she does and how she still maintains her mass appeal: "DEREK. She's had a frightful life… she's been stepping on broken glass since she could walk. She is pure survival- which could be why she moves you" (2009, p. 214, Act. I). While it may be the financial risks of a film not being completed, and the potential doom to their own careers that the director and producer fear, Miller portrays Ochsner as caring for Kitty and "deeply disturbed", but this otherwise intelligent man ignores, misunderstands, or cruelly dismisses signs of her serious depression:

> "OCHSNER. (deeply disturbed) [...]. I still can't understand this!- She's the envy of half the world" (2009, p. 229, Act. I).

Ochsner seems unable to get beyond a surface understanding of Kitty's interior life, her hopes, her dreams, her challenges, and her fears, as does society at large. Yet another character, Edna, Kitty's personal assistant, attempts to shed light on Kitty's behavior. Edna seems to parallel Mrs. Eunice Murray, Marilyn's real-life housekeeper and aide who also unbeknownst to Marilyn served as a psychiatric nurse that Marilyn's psychiatrist, Dr. Ralph Greenson, had suggested she hire. Edna explains to Derek what causes Kitty's immobility, her inability to sleep without medication, and her prolonged delays on arriving to the set in her perfect image of seductive whiteness for filming:

> EDNA. [...] It's fear, Derek, it's terror! The bottom drops out; she's afraid she's going to be ridiculous; she has no... no... what the hell is the word? – *resources*! She is like a sensitive poet! [...] But you must hold on, try to be as kind [...]. (2009, p. 256, Act. III)

Edna identifies Marilyn's deep insecurities in such a highly competitive world that flourishes on an ongoing, ever-turning mill of beauty, youth, talent, and demands for perfection. Edna's suggestion "Try to be" intimates the lies and pretense that surround the fragile, poetic Kitty in this world of ever-changing teams, crews, relationships, and allegiances, an environment of masks, screens, and constructed images. If Kitty, a lens into Marilyn, were alive today, she might find company among other women who courageously have begun to speak out in the *Me Too* movement about their having been abused in many professional and personal environments to maintain their presence in them. They have been victims of predators in their relationships and in the movie industry. They have been victims of gaslighting.

Through the dialogue among the characters behind the set of *Finishing the Picture*, we begin to understand how Kitty is perceived by others. She is their profit-making machine who keeps them all employed, yet she is burdened by serious sorrow and depression that Miller's play neglects to reveal beyond the obvious—her estranged relationship with her husband and her need for unconditional support from her adoring drama coach, Jerome. Kitty though in this drama remains silent, an elusive shadow to the entire production, a character without a say, without any control over her life except to resist showing up ready when possible to project flawless, white beauty, and to recite the ongoing-heavily-edited lines. This inaction is the only means by which she exerts control and a degree of power over others. The play itself ends quite dramatically, poetically with reference to the devastating fires in California that the crew senses even at a great distance in the Nevada desert. Edna tells Kitty what the cameraman, Terry Case, understands about a positive effect of such seeming devastation and destruction upon the environment: "EDNA. [...] But Terry says it makes the seeds germinate. (*She turns upstage.*)- The fire, darling... the heat opens up the seeds" (2009, p. 263, Act. III).

Miller leaves the play open-ended, poetic for the audience to interpret. In the Pinelands and other environments with moist conditions, seeds may germinate; however, without particular environments, such raging fire could cause mass destruction. Possibly the creative process with its tensions in the right environment cultivates the energy of the crew, providing in some mysterious way the anima, or spirit that lies latent within the actors and crew for the production to coalesce into a good film. Ochsner adds how film production likens to another creative process—the struggles of the birthing process:

> "OCHSNER. The baby I cleaned up, the sheets are changed, the mother is bathed... and everybody forgets the screaming" (2009, p. 262, Act. III).

Ochsner seems unaware that some mothers after the birthing process experience postpartum depression that when left untreated has severe consequences. With each hopeful belief about the creative process, the men neglect to consider several major risk factors for each, such as particular fire regimes in different ecosystems and the varying adaptations of trees, plants, animals, and humans to different situations. While *Finishing the Picture* ends with Kitty's still being alive, as honorable to her word and to her commitment to complete the film, as Paul claims, severe warning signs of her life being held together by a thin thread are evident.

Psychoanalysis has evolved since the 1950s and 1960s. Lisa Appignanesi, author of *Mad, Bad and Sad: Women and the Mind Doctors* (2011), reveals in an interview conducted by Brenda Webster in 2009 that Marilyn was "trapped in excess, a fuddle of pills, and a sexual image which rebounded on her own sense of her sexuality" (p. 793). Her experiences as a child, Appignanesi explains, "left her with scars that were constantly re-opened in her experience of men" (2009, p. 793). Her quest for her father was never satisfied nor was that figure of unconditional love from a father figure ever "found again in the men in [her life]" (2009, p. 793). Rather than depression as a diagnosis for Marilyn, Appignanesi identifies borderline personality disorder as the classification for understanding her aberrant behavior.[3] A different course of treatment by her doctors, her psychiatrist, and the studio's doctors might have allowed Marilyn a chance to survive.

Death by overdose—accidental or intentional—by famous performing artists has become commonplace since Marilyn Monroe's death. Prince, Amy Winehouse, Margeaux Hemingway, Judy Garland, Janis Joplin, Whitney Houston, River Phoenix, Philip Seymour Hoffman, Michael Jackson, and Heath Ledger, to name just a few famous performing artists, have become victims, like Marilyn, to effects of excess with drugs. Robert Dorfman, Emily Berquist Soule, and Sukumar Desai (2018, p. 32) explain how "Marilyn Monroe's life and death previewed the opioid epidemic." They highlight how "Abuse of prescription drugs has only risen since then [1962]. Now anyone can die like Marilyn" (2018, p. 32). Marilyn's access to barbiturates and amphetamines was chronicled throughout her adult life, yet her using never became a criminal activity. In the 1950s, Hollywood was known for the ease of access to drugs for those in the competitive performing arts to reduce anxiety, lose weight, and sleep: "By mid-century, drug companies were marketing no fewer than 30 barbiturates, with Amytal, Nembutal, and Seconal the most popular. After World War II, 'goofballs' were everywhere-and cheap. A dozen pills went for about $1" (Dorfman et al., 2018, p. 35). Marilyn had prescriptions from the studio doctors, as well as her own psychiatrist, who had diagnosed her as a "borderline paranoid schizophrenic" (qtd. in Dorfman et al., 2018, p. 38).

Society at large has little understood mental illness, such as borderline personality disorder, schizophrenia, paranoid schizophrenia, or borderline paranoid schizophrenia. Without understanding the fragility of persons with these mental illnesses, the medical community unintentionally overprescribed addictive medicines, as was the case with Marilyn. She relied on pharmaceuticals to ease all pains: "[She] was an addict, and addiction killed her, intentional or not" (Dorfman et al., 2018, p. 35).

[3] According to the National Alliance on Mental Illness (NAMI), a person with borderline personality disorder might experience "wide mood swings and can feel a great sense of instability and insecurity" (NAMI, 2020). *The Diagnostic and Statistical Manual Diagnostic* framework identifies several indicators that may include the following: (i) Frantic efforts to avoid real or imagined abandonment by friends and family; (ii) unstable personal relationships that alternate between idealization ("I'm so in love!") and devaluation ("I hate her"). This is also sometimes known as "splitting"; (iii) distorted and unstable self-image, which affects moods, values, opinions, goals, and relationships; (iv) impulsive behaviors that can have dangerous outcomes, such as excessive spending, unsafe sex, substance abuse, or reckless driving; (v) self-harming behavior including suicidal threats or attempts; (vi) periods of intense depressed mood, irritability, or anxiety lasting a few hours to a few days; (vii) chronic feelings of boredom or emptiness; (viii) inappropriate, intense, or uncontrollable anger—often followed by shame and guilt; (ix) dissociative feelings—disconnecting from your thoughts or sense of identity or "out of body" type of feelings—and stress-related paranoid thoughts. Severe cases of stress can also lead to brief psychotic episodes.

Nevertheless, Marilyn transformed in front of a camera, as best described by photographer George Barris, who recalled how when she posed in front of the camera, she always projected joy. She was recognized for her wit, her identity as a comic actress whose hair, her pouty, breathy childlike voice, and her alluring figure inevitably would steal the gaze of the camera crew and the audience. As she secured some fame in alluring roles, even in some songs that she popularized, such as "I wanna be loved by you,"[4] she aligned with powerful men in her sexual relationships. Some knew of her mother's institutionalization for paranoid schizophrenia, and Marilyn's personal history of being legally prescribed medicines to sedate her, or to energize her to meet the demands of controlling men in the film industry and in her life, but few recognized her fears of becoming another family member who had been deserted by men and who had experienced depression: "Ironically she became famous with the family name of both her maternal grandmother and her mother, whose shared fate of desertion by men and depression would be continued to the third generation" (Steinem, 1986, p. 56). Through analysis of four mental scripts that Norma Jeane conjures throughout her life, as explained by the fiction writer, Joyce Carol Oates in her novel *Blonde*, the psychological needs of Norma Jeane are revealed—the need to be understood, to be unconditionally loved, and, as she herself explained to Pete Martin, a journalist who was writing a book about her in the 1950s, to be able "to be wonderful" (qtd. in Steinem, 1986, p. 63).

Her *magic friend* in the mirror allows her to transform from the ordinary orphan or the lonely woman into the expected sexy, sultry, flawlessly white Marilyn identity, America's pin-up and sensational star. Her fairytale script of her own evolution from a beggar maid into a fair princess surfaces throughout her relationships with numerous men over time, men whom she desires will fill the emptiness caused by her own biological father's[5] lifetime silence and rejection of her and her mother. Norma Jeane, her name throughout this novel, pursues her elusive desire to be whole as an actress by imagining herself as one who projects serious women in dramatic theatrical productions, such as those by William Shakespeare and Henrik Ibsen. Finally, she desires a life with baby—her idealized notion of her child, one of several she lost through miscarriages, and others who were aborted. Norma Jeane sees in her creative endeavors wholeness and her destiny to be the finest actress. With numerous attempts at suicide throughout her life, Marilyn's death in the end at age 36,

[4] "I Wanna Be Loved by You," written by Herbert Stothart and Harry Ruby with lyrics by Bert Kalmar was sung by Marilyn Monroe in Billy Wilder's 1959 classic farce *Some Like It Hot*.

[5] Gloria Steinem notes that C. Stanley Gifford, a salesman at the film lab where Gladys, Marilyn's mother had worked, is Marilyn's biological father (1986, p. 44).

as Oates describes it through her fictionalized character, shows the truth about her vulnerability to an industry that little understood or respected the range to her creativity, her desires for a family of her own, and her needs to be free of damning dependence on pharmaceutical fixes to her emotional pain.

A Magic Friend in the Mirror

In Ovid's telling of the myth of Narcissus, the young lad after having rejected pursuit by Echo is punished by the goddess Nemesis with the fate of falling in love with his own reflection in the pool of water. When his love for the image he sees cannot be reciprocated, Narcissus feels the pain of unrequited love and, ultimately, dies. At the site of his death, Narcissus is transformed into a thing of beauty—the narcissus flower. Like Narcissus, the lonely seventh grader Norma Jeane finds solace in the image she conjures of her magic friend in the mirror:

> Her magic friend was not fearful. Only Norma Jeane was fearful. Her friend-in-the-mirror who pirouetted in nakedness, did the hula, wiggled her hips and breasts, smiled smiled smiled, exulted in nakedness before God as a snake exults in its sinuous glittery skin. (Oates, 2009, p. 93)

Her self-image of the sex goddess, for whom people would turn to gaze, Oates identifies as surfacing for Norma Jeane as an adolescent when she experiences loneliness after being separated from her mother when she was institutionalized and, again, when she moved from her mother Gladys' friends' home to several foster care homes, and then to the Los Angeles Orphans Home Society:

> In secret Norma Jeane often crept into the lavatory in the middle of the night. The other girls in the dorm sleeping. [...] At such times the dingy foul-smelling lavatory was a place of excitement like a theatre before the lights darken, the curtains part, and the movie begins, if Norma Jeane believed herself safely alone. Removing her nightgown, as capes, cloaks, clinging garments are removed in movies, and a subtle pulsing movie music beneath as her Magic Friend is revealed, as if hiding inside the drab garment only just waiting to be revealed. This girl-who-was-Norma-Jeane yet not-Norma-Jeane but a stranger. A girl so much more special than Norma Jeane could ever be. (2009, p. 94)

This child escapes into her fantasy of solace where ordinary girls are transformed into princesses and beauties: "Her arms across her breast she laid; / She was more fair than words can say: / [...] 'It is no wonder,' said the lords,

/ 'She is more beautiful than day'" (Tennyson, 1842, lines 1–2, 7–8). Like Cinderella, too, the child dwells in romantic fantasies and dreams of her being transformed from the unloved and neglected girl into the beautiful princess for whom the charming prince does all he can to find her. In yet another fairy tale, Snow White's cruel stepmother asks "Mirror, mirror on the wall, who is the fairest of them all?" Of course, Snow White is identified. But in 1950s Hollywood, the "fairest of them all" would be Hollywood's iconic image of glamour in the guise of Marilyn Monroe, Norma Jeane's magic friend.

The narrator tells the reader that Norma Jeane recalls some distorted details from the day when her mother's friends, Clive Pearce and Jess Flynn took her, the eight-year-old, to the orphanage: "One day when Norma Jeanne would come permanently to dwell in the Kingdom of Madness she would recall how logical, if still hurtful, was this day" (Oates, 2009, p. 69). At other times she feels abandoned. By the time she turned 16 and quite alluring to the eye, she is married quickly to Bucky Glazer, "Daddy," after other foster guardians (Elsie and Warren Pirig) decide it is time for Norma Jeane to move into her own home with her own husband. The narrator explains how Elsie had observed her husband's gaze on Norma Jeane and decided that the 15 year old with the beautiful figure had to become engaged or return to the orphanage: "It's a man's world and to survive a woman must betray her own kind" (Oates, 2009, p. 111).

Tanya Horeck (2010, p. 26) identifies how Oates provides the "internal thoughts and feelings of lost girls, their dreams, their desires, and ambitions." Interspersed throughout *Blonde*, televised news reports about missing young girls who have been mutilated and raped also surface. Norma Jeane becomes very aware that these young victims could have quite possibly been her. As readers we know that Norma Jeane had died, either as a victim of murder or by suicide, yet she reveals her thoughts about these victims from beyond her grave. These young victims of violence, abuse, and rape surface as uncanny doubles of herself.

It is in her fantasy world, though, that Norma Jeane constructs beauty and her joy. It is in her life in front of a camera when the illusion of joy and of a woman in control of the scene surfaces, especially when as Marilyn, she played Roslyn in *The Misfits*. The magic friend in the mirror emerges despite her prolonged delays in conjuring the character Roslyn before arriving on the set:

> Roslyn was like a beautiful vase that has been broken and shattered yet by patience, craft, and cunning meticulously restored, fragment by fragment, bit by bit, with tweezers and glue, you see only the restored vase and have no knowledge of the shattered vase, still less of the monomaniacal energy that has gone into the restoration. (Oates, 2009, p. 662)

Norma Jeane depends upon her trusted cosmetologist, Whitey, and her hairstylist to help maintain her camera-ready beauty, but she relates to her magic friend in the mirror for that confidence to face the world: "[…] she dared not tell him how longer and longer each morning it was required to summon her Magic Friend out of the mirror" (Oates, 2009, p. 556).

Like Narcissus, Norma Jeane turns away from lovers. She experiences loss of freedom with her perceived equals, having attempted relationships with Cass and Eddy G., who were children of famous male leading actors in films, marriage to the iconic ex-athlete, and then the award-winning intellectual American playwright, and, finally, affairs with famous politicians, the President, and his brother. She lives forever though in images and representations of her, especially the iconic image of The Girl (no special name) in that white dress standing over the subway grating in New York City in the film *The Seven Year Itch* (1955) that can be likened to the image of Venus in Sandro Botticelli's *The Birth of Venus* (1486; Virtual Uffizzi Gallery, n.d.). In each image, the sensual beauty, a goddess of love, attempts to cover her exposed body, yet her simultaneous beauty and consternation capture the gaze, desire, and delight of viewers in all kinds of media. This Girl in the film played by Marilyn becomes the twin to the model, Simonetta Cattaneo Vespucci, the other beautiful blonde in Botticelli's painting where, as Venus, she represents the goddess of beauty.

Beggar Maid into Fair Princess

Contemporary women writers, such as Anne Tyler, Alice McDermott, and Jane Smiley, re-envision traditional fairy tales in their stories about women. Unlike the ending in traditional fairytales where the initially perceived woman as victim or societal underdog triumphs, such writers, including Joyce Carol Oates, create more realistic endings that bespeak social injustice and society's privileged structures that seem insurmountable, as in the case with Norma Jeane who seems unaware and powerless; in effect, she attempts to reinvent herself, but she remains victim to patriarchal structures in the film industry and ongoing misogynistic treatment by men. For *Blonde,* Sharon Oard Warner identifies the following fairytales interspersed in the storyline: "The Beggar Maid," "Rumpelstiltskin," "Red Riding Hood," "Sleeping Beauty," and "Beauty and the Beast" (2006, p. 520). Oates' choice of details and fictionalized representations of real persons and incidents from Norma Jeane's life reveals the woman attempting to navigate through pervasive patriarchal structures. Through Oates' focus on historic moments and cultural contexts, as a feminist, she subverts the pop culture narrative of Marilyn Monroe's life and death and, as Henry Louis Gates comments, "Find[s] just where it hurts and then press[es], *hard*" (qtd. in Warner, 2006, p. 518). As an effect of Norma Jeane's "anxious attachment" to others throughout her life, similar to the experiences of even more contemporary women, as explained by feminist psychologists, her the voice of experience seems to have been disabled which repeatedly prevents her one from any "protest against experiences of violation or subordination" (Gilligan & Snider, 2019, p. 90). There is no fairy godmother or prince charming for Norma Jeane, just fiction writer, Joyce Carol Oates.

The beggar maid seems to project Norma Jeane's desired self-identity. In the legend of *King Cophetua and the Beggar Maid*, as retold by Horace Scudder in 1900 and then republished in 2006, the rich and powerful bachelor king who lived in Africa had all beautiful things, but he had not yet met a woman to be his wife. This generous and kind young man sought to find his mate, but his counselors could not find a princess to their liking for their king. He remained lonely until one day as he went out riding for a hunt along with other nobles, he noticed a blind old beggarman with his daughter by his side. When the King asked the girl her name, she responded, "Penelophon" without adding the words of respect, "Your Majesty." Also, without knowing correct protocol, she looked at the King directly in the eye. As legend goes, King Cophetua could see through her eyes her trusting soul, and instantly, impulsively, he asked her to marry him. Racialization or whiteness is absent in this story. And so they lived, happily ever after. Other storytellers have told the story of the poor girl and the prince. as in *Cinderella*. These are rags-to-riches stories and manifestations of other stories where prince charming or the knight in shining armor comes to the rescue of the fair maiden, and in which they each experience unconditional love.

Another fairytale character surfaces in *Blonde*—Rumpelstiltskin in the guise of Shinn, her agent who attempts to place Norma Jeane in *Don't Bother to Knock* (1952) as Nell, the psychotic babysitter who attempts to seduce a man. The plot seems centered around a schizoid young woman who seems somewhat suicidal and, by the end of the film, is taken to what Shinn calls, "a loony bin" (Oates, 2009, p. 289). The reader then sees inside Norma Jeane's mind as she wonders if her agent disregards her need for the story of transformation from rags to riches, not the tragic ending of loss and misery: "What had happened to fierce Rumpelstiltskin? Had Norma Jeane imagined his magic? And what of the Fair Princess, his creation, if Rumpelstiltskin was losing his power? *He knew me: the Beggar Maid. They all knew me*" (Oates, 2009, p. 289). Later in the novel, soon before her death, her fantasy of herself as the beggar maid turned fairytale princess turns on itself. The experience, as described, has her transform into a demeaned and abused whore. As she is flying first class as "P. Belle" from the West Coast to the East Coast, she perceives this flight as special; she is "traveling incognito lost in dreamy reverie of *A rendezvous. With him*" (Oates, 2009, p. 701). She feels as if she is making history by engaging in this romantic date with one of the most powerful men in history, the President. She so much believes that this encounter will be transformational for both him and her. By the end of their brief encounter though, with the man engaging in phone conversations, and disregarding her as that fair princess, the narrator describes how this experience seems like a soft porn film being spliced together with different sexual acts for complete gratification of the male. Marilyn struggles to make some sense of this debasing encounter with its lack of intimacy. The reader understands it as his the powerful male's act of blatant misogyny without her having words to understand her idol's consumption of her beauty for his own satisfaction. The experience caused her to lose consciousness, possibly caused by a drug in her drink or quite possibly by the extreme shame she experienced.

Method Actress

> The acting area is a sacred space [...] where the actor cannot die.
> Michael Goldman, *The Actor's Freedom.* (1975)

In real life, Marilyn had studied method acting for a time with founding director, Lee Strasberg and his wife, Paula, of the Actors Studio in New York City. Through strategies of this method, actors discover from within how to get into character. Norma Jeane recognizes that in her own life she has many women whose mannerisms and overall demeanor she can conjure when playing diverse roles. When she is playing the role of Nell, a psychotic babysitter in *Don't Bother to Knock* (1952), for example, Norma Jeane recalls her own mother's restless, shaking hands, and through her method acting, she uses this body language to project Nell's inner turmoil and her madness. Norma Jeane also recalls her relationship with the detective from her youth, Frank Widdoes (Oates, 2009), as she tries to make Nell become real in the film. Through experiences of persons in her own life, she is able to project Nell's madness and her suicidal tendencies.

In yet another film, *The Misfits* (1961), Marilyn gets into character beyond expectations of others on the set. When Marilyn screams, "Liars! Killers! I hate you" at the men who in the film attempt to capture and kill the small herd of wild mustangs, she seems to be tapping into her own true feelings of rage. Oates explains that "The Blond Actress was expressing anger, rage. At last [...] general passion ripping through the woman's body like an electric current" (2009, p. 668). This film was produced at a time in Norma Jeane's life when her marriage to the intellectual playwright was failing and she had experienced at least three unsuccessful pregnancies. She could tap into her own anger against her own body—voluptuous and as sexually provocative as she was, her body miscarried at least three times with one being an ectopic pregnancy. Norma Jeane knew the pain of loss—loss of her mother, loss of her wanted children, and loss of her husband to whom she was married the longest. She knew how to rage against the ranchers who were about to kill the wild horses, including the foal. Norma Jeane must have empathized with these wild creatures who travel together in their small community. As one of the three epigraphs at the beginning of *Blonde*, one by the founder of method acting, we begin to understand how Norma Jeane was advancing in her roles as an actress, and she was projecting her own love for this wild, free, family of horses, a family the likes of which she longed to belong. She succeeds in emoting her singular anger:

> In the circle of light on the stage in the midst of darkness, you have the sensation of being entirely alone [...] This is called solitude in public. [...] During a performance, before an audience of thousands, you can always enclose yourself in this circle, like a snail in its shell. [...] You can carry it wherever you go. (Stanislavski, 1963, p. 115)

This method of tapping into one's feelings and experiences to improvise in some ways what the character being portrayed feels strengthened Norma Jeane's performances in front of the camera.

Mother with Her Baby

George Barris, the last photographer to take professional photos of Marilyn when alive in June and July 1962, as a photojournalist, also interviewed Marilyn. She explained to Barris that what she wanted most was children—her own and others that were adopted, but she qualified her statement by adding, "'But I don't think a single person should adopt children. There's no Ma or Pa there,' she said sadly, 'and I know what that can be like'" (qtd. in Steinem, 1986, p. 2).

When married to Arthur Miller, Marilyn had desired children. Oates describes the three miscarriages, and Norma Jeane's attempts at becoming a mother. It was not fated to be. Even in the novel, Norma Jeane from beyond her life explains another possible theory about how, toward the end of her life, she was stolen from her house due to a pregnancy that could cause such scandal to the White House:

> she was borne away to an operating room where a surgeon removed the President's baby (under the pretext it was misshapen & could not survive & when she awoke fifteen hours later exhausted & bleeding from the womb thick brackish blood soaking the sheet & mattress where she slept naked & her lower body throbbing with cramps her first thought was *Oh Christ what an ugly dream* & her second thought was *It had as well be a dream, no one would believe me anyway*). (2009, p. 731)

Conspiracy theories have contended that Marilyn may have had an abortion but held secrets about her relationships in a little red diary that went missing from her home after her death.

As explained in "Marilyn Monroe and Charitable Causes" (n.d.), Marilyn's final charitable donation was her largest. It is explained in her will that she left 25% of her estate to former psychiatrist, Dr. Marianne Kris. It was her intent that Dr. Kris decides how the funds would be used, and as explained on this site, "Kris chose the Anna Freud Children's Clinic of London," a clinic that specializes in treatment of children with mental illnesses.

Conclusion

Tanya Horeck concludes that *Blonde* in its blending of fact with fiction unearths the emotional truth at the heart of Norma Jeane's story:

> [It] splits open the fantasies that individuals- and the culture at large- spin around the figure of the lost (white) girl and the terrible violence that underpins those fantasies. In so doing, Oates reveals the personal and cultural investment in archetypal roles and narratives regarding masculinity and femininity, and the ways in which that investment leads, all too unavoidably, to moments of awful, unalterable violence. (2010, pp. 36–37)

The range to violence in Norma Jeane's life included cruelty to her by both her mother and biological father, abuse and rape by at least one trusted adult when she was a child, abandonment to an orphanage when friends of the family could no longer care for her, the film industry's abuse of power over hungry and anxious aspiring actors, such as her, overall misunderstanding of the woman's psychological needs even by those in the medical community, and social dominance when male partners coerce beautiful women, such as Norma Jeane, into forceful submission to them and their sexual fantasies. Throughout the novel, news commentators report on the brutality toward beautiful women that seems out of control, yet by the time Norma Jeane was 30, she seems to have escaped such murder:

> But no harm had come to Norma Jean. Each of the eight or nine or ten raped-and-mutilated girls was known to her, or might've been known to her, sister starlets at the Studio or sister models at the Preene Agency, or models of Otto Öse's, yet were not ever *her*. (Oates, 2009, p. 489)

These mutilations and murders of other young models and hopeful starlets pervade the telling of Norma Jeane's story, almost as a fatalistic template of what seems doomed to occur despite her having escaped random acts of violence in Hollywood and its surrounding areas.

Norma Jeane, the beautiful pin-up trying to succeed in Hollywood, the land of fantasies and dreams, escapes into what Oates describes as her own inner world: She conjures her fantasy of her magic friend in the mirror as she puts on her mask of beauty; she indulges herself with another fantasy of herself as the beggar maid who will transform into the princess; she engrosses herself in intellectual pursuits by reading a vast array of literature and by studying method acting along with some of the greatest actors of the twentieth century; and finally, she herself acts as the mother of her own mother with whom she has never really felt secure. Marilyn had relocated her mother to a private mental institution, and until her mother's death in 1984, 22 years after Marilyn's own death, the abandoned daughter's estate paid for her mother's caretaking. Marilyn becomes the nurturer and provider for her own mother, Gladys.

Norma Jeane's story becomes a curious variation on the myth of Persephone and Demeter, the story of the relationship between mother and daughter that gets compromised by Hades, the god of the underworld and death. Demeter was the goddess of fruitfulness with crops and fertility. One day when Persephone was playing with her friends in a field, she is drawn to a beautiful narcissus plant. At that point, the earth splits open, and Hades, the god of the underworld kingdom, emerges to steal Persephone away as his wife. Hades had arranged with Zeus to abscond with Persephone as his wife to the underworld, but her mother, Demeter, the goddess of the earth grieves, and rebels, by neglecting to function in her role as caretaker of the earth. As an effect, crops fail, and people suffer and die. After some time passes, Hades relents to Zeus' persuasion and to Demeter's pleas for the return of her daughter, but he forces Persephone to eat some seeds of the pomegranate which then requires her to return each year after several months with her mother. This time with her mother allows Persephone to experience joy, as too, does the mother, Demeter, with the well-being of earth restored.

Carol Gilligan identifies this particular myth as holding deeper insight into woman's psychological development:

> The elusive mystery of woman's development lies in its recognition of the continuing importance of attachment in the human life cycle [...]. The myth of Persephone speaks directly [...] by reminding us that narcissism leads to death, that the fertility of the earth is in some mysterious way tied to the continuation of the mother-daughter relationship, and that the life cycle arises from an alternation between the world of women and that of men. (1982, p. 23)

Unlike Persephone, though, Norma Jeane's mother remains indifferent, even callous to the needs for approval that her daughter seeks, as her own psychological needs take precedent throughout her life. Despite attempts by Norma Jeane to rescript her life and to sustain the fantasy of the fairy princess, she succumbs to death by suicide, either intentional or unintentional, or set up to appear as suicide. Yet Marilyn Monroe, the legendary and iconic beauty of Hollywood films and media, flourishes in her afterlife.

References

Appignanesi, L. (2011). *Mad, bad and sad: A history of women and the mind doctors from 1800 to the Present*. Hachette.

Baker, R. W. (Director). (1952). *Don't bother to knock*. Twentieth Century Fox Studios.

Botticelli, S. (1486). *The birth of Venus*. Galeria degli Uffizi.

Dorfman, R., Soule, E. B., & Desai, S. (2018, August). Dying like a star. *American History Magazine* 32–39.

Gilligan, C. (1982). *In a different voice: Psychological theory and women's development*. Harvard University Press.

Gilligan, C., & Snider, N. (2019). *Why does patriarchy persist?* Polity Press.

Goldman, M. (1975). *The actor's freedom: Toward a theory of drama*. Viking Press.

Horeck, T. (2010). Lost girls: The fiction of Joyce Carol Oates. *Contemporary Women's Writing, 4*(1), 24–39. https://doi.org/10.1093/cww/vpp002

Huston, J. (Director). (1961). *The misfits*. Seven Arts Production.

John, E., & Taupin, B. (1973). Candle in the wind. In *Goodbye yellow brick road*. MCA.

Kähkönen, L. (2009). Anxiety about whiteness in Joyce Carol Oates's novel *Blonde*. *Nordic Journal of Feminist and Gender Research, 17*(4), 289–303. https://doi.org/10.1080/08038740903257475

Marino, S. (2005). Language and metaphor in Arthur Miller's *After the fall*. *South Atlantic Review, 70*(2), 41–56.

The Marilyn Monroe collection. (n.d.). Marilyn Monroe charity and charitable causes. *The Marilyn Monroe Collection*. https://themarilynmonroecollection.com/marilyn-monroe-charitable-causes/. Accessed 2 August 2021.

Miller, A. (2009). *Finishing the picture*. Methuen Drama. (Original work published in 2004).

Miller, A. (2015). *After the fall. Arthur Miller: Collected plays*. Penguin Classics. (Original work published in 1964).

NAMI. (2020). Borderline personality disorder. *NAMI*. https://www.nami.org/Learn-More/Mental-Health-Conditions/Borderline-Personality-Disorder. Accessed 28 Jul 2020.

Oates, J. C. (2009). *Blonde*. Ecco.

Kennedy, R. F. (n.d.). *John F. Kennedy Presidential Library and Museum*. https://www.jfklibrary.org/learn/about-jfk/the-kennedy-family/robert-f-kennedy?gclid=CjwKCAiA6bvwBRBbEiwAUER6JQ1WOxHvqCmQJHb2U7BEBs-r2XdhFASTEtL875VwZlTP-fByuwTtyRoCa2gQAvD_BwE. Accessed 9 Jan 2020.

Scudder, H. E. (2006). King Cophetua and the beggar maid. In H. E. Scudder (Ed.), *The book of legends* (pp. 17–19). Yesterday's Classics. (Original work published in 1900 by Houghton Mifflin).

Smith, M. (2004). *Marilyn's last words: The secret tapes and mysterious death*. Carroll & Graf Publishers.

Stanislavski, C. (1963). *An actor's handbook: An alphabetical arrangement of concise statements on aspects of acting*. Theatre Arts Books.

Steinem, G. (1986). *Marilyn* (G. Barris, photographer). Henry Holt and Company.

Stinson, J. J. (1967). Structure in *After the fall*: The relevance of the Maggie episodes to the main themes and the Christian symbolism. *Modern Drama, 10*(3), 233–240. https://doi.org/10.1353/mdr.1967.0019

Stothart, H. (Composer), Kalmar, B., Ruby, H. (Lyrics), & Monroe, M. (Singer). (1959). I wanna be loved by you [1928]. In B. Wilder (Director), *Some like it hot*. Ashton Production and the Mirisch Corporation.

Sullivan, R., & Daspin, E. (Eds.). (2017). Remembering Marilyn. *Life, 7*(14), 1–128.

Tennyson, A. L. (1842). The beggar maid. *The Literature Network*. http://www.online-literature.com/tennyson/the-early-poems/85/. Accessed 1 Dec 2019.

Virtual Uffizzi Gallery. (n.d.). The real name of the *Birth of Venus - Botticelli*. *Virtual Uffizzi Gallery*. https://www.virtualuffizi.com/botticelli%E2%80%99s-venus-and-some-love-stories.html. Accessed 9 Jan 2020.

Warner, S. (2006). The fairest in the land: *Blonde* and *Black water*, the nonfiction novels of Joyce Carol Oates. *Studies in the Novel, 38*(4), 513–524.

Webster, B. (2009). An interview with Lisa Appignanesi, author of *Mad, bad and sad: Women and the mind doctors. Women's Studies., 38*(7), 791–798. https://doi.org/10.1080/00497870903155972

Wilder, B. (Director). (1955). *The seven year itch.* Charles K. Feldman Group, Twentieth Century Fox.

Wilder, B. (Director). (1959). *Some like it hot. Mirish Company.*

Gail Shanley Corso Ph.D., Professor of English and Humanities at Neumann University in Aston, Corso teaches courses in American literature, drama, and writing. Her most recently published book is an edited volume entitled Alice McDermott's *Fiction: Voice, Memory, Trauma, and Lies* (Peter Lang, 2018). Her articles have been published in *Studies in Arts and Humanities, The International Journal of the Literary Humanities, Teaching American Literature: A Journal of Theory and Practice, The International Journal of Teaching and Learning,* and *Kairos, A Journal of Rhetoric, Technology, and Pedagogy.*

Suicide Is Not for the Poor: Self-Death in Veristi Authors, Luigi Capuana and Giovanni Verga

Anita Virga

Contents

Suicide as a Downside of Modernity ... 97
Capuana and Verga's Elite Suicides ... 100
Capuana and Verga's Suicides Among the Poor ... 104
Conclusion ... 106
References ... 107

In the second half of the nineteenth century, after the unification of Italy, the eruption of *verismo* brought into literature a completely different approach to the making of art. Once a unified Italy was—more or less—achieved, the urgency shifted from the passion of creating the new nation to the need to analyze this new state:

> The ruling class that came to power after the unification of Italy does not need patriotic songs and hymns any longer, nor does it need historical novels. Other problems have to be faced; other energies and resources thus need to be employed. (Spinazzola, 1977, p. 250)

A. Virga (✉)
University of the Witwatersrand, Johannesburg, South Africa
e-mail: Anita.Virga@wits.ac.za

J. Ros Velasco (ed.), *Suicide in Modern Literature*,
https://doi.org/10.1007/978-3-030-69392-3_6

In a moment of great changes, the *veristi* were very preoccupied with the description of what was happening before in front of their eyes: New social forces were emerging, new laws and legislations were turning customs and traditions upside down, and new economic structures were reshaping the social organization of society.

Luigi Capuana (1939–1915) and Giovanni Verga (1940–1922) are the two main *veristi* authors; both came from the same area of Sicily, the countryside of Catania. If at the outset of the newly formed state, Capuana still paid tribute to the enthusiasm for the recent political events, with a non-impressive poem called *Garibaldi. Leggenda drammatica in tre canti* (*Garibaldi. Dramatic Legend in Three Songs*) (1861), he soon abandoned political subjects and turned his attention to the investigation of reality with a specific preference for *pathological cases* or what was otherwise extraordinary. Similarly, Verga's literary debut was dominated by patriotic and romantic motifs, before turning to the description of local reality with the intention of adopting a *scientific* approach to his literary subjects. In both cases, the reality the authors wanted to describe was not only that of the gentry but of people of all classes: Peasants, fishermen, and miners. That is, once Capuana and Verga turned their eyes toward their society without idealization, they realized that the very same society they now wanted to elect as subject of their works was composed not only of aristocrats and bourgeois like themselves but also of simple workers of the land and humble folk.[1]

Probing the whole social spectrum in all its manifestations was thus their new goal. Capuana, as the eclectic writer that he was, would have accomplished the *task* by switching easily from one literary genre to another and from one social class to another. Verga, on the other hand, intended to accomplish this feat by drafting the cycle of *I Vinti* (*The Doomed*) (2020), a series of five novels each of which would investigate a different social class starting from the lowest strata of the population. In this undertaking, of course, the theme of suicide does not remain alien, being both one of the expressions of human behavior and a typical example of the *documenti umani*[2] so dear to

[1] The introduction of the humble people as protagonists of literary works was perceived as a new development in Italian literature, something for which Capuana was praising his friend Verga when the latter published his novel *I Malavoglia* (*The House by the Medlar Tree*) (1881 [2014; 1983]), completely dedicated to a family and an entire village of fishermen: "the once romantic chronicler of elegant lifestyles has returned to the fields of his native Sicily, to that corner of the island which is between Mount Lauro, the hills of Vizzini and the vast plain of Mineo. And oh how inspired it was of him to pick up the thread of what he had started when writing the short story Nedda!" (1882, p. 122).

[2] The *documenti umani* are real facts on which literature, according to Capuana who derives his ideas from the French writer Zola, should be based. In response to those who were accusing the *veristi* of reproducing a folkloristic version of reality, Capuana claimed that Verga's and his own stories were always exact repre-

Capuana. Yet, and this is what I intend to show here, what transpires from Capuana and Verga's literary works is that suicide does not occur equally in all social classes but is rather a prerogative of the upper ones.

Although no critical attention has so far been given to its recurrence, this extreme gesture appears many times both in Capuana's and Verga's texts, usually as the ultimate outcome of the story. In Capuana's works, suicide is present in three of his five novels: *Giacinta* (*Jacinta*) (1879 [2011]), *La Sfinge* (*The Sphinx*) (1895), and *Il Marchese di Roccaverdina* (*The Marquis of Roccaverdina*) (1901 [2001]); the first two in fact end with this final gesture being carried out by the main character. On Verga's side, two of his youthful novels, *Una peccatrice* (*A Sinner*) (1866 [1965]) and *Eros* (1875 [1976]), and the short story "L'ultima giornata" ("The Last Day") (1883 [2011]) are also marked by the main character's suicide. Out of all these, only in *Il Marchese* and "L'ultima giornata" is the character who commits suicide from a lower class, but—as I intend to demonstrate—the gesture does not suggest that suicide is an option for the poor.

Suicide as a Downside of Modernity

Commenting the work of the first naturalist Spanish writer, Emilia Pardo Bazán, Capuana in *Ismi* focuses on the method utilized by the author in creating her work, *La tribuna* (*The Grandstand*) (1981), and says:

> Shortly afterward, the newspapers reported that a girl from the Tobacco Factory had committed suicide for love: she was the very girl seen about dressed like a bohemian student, cheerful and chirpy like a sparrow. [...] With her savings she had gone to buy a revolver, saying it was a gift for a cousin. The gunsmith initially hesitated; then seeing her lively, cheerful face, he had sold her the revolver. And she had put a bullet straight through her heart. [...] And the writer, narrating this fact, reflects: - «that no peasant woman would be able to kill herself in that way; the mediocre culture of factory-workers, the strain on the nerves, the thinning of the blood and the continuous unhealthy contact with city life create a new type of woman, more complicated and consequently more unhappy than any peasant woman.» (1898, pp. 243–244)

Pardo Bazán's comment on life in the city reported by Capuana was not an uncommon view held at that time. It is quite clear that Capuana too, in

sentation of their lands and the people who were living there (see "Polemica" in *Gli "ismi" contemporanei* [*Contemporary "isms"*], 1898).

quoting her, agreed with the idea that the life of a peasant was a simpler and happier one compared to that of those who lived in the city. Modernity is identified as being the main cause of psychological instability. As Fusaro (2007, p. 106) notices, speaking about Capuana and the neurosis: "Neurosis appears as the disease par excellence of the most refined men of civilization, furthest from the state of nature, especially aristocrats and artists." Capuana uses one of the characters in *Fausto Bragia* to express this idea: "The disproportion between intellectual and physical work gets bigger day after day. We are all already sick, neurotic, cachectic. The reproduction of the human species is left in full to the discretion" (2019, p. 80).

Capuana had a rather idealized idea of peasants,[3] as shown in this passage from the speech he gave in Bologna at the Dante Alighieri Society in 1894:

> Certainly my sadness derived from the great and profound transformation effected by the passing years and the processes of civilization; but I didn't miss my farmyard; and the filthy little houses, and the illiterate poets, and the songs, and the often fatal challenges to a duel with a bite on the earlobe, and the legends about brigands, and the rough stubborn character of the people [...]. I did not regret them on account of a misunderstood archaeological / deep-rooted predilection, but because they seemed to me more beautiful, better people, more authentically typical of all that has replaced them; because even in superficial, accidental things, I could see a substantial transformation and it did not make me happy. (1988, pp. 95–96)

Back in Sicily after a period of absence, Capuana finds his land very different from how he had left it. Modernity was changing for the worse, not only the society in general but more specifically the lower classes, which, according to the writer, are the true custodians of Sicilian culture.

Equating the poor with a simpler, happier life is a recurrent idea in Capuana. In one of his articles, he explained why it was necessary for contemporary art to start from the easier description of the lower classes than writing directly about the higher classes, implying that there was a correspondence between the simplicity of the subject and the simplicity of the form of art. He wrote:

> The predilection of modern artists for a more instinctive animalistic type of art, and for the passions and more sensual pleasures of the dregs of humanity perhaps comes a bit from the difficulty they encounter when attempting to rise to higher levels; it is almost as if (and this is my opinion) some inescapable laws regulate the process of art like the process of nature itself. It goes from the more

[3] On the idealization of Sicilian peasants in Capuana, see Virga (2019).

material to the more spiritual, in the same way as in nature things evolve from simpler inferior forms to richer /more complex and superior ones. (1880, p. 85)

Although never directly discussed by Capuana, a reading of his literary works shows that for the writer, self-killing does not belong to the realm of the poor; it is more a consequence of the complications of modern societies that affect middle and upper classes the most. In Capuana's view, an extreme gesture like suicide does not even cross the minds of the poor, when they remain in their *place* and are faithful to their role of custodians of the *original* culture.

Unlike Capuana, Verga did not write critical essays; nevertheless, his ideas on modernity are directly derivable from his literary works and from the prefaces he wrote for the first novel of *The Doomed* and *Eva* (1873 [1965]). Humble people, according to Verga, are psychologically simpler: Their needs as well as their feelings are less complicated and, therefore, easier to describe.[4] In *Eva*'s preface, the writer more explicitly attacks the bourgeois way of life, an expression of modern society ruled by businesses and banks and in which art is just a luxury for those who do not have anything better to do.[5]

Capuana and Verga's views on the poor and the connection between modernity and suicide are in line with trends transpiring at the time from the literature on suicide. The matter was one of the privileged subjects within the ambit of the emerging social sciences. Right in Italy in those years, the positivist researcher, Enrico Morselli, wrote one of the first treatises on suicide, *Suicide: An Essay on Comparative Moral Statistics* (1881). By analyzing the statics available at the time, Morselli showed an inverse relationship between suicide and crime, claiming that where societies were most advanced—like in northern European countries and the north of Italy—crime was less and suicide cases more prevalent and vice versa in less modernized countries. The suicide rate was thus taken as an indication of society's advancement and as an aspect of the theory of evolution.[6]

---

[4] In the preface to the first novel of *The Doomed* cycle, *I Malavoglia* (*The House by the Medlar Tree*), he wrote: "The motive force of human activity that propels the current of progress is here caught at its source, in its most modest, material expressions. The mechanism of the passions acting as determinant in these low spheres is less complex and can therefore be observed with greater precision. All one need to do is leave the picture its clear, calm colors and its simple design" (1983, p. 3).

[5] "Art was once an expression of one's culture, today it is a luxury item: or rather a luxury for the idle to indulge in. [...] We live in an environment dominated by banks and industrial companies, and the feverish pursuit of pleasure is the exuberant manifestation of such a life" (Verga, 1965, p. 225).

[6] "Homicide, theft and deceit are, he continued, immoral acts performed to satisfy some instinct or want, «the morbid weapons of the competition for life.» However, in civilized societies, the struggle for survival tended to manifest itself intellectually. Under the excessive weight of a struggle to which their faculties proved unequal for some, brain deterioration induced madness or frustrated aspirations, which in turn led to despair and thoughts of suicide. «[H]e [...] in whom education instilled the sentiment of duty, will

Morselli's study (1881) was very influential on a later and more famous study on suicide, namely, on Émile Durkheim's seminal work, *Le Suicide* (*The Suicide*) (1897 [1951]). The French sociologist concluded his study with the comment: "The exceptionally high number of voluntary deaths manifests the state of deep disturbance from which civilized societies are suffering and bears witness to its gravity" (1951, p. 391). Capuana and Verga seem to fully embrace the notion and represent in their respective works the correlation between the advancement of civilization and suicide as a deviant answer to it.

Capuana and Verga's Elite Suicides

In both the novels *Giacinta* and *La Sfinge*, the protagonist, who takes her or his life, belongs to the upper-middle class, and in both cases Capuana is interested in narrating the story of progressive deviation from established norms that ends in an extreme way.

In *Giacinta*, what seems at stake is an "infringement of the social norms, in this case supported by the papers, which dictate our code of conduct" (Michelacci, 2015, p. 71). Giacinta, the protagonist, is born to a wealthy family but lacks love especially from the mother, Teresa. In her early adolescence, she is raped by the factotum of the family, Beppe, whose description mirrors that of those doomed to be criminals according to Lombroso's theories. As much as the rape negatively affects the girl, it is not the event itself that determines Giacinta's future difficulties but rather the stigma it leaves on a social level: According to a typically patriarchal mentality, what is compromised in the rape is the protagonist's reputation. This view is so ingrained that at one point even Giacinta will develop a kind of sympathy for Beppe, not seeing him at all as the cause of her troubles.

Giacinta falls in love with Andrea, a rather mediocre and inept man, but she marries a rich man who will have her but whom she does not love. She then continues an adulterous relationship with Andrea from which she will have a baby girl. Giacinta convinces Andrea to leave his job and live off the money that she is going to give to him; however, at this point, he realizes that he does not love her anymore and he starts keeping away from her. When the baby dies because of an illness, he remains indifferent to the tragic event. Left with nothing to live for, Giacinta decides to commit suicide: "«Yes, die!» her

---

cut the thread of existence with his own hands rather than make use of [...] [the] homicidal weapon»" (Brancaccio, 2013, p. 709).

heart said, with sweet allure. «Your love has gone! There is no purpose to your life! Yes, die! die!»" (Capuana, 2011, p. 197).

In the same way that from the beginning Beppe is described as predetermined to commit crimes, Giacinta too seems doomed to succumb, to the extent that she forges her own destruction as if she was compelled to do nothing else but that. Her suicidal resolution follows the same pattern; it comes as the final gesture of a linear trajectory:

> «To die! To die!» Feeling light-headed and rid of everything, she had no other thought. People with this character trait, having made a decision, feel real relief. They know that now they must reach their goal and they do not look back or sideways. They forge straight ahead, with their heads held high, fleet-footed and sure, seeing only that final goal. (Capuana, 2011, p. 198)

Suicide comes to her mind as the only possible solution to her *inability* to live. However, more than being a philosophical or existential decision, it is depicted as the answer to the lifestyle of this affluent middle-class society with all its hypocritical constrains.

As Scalessa notes, there is a strong connection between suicide and class belonging:

> Suicide may be interpreted both as a reaction against the narrow rules of a hypocritical and patriarchal society and as the result of an egotistic girl exasperated by the insults to which life has exposed her (according to a nineteenth-century male perspective, egotism is an integral part of several female personalities). It has to be added, too, that such a character as Giacinta might have developed only within a bourgeois context and we could not conceive a similar affair occurring among those peasants or miners featured in *Verismo*'s narrative. In some sense, therefore, Giacinta's *caso patologico* may also be referred to as a kind of bourgeois suicide, providing an example bound to be followed by later authors. (2013, p. 164)

Although rape, adultery, loss of a lover, and a child's death are also very much part of the life of a peasant, in a typical *verista* scenario, they would not lead the protagonist to suicide. It seems, as we will see, that peasants are far too concerned with surviving that they do not have time to think of dying. In Giacinta's case, suicide is also the product of a pathological situation, which, again, derives from modernity and from the complexness of high society. Interpreted as being simple people by *veristi*, peasants do not have in their mental makeup the complexity of thought that can lead them to take their own life. Suicide, in this novel, is the inevitable consequence of a neurotic character's defeat by social conventions.

In this sense, the less known but critically appreciated short novel, *La Sfinge*,[7] is constructed in a similar way in so far as it brings to the extreme consequence the inability of the protagonist to navigate reality. Here, even more than in *Giacinta*, everything seems construed to prepare the ground for the final act.

Giorgio Montani, the protagonist, is a writer in the middle of a creative crisis. He has never really loved anyone until he meets Fulvia, a widow with a sickly child. After casually noticing her a year earlier, Giorgio finds out that the woman and child live in front of his house. They meet again and they start a relationship in which for the first time he feels strong emotions. Surprised by his own feelings, he begins to think that the best work of art is the one that you can live, thus replacing his failure as a writer with the love story he is experiencing. When doctor Butironi, the child's doctor and a family friend, appears on the scene and starts visiting Fulvia very often, Giorgio's jealousy erupts to the extent of compromising his relationship with the woman. At the same time, Fulvia ambiguously makes Giorgio understand that their relationship is not as real as it seems to him; it is more like an *artistic* creation, which cannot last long nor be approved by society. Completely blinded by jealousy and the impossibility of fully living his love story, Giorgio commits suicide.

Capuana puts the reader again in front of a situation in which middle-class rules determine the boundaries of the character's actions. As in *Giacinta*, we are dealing with a pathological case in which the protagonist is unable to manage real-life situations. According to Pagliaro (1988), the real reason for the suicide is Giorgio's own literary failure; however, Burnaby claims that "Montani's suicide is less an acknowledgement of failure as a desperate attempt to safeguard his living masterpiece" (2004, p. 26). Moreover, the critic also notes that "Montani by no means kills himself at an emotional peak" (2004, p. 22). In fact, the protagonist's suicide is long meditated and not the consequence of an impetuous decision.

The seed of self-death is there from the very beginning, since Giorgio's sadness and pessimism are linked to the passing of his beloved mother and the suicide of his brother for unknown reasons. When Giorgio feels so happy with how his relationship with Fulvia is going, he starts to think of dying to preserve this unique moment of his life:

[7] For a summary of the critical debate around *La Sfinge*, see Zuccala (2019).

> Until yesterday I either did not dare to believe, or I doubted, or I did not believe at all, according to the circumstances, the appearances of things and the state of my mind; today I believe. And before my dream—this reality is so beautiful that I can't call it otherwise—and before my dream fades away, before you, still so young, find that your love for Giorgio has worn away and died and life has enticed you and invited you to feel other emotions (everything changes, everything causes sorrow, everything withers away and dies here!), I would like to die, to die loving you, without ever waking up from this sweet dream. (1895, p. 118)

When he finds himself at the opposite end of the emotional scale and now has doubts about Fulvia's love for him, his response is the same: He contemplates committing suicide as his brother had done six years earlier. He regrets not having killed himself when he was still happy—"He would die happy, deluded to be loved! While now..." (1895, p. 158)—for now, the motivation is the exact opposite. Interestingly enough, what changes is the reason why the protagonist should kill himself and not whether he should. All Giorgio's internal debates around suicide always go hand in hand with physical manifestations designed to show the alterations in the character's state of mind, as in the following examples: "He would feel as if suffocating; and would grip his temples for as his head felt about to burst" (1895, p. 47); "wringing his hands, biting his lips so as not to shout, always with that hideous scene playing out before his eyes, always with those stabbing pains at the heart which made him anxiously count the minutes" (1895, p. 51):

> He sprang from the armchair where he had been curled up to ponder better in the dark, he sprang up (he didn't know whether out of fear of himself or savage joy) as the idea flashed in his mind like lightning. He was in a cold sweat. He passed his hands over his forehead again and again, now to brush away that idea, now to better see it through the fog that clouded his mind. (1895, p. 159)

Giorgio's suicide appears, even more so than Giacinta's one, the result of a sophisticated overactive mind and a twisted way of thinking. Giorgio right from the beginning seems destined to commit this extreme gesture. If one views the general consensus of critics reading the novel as a response underpinned by the advance of Decadentism, embodied by D'Annunzio (Pagliaro, 1988; see also Barnaby, 2004), once again we find Capuana's idea regarding modernity being confirmed claiming its pledge; that is, the popularity of Decadentism, the most modern approach to literature and life at the time, was the result of the changing ethos away from tradition, and it is this that sets the tone to the plot. Capuana's protagonist is created almost to *mock* contemporary decadent characters, similarly burdened by modernity, and he pays the toll.

Verga's suicidal literary cases move in the same social sphere as Capuana's ones. Pietro Brusio, the protagonist of *Una peccatrice*, is a law student with a passion for literature, while Alberto Alberti, the main character of *Eros*, is a marquis. Passion and love are again the motives for their actions and suicide. Pietro, in love with Narcisa Valderi, wife of a count, is able to conquer her thanks to the success of one of his theatrical plays. After a period of intense happiness, Narcisa realizes that Pietro does not reciprocate her love anymore and commits suicide. Pietro is shocked by the event but carries on conducting a dissipated mediocre life:

> The promise of the splendid heights his creative genius would reach, which love in one day had elevated to match his ardent soul, had fallen away with this love itself. Pietro Brusio is now less than a mediocre being, who drags out his days in his native town, composing a few sterile verses for his relatives on their feast days, and dissipating his sparse patrimony as merrily as possible. (1965, p. 128)

In *Eros*, it is the protagonist, Alberto, who commits suicide after a debauched life. He spends his youth passing from one relationship to the other until he gets married to Adele, his first love. When she finds out that he is meeting one of his previous lovers, the couple faces a crisis that Alberto does not know how to handle and therefore leaves. During his absence, the wife becomes ill and he returns to her only to see her dying. Realizing how he has wasted his own life, Alberto commits suicide.

Eros is the last of the Verga's pre-*verista* novels, characterized by upper-middle-class settings and generally located in the north of Italy. In these, Verga shows his critique of such a society by portraying dissolute lives like Alberto's one: "in Verga's anti-bourgeois protests, and more specifically his youthful novels, one finds traces of a return to 'healthier' values emerging, which presented an alternative to bourgeois degeneration of a cleaner bourgeois lifestyle" (Masiello, 1970, pp. 58–59).

Capuana and Verga's Suicides Among the Poor

While in Capuana and Verga's representations, rich and upper-middle-class people are fighting or succumbing to the evil of modernity, poor people are left with no choice but to accept their condition or perish. Verga's *Malavoglia* clearly depicts the effect of modernity on the poor and how it engulfs and sweeps such people away after they have been exposed to alien lifestyles. The novel focuses on the Malavoglia family to show different responses to modernity. One of the sons, 'Ntoni, faces his downfall after trying to make a better life for himself outside his village and away from his family's traditions; whereas the youngest son, Alessi, accepts his condition and is able to build a decent and stable life. Other characters are doomed to succumb as well, but none of them ever think of committing suicide. All the misfortunes that befall them, brought on by the novelty of modernity, are faced with either resignation or rebellion. Even in the moment of greatest misfortune, the characters, regardless of their choices, are supported by an inspired almost epic tenacity and the simplicity of thought which do not allow them to think of ending their own lives.

Only two characters from lower classes commit suicide in Capuana and Verga's works. In Verga's short story, "L'ultima giornata," an unknown worker in the northern region of Lombardy lies down on the railway tracks and waits for the passing train to kill him. Being unemployed, without money, family or friends, or even a place to stay, he wanders desperately through the countryside until he reaches his final solution. The other characters—mostly a crowd that chorally comments on the suicide—have no empathy for him nor do they display sincere sorrow. The distance between the dramatic gesture and the emotions of those who witnessed it only heightens the sense of despair and loneliness of the anonymous protagonist might have felt: "Nobody knew anything else. He had come from afar. He had been told: In Milan, which is a big city, you will find [what you are looking for]" (2011, p. 418).

It is precisely the fact that the suicidal person has no name that makes him a universal figure; he is more of a symbol standing for desperate humanity affected by the effects of modernity (he had gone to the big city in the hope of finding work) than an example of the tragic living conditions of the working class that can drive one to suicide. It is more of an existential story rather than one of denunciation. The *hermeneutic* narrator, as Contarini (2008) notes,[8] is the only one capable of giving meaning to the protagonist's desperation and of recognizing his humanity among the indifferent group of characters that surrounds him and his death.

[8] "In Verga it is not unusual to have a narrator interpreting events as part of the story, and furthermore who undergoes a progression as the text advances; if in *Bastione di Manforte* he only imagines the «sighs of love or pangs of hunger» that filter through «the thin walls of those small rooms», in the short story that symbolically closes the collection, *L'ultima giornata* (*The Last Day*), his voice gives meaning to the action of the desperate, misunderstood, long-suffering man who committed suicide, which otherwise was passively witnessed by casual passers-by" (Contarini, 2008, p. 337).

Likewise, Capuana depicts a suicide from the lower class in his novel *Il marchese di Roccaverdina* (1901 [2001]). Compare Santi, a peasant farmer, is forced to sell his little piece of land to the Marquis, who already owns all the land around it. After the deal, he is left with nothing and commits suicide by hanging himself on the same piece of land that once was his. Before dying, the Santi character, already in dire poverty, appears three times in the novel, always to obsess with his presence the Marquis, responsible for his fall. However, after the suicide, the peasant comes back to haunt the Marquis and challenges his psychological stability, already compromised by the memory of the murder he committed of another farmer, who had been his right-hand man. This homicide is part of the main plot of the novel, whereas comparing Santi's story is a secondary thread that interweaves with the main one and is functional to its unraveling. The Marquis' madness, in fact, will be exacerbated by different episodes among which there is that of Compare Santi's suicide. In one of the crucial moments that determine the progressive fall into madness, the Marquis in his mental nightmares conflates the murder of the farmer with the suicide of Santi:

> The Marquis had fallen back into that intermittent state of lucidity from which he had awakened a moment earlier; only his cousin's faint, almost indistinct words rang in his ears: «Those you were prompted to kill! These were driven to kill!» Yes! Yes! The devil, alas! had whispered the terrible word to him for a whole week [...] And he had killed! [...] So, later, the devil had suggested to Santi Dimauro: «Go hang yourself! Hang yourself!». And he had hanged himself! [...] Would he never be rid of these nightmares?. (2001, p. 234)

It is evident that the suicide of this poor peasant is subordinated to and has more to do with the Marquis' story rather than with it being included to denounce the unbearable difficulties the poorer classes have to contend with; in other words, Santi's death counts more for the influence it has on the Marquis' mental stability than for itself.

Conclusion

Through a close reading of the suicide cases present in Capuana and Verga's writing, it becomes clear that self-death, seen as a consequence of modernity, is an option only for the middle and rich classes who are an expression of that modernity, while the desperation provoked by the hardships and living conditions of the poor is not necessarily a trigger for taking one's own life. In treating suicide as a by-product of modern living and as a matter affecting the privileged classes, the two Sicilian authors follow the dominant discourse emerging from social science, which was claiming precisely the existence of a link between the degree of so-called civilization and the suicide rate.

References

Burnaby, P. (2004). The riddle of the Sphinx and Ariadne's thread: The critique of positivist and decadent sexual myths in Capuana's *La Sfinge*. *Spunti e ricerche, 19*(1), 13–28.

Brancaccio, M. T. (2013). The politics of suicide: Historical perspectives on suicidology before Durkheim. *Journal of Social History, 46*(3), 700–715.

Capuana, L. (1861). *Garibaldi. Leggenda drammatica in tre canti*. Galatola.

Capuana, L. (1880). *Studii sulla letteratura contemporanea*. Brignola.

Capuana, L. (1882). *Studii sulla letteratura contemporanea. Seconda serie*. Giannotta.

Capuana, L. (1895). *La Sfinge*. Brigola.

Capuana, L. (1898). *Gli "ismi" contemporanei. Verismo, simbolismo, idealismo, cosmopolitismo, ed altri saggi di critica letteraria e artistica*. Giannotta.

Capuana, L. (1988). La Sicilia nei canti popolari e nella novellistica contemporanea. In M. Freni (Ed.), *L'isola del sole* (pp. 75–97). Edizioni del Paniere.

Capuana, L. (2001). *Il Marchese di Roccaverdina*. Garzanti. (Original work published in 1901).

Capuana, L. (2011). *Giacinta*. Mondadori. (Original work published in 1879).

Capuana, L. (2019). *Fausto Bragia e altre novelle*. Nerosubianco.

Contarini, S. (2008). La fantasmagoria del reale: una lettura delle 'novelle milanesi' di Verga. *Lettere Italiane, 60*(3), 323–351.

Durkheim, É. (1951). *Suicide: A study in sociology*. The Free Press.

Fusaro, E. C. (2007). *La nevrosi tra medicina e letteratura: Approccio epistemologico alle malattie nervose nella narrativa italiana 1865–1922*. Polistampa.

Masiello, V. (1970). *Verga tra ideologia e realtà*. De Donato.

Michelacci, L. (2015). *Il microscopio e l'allucinazione. Luigi Capuana tra letteratura, sceinza e anomali*. Pendragon.

Morselli, E. (1881). *Suicide: An essay on comparative moral statistics*. C. Kegan Paul & Co.

Pagliaro, A. (1988). Aspetti tecnici e continuità tematica in *La Sfinge* di Luigi Capuana. *Spunti e ricerche, 4–5*, 63–82.

Pardo Bazán, E. (1981). *La tribuna*. Library of Alexandria.

Scalessa, G. (2013). Representations of suicide in Italian narratives from the 1860s to the early twenty century. In P. Bernardini & A. Virga (Eds.), *Voglio morire! Suicide in Italian literature, culture, and society 1789–1919* (pp. 159–176). Cambridge Scholars Publishing.

Spinazzola, V. (1977). *Verismo e positivismo*. Garzanti.
Verga, G. (1965). Una peccatrice. Storia di una capinera. *Eva. Tigre reale. Milan*. (Eva original work published in 1873).
Verga, G. (1976). *Eros*. Milan.
Verga, G. (1983). *The house by the medlar tree*. University of California Press.
Verga, G. (2011). L'ultima giornata. In G. Verga (Ed.), *Tutte le novelle* (pp. 415–420). Einaudi.
Verga, G. (2014). *Malavoglia*. Interlinea.
Verga, G. (2020). *I vinti di Verga*. Independently Published. (Original work published in 1873).
Virga, A. (2019). Orientalization and romanticization of the sicilian people in Capuana's work: A postcolonial reading. In A. Pagliaro & B. Zuccala (Eds.), *Luigi Capuana: Experimental fiction and cultural mediation in Post-Risorgimento Italy* (pp. 95–107). Florence University Press.
Zuccala, B. (2019). Gendered self-reflection and theory of form in Capuana's *La Sfinge*. In A. Pagliaro & B. Zuccala (Eds.), *Luigi Capuana: Experimental fiction and cultural mediation in Post-Risorgimento Italy* (pp. 157–180). Florence University Press.

Anita Virga is Senior Lecturer in the Italian Department at the University of the Witwatersrand. She completed her Ph.D. at the University of Connecticut in 2015. Virga has published various book chapters and papers on Italian cinema and literature in academic journals such as *Italian Studies in Southern Africa, Spunti e Ricerche, Italica, LEA, English Studies in Africa, JICMS*, and *Tydskrif vir Letterkunde*. She is the author of the monograph *Subalternità siciliana nella scrittura di Luigi Capuana e Giovanni Verga* (Firenze UP, 2017). Virga was the President of the Association of Professional Italianists (API in South Africa) from 2015 to 2017, and she has been the Editor of the journal *Italian Studies in SouthernAfrica* since 2018. She is the co-founder of BLOSA (A South African Platform for Blended Learning). Her research interests are postcolonialism, migration, black identity, blended learning, Sicilian literature and cinema, and the works of Luigi Capuana and Giovanni Verga.

Irony, Suicide, and Social Criticism in Margarita Nelken's Short Novel: *Mi suicidio* (1924)

Juan A. Godoy Peñas

Contents

Introduction.......... 109
Irony, Suicide, and Social Criticism.......... 112
Conclusion.......... 117
References.......... 118

Introduction

The loss of the last colonies in America in 1898 caused Spain to engage in deep social and cultural reflection as a society, which, in addition to increasing industrialization and internal displacements from rural areas to the cities (and the socioeconomic changes related to it), contributed to the creation of literacy institutions to make education more accessible to workers. This educational transformation contributed to the proliferation of readers of newspapers and short novels, seeking to satisfy their new literary pastime. At the same time, this led to a revolution of the publishing market as more writers found

J. A. Godoy Peñas (✉)
University of Cincinnati, Cincinnati, OH, USA
e-mail: godoyjo@ucmail.uc.edu

J. Ros Velasco (ed.), *Suicide in Modern Literature*,
https://doi.org/10.1007/978-3-030-69392-3_7

an audience for their texts, and new, low-price journals needed to be created in order to host these works. The formats of serialized novels and sagas, which were very successful during the nineteenth century, gave rise to a genre that had been popularized many years previous by Miguel de Cervantes and María de Zayas y Sotomayor: The short novel.

The first publication where a short novel can be found came to light in 1907 under the title *El Cuento Semanal* (*The Weekly Tale*). The increase in cultural interest of the readers, the low price of these journals, and the *political tranquility* of that moment favored the reception of this kind of publication. Other critics, such as Pascual Martínez, have also noted that the increase of the population, the entry of women into cultural and social life, and the growing erotization of the genre as reasons to explain the success of this editorial revolution (2000, p. 71). However, *El Cuento Semanal* is not the only journal that emerged. The labors of Sonia Thon, Pedro Pascual, Ángela Ena Bordonada, Alberto Sánchez, and Julia María Labrador were essential, as they researched all new publications that arose and reclaimed their role in the cultural and intellectual outlook of the first third of the twentieth century. After *El Cuento Semanal*, Eduardo Zamacois, who had lived in France and knew the French *nouvelle* very well, created *Los Contemporáneos* (*The Contemporaries*) in 1909, which lasted until 1926. Three years after the origin of *Los Contemporáneos*, we can find *El Libro Popular* (*The Popular Book*) (1912–1916). *La Novela Corta* (*The Short Novel*), *La Novela Cómica* (*The Comic Novel*), and *La Novela Teatral* (*The Theatrical Novel*) were published for the first time in 1916. Other important collections of this period were *La Novela de Hoy* (*Today Novel*) (1922–1932), *La Novela Ideal* (*The Ideal Novel*) (1925–1938) with a total of 521 numbers, *La Novela Ilustrada* (*The Illustrated Novel*), by Vicente Blasco Ibáñez, or *Revista Literaria Novelas* (*Literary Magazine Novels*) *y Cuentos* (*Tales*), which survived until 1966.[1] These publications counted on writers as important as Miguel de Unamuno, Emilia Pardo Bazán, Benito Pérez Galdós, Carmen de Burgos, Jacinto Benavente, Magda Donato, Margarita Nelken, and other less popular writers, such as Juan Pérez Zúñiga, Alberto Valero Martín, Alfonso Vidal y Planas, or Eugenio Noel.

On December 27, 1924, Margarita Nelken published her short novel entitled *Mi suicidio* (*My Suicide*) in the collection *La Novela Corta* (1924a). It was in the number 474, though *La Novela Corta* would not survive much longer as it came to an end in 1925 after 499 weekly collaborations. According to

[1] To see a full list of the collections and journals published, see "Las escritoras de novela corta," by Pedro Pascual Martínez (2000).

Alberto Sánchez Álvarez-Insúa and Julia María Labrador Ben, *La Novela Corta* was the journal that actually transformed the publishing market of that time:

> But, with the publication of *La Novela Corta*, an authentic editorial revolution and a profound change in the content of readers' class will take place. The late century model: coated paper, photochromes, double column, tabloid, etc., is definitely abandoned and replaced by newsprint; at five cents for delivery, although soon to rise to ten, the lower bourgeoisie and the proletariat immerse themselves once and for all in reading. (2002, p. 215)

La Novela Corta, founded and directed by José de Urquía in 1916, aimed to raise the cultural level of Spain, as stated in its first numbers:

> The artisan, rather than bulls, will talk about letters: and the worker, when leaving the workshops, will discuss who writes best, whether it is Benavente or Galdós, whether it is Blasco Ibáñez or Baroja, whether it is Dicenta or Valle Inclán. This is the true way of making the Homeland, of raising the cultural level of a country, of dignifying the worker. (qtd. in Álvarez-Insúa & Labrador Ben, 2002, p. 2)

In 1924, a few months before *Mi suicidio* was published, Margarita Nelken wrote two other short novels for *La Novela Corta* entitled "Una historia de adulterio" ("A History of Adultery") (1924b) and "Pitimini Etoile" (1924c). They were not the first short novels that Margarita Nelken signed, as she had already published a short story in *La Novela de Hoy* entitled "La aventura de Roma" ("Roman Adventure") in 1923. After *Mi suicidio*, she published another short story in *La Novela Corta*, "El viaje a París" ("Travel to Paris") (1925), and few more in other publications, such as *La Novela Femenina* (*The Female Novel*), *Los Contemporáneos*, and *La Novela Roja* (*Red Novel*).[2]

Born in 1894, of Jewish origins, Margarita Nelken played an important role for close to four decades of the early twentieth century. Her wide range of interests (art, journalism, literature, and politics), her political ideology, and her social commitment gave her an active position in Spanish society for her time. She was the only elected Congresswoman during the three legislatures of the II Republic. Proof of her social commitment is the foundation of La Casa de los Niños de España (The Spanish Children House) in 1919 to host the children of single or married women workers and the publication of *La condición social de la mujer en España* (*Women Social Condition in Spain*)

---

[2] For more details, please see *Una posición ante la vida. La novela corta humorística de Margarita Nelken*, by Sonia Thon (2010).

two years later (2013). Among her journalistic work and the short novels abovementioned, she also wrote *La trampa del arenal* (*Sand Trap*) (1923) (Nelken & Ena Bordonada, 2000) and *El orden* (*The Order*) (1931). However, after that, she seemed to be more engaged with social activism and placed her literary creativity in second place. In 1939, she went into exile in Mexico where she earned prestige due to her work as a journalist and art critic. She died of cancer in 1986, without ever returning to Spain.

Despite the small quantity of literary works, her short story *Mi suicidio* allows us to reflect on her vision of society. In the novel, Juan López, later known as "Juan de la Cumbre," a man of a low social class who had arrived in town ten years prior to become a writer, is struck by a car operated by "el Sr. Duque de las Siete Partidas," an illustrious figure of the nobility. However, what seems to be a simple car accident becomes a suicide attempt according to the Duke. While in the hospital, Juan López discovers that the Duke has changed the version of the story and has made everyone believe he tried to commit suicide. After leaving the hospital, Juan López starts to be called "Juan de la Cumbre," as all newspapers and journals want to publish his works. Celes, his ex-lover, learns the situation and decides to take advantage of it. During the time Juan López spends in the hospital, Celes talks to the Duke and explains to him that Juan López tried to commit suicide because she broke his heart. Her goal was to make him move his contacts and give her a paper in a zarzuela. In this way, Celes sees Juan López as an opportunity for her to climb in social status. Therefore, Juan López becomes a victim of the circumstances to the extent that he has lost the control of his life, making the reader believe that a real suicide is his only way to escape this situation.

Therefore, Nelken uses a *fake suicide* to show us the division of social classes, the Europeanization of Spain as a result of the industrialization, the phenomenon of the *tertulias*, and the new publishing market. She accomplishes all of this through the use of irony. Therefore, the goal of this chapter is, firstly, to analyze the *fake suicide* as a leitmotiv of her social criticism and, secondly, to establish the connections between the irony and the suicide in order to deepen her understanding of the recent changes Spain was suffering.

Irony, Suicide, and Social Criticism

As Simon Critchley has described: "Humor is produced by a disjunction between the way things are and the way they are represented in the joke, between expectation and actuality" (2002, p. 1). However, the use of this disjunct image may vary depending on the goals of the humorist. Regina

Barreca, defining features of comedy in women's writing, affirms women write comedies to destroy a social order, but not always to propose a new and different one. Besides, she asserts that women "use comedy not as a safety value but as an inflammatory device, seeking, ultimately, not to purge a desire and frustration but to transform it into action" (1988, p. 8).

In the case of *Mi suicidio*, Margarita Nelken does not set out a new social hierarchy, but definitely criticizes the existing one. The first part of the short novel is focused on two male characters: Juan López and the "Duque de las Siete Partidas." Although one of the characteristics of this genre is the schematization of the characters and the lack of a psychological draw to them, Margarita Nelken provides enough details about their social status in order to criticize the social division that Spain suffers during the first third of the twentieth century. The story starts using the first person singular: "I do not suffer" (1924a, p. 1). Behind this "I," the reader identifies Juan López y García, whose name we know, for the first time five pages later. Not only is his name very popular, but his two surnames are as well, which proves that he is ordinary. However, the other male character holds a very distinguished name and nobility title: "Duque de las Siete Partidas." Besides these two characters, we find a third one, a woman, who does not even have a surname, which places her in an even lower social rank. The only name of her the reader knows is "Celes."

Though the differences between their names already allow the reader to clearly identify them in their respective social class, Margarita Nelken also provides other information to dispel the doubts. In relation to Juan López y García, she writes: "One night that I have, by chance, a penny in my pocket, he forced me to change it to give him two pesetas" (1924a, p. 4). Therefore, the reader is aware of the lack of wealth of this character, which is reinforced by his humble origins: Guadalajara. Also, in another part of the story, Nelken describes him as someone who "doesn't have a penny to his name" (1924a, p. 8). We also know about his social status because of the type of texts he had to write to make a living: "To pay the subscription of two pesetas a day to 'Gourmets' Kitchen' ['La cocina de los gourmets'] (what a concoction, Holy God!) I had to devise verses for advertisements for oil stoves and toothpaste" (1924a, p. 8).

In contrast, "Duque de las Siete Partidas" is presented as an upper-classman, owner of a car driven by a chauffeur, and whose financial situation allows him to be generous with Juan López y García, offering to pay the expenses of such a terrible accident:

> The renowned hero, who is proud to play the role in our society never quite praised of Maecenas, announced upon learning about the victim's personality

> that he would take on all the expense that must originate from the stay in the "Juan de la Cumbre sanatorium." (1924a, p. 5)

Through the opposition of these two male characters, Nelken denotes the prevailing social class distinction.

Although Nelken's contribution to the women's rights movement and the defense of the role of women in society has been very well documented in recent years, Nelken not only fought for women but also for the proletariat. As Ángela Ena Bordonada states (2000), during the 1920s, she had become increasingly involved with worker's conflicts. She led the first women's cigar-makers strike and gave multiple conferences and rallies for the sake of the proletarian cause. During Primo de Rivera's dictatorship, she participated in multiple talks at Casa del Pueblo and "Ateneos obreros" all around Spain (2000, pp. 15–16). In fact, in 1931, she published her novel *El orden*, which, among other topics, denounced the social and political circumstances of Spain. Besides, Vicenta Verdugo Martí has pointed out Nelken's fight for land reform to improve the situation of the peasantry from Andalucía and Extremadura (2012, p. 58). Verdugo has also highlighted Nelken's active role in the revolution of Asturias in 1934, as she supported the miners in her role as socialist deputy (2012, p. 59). Her social and political commitment allows us to interpret the humor and the irony explicit in the "fake attempt" as central to social claim. Nelken parodies the counterfeiting of a car accident, which suddenly becomes a suicide attempt, in order to benefit "Duque de las Siete Partidas" without considering the detriment this could cause to Juan López y García. However, Nelken reversed the situation through the use of humor; something as traumatic as a suicide attempt becomes the beginning of a successful literary career.

However, Nelken reverses this success again when Ceres appears in the story. Ceres is a stereotyped feminine character, who seems to have a cloudy life and is willing to do anything to become a popular singer of zarzuela, even taking advantage of as poor a man as Juan López y García. With regard to her, Nelken writes from the lips of Juan:

> To such an elegant, made up, and perfumed "young lady," whom I had a hard time recognizing as Celes, the Celes who, for a couple of months, made my misery even gloomier with her hubbub and her impossible temper, and that one day decided to give me the greatest happiness possible, obeying, at last, my plea to go to hell and leaving our garret with the two pairs of stockings, the shirt, the suit, the two scarfs, and the shoes with insoles that made up all her trousseau. (1924a, p. 10)

In fact, Celes takes advantage of the situation and becomes an accomplice of "Duque de las Siete Partidas" when she tells him that Juan López y García tried to commit suicide because she left him alone. As Celes' story fits together with the Duque de las Siete Partidas' version of the accident, he promises to help her to find a job in a zarzuela. Therefore, Celes comes back to Juan López y García and promises not to leave him alone anymore. Within this context, he is again a victim and loses his freedom when he tries to run away from her. Celes replies to him: "Because your life is mine, you know? Mine. And, being mine, you have no right to «threaten it»!" (1924a, p. 15). Those are the last words the audience can read. That way, the social division between the three characters suddenly disappears, as Juan López y García becomes Juan de la Cumbre and Celes becomes a zarzuela star. The three characters now belong to the upper class, "erasing" any trait of disparity caused by his origins. At the same time, it allows the reader to think about the different backgrounds of those that belong to the upper class and the various potential ways they obtained this socioeconomic status.

However, it is necessary to wonder why Nelken makes such a negative portrayal of women when she advocated for their rights her whole life. As Josebe Martínez has explained, Nelken's understanding of the feminine gender is based on her opposition to the traditional dichotomy between the social construction of the woman and her biological function (1997, pp. 19–20). Besides, she advocated for the economic independence of women, as well as for their access to education. In fact, Nelken considered education as a key factor before women could opt to vote and that is why she was opposed to women's suffrage. Like many other intellectuals, she thought that, without education, the women's vote would be under the control of the church or their husbands and/or fathers. The reason to understand why Nelken draws such a stereotyped portrayal may be behind Joane Gilbert's theory about the politics of performing marginality. In her analysis of the humor and the social criticism in the Spanish novel after Franco's death, Pilar Martínez-Quiroga has pointed out that, although parodying one's own group contributes to reinforcing a sense of community (based on a set of features, traditions, and behaviors that its members are supposed to have in common and, therefore, to strengthen a stereotype), writers may also use the parody as an appropriation for subversive use (2015). In fact, Gilbert affirms that: "Female comics, like so many others, perform their marginality in an act simultaneously oppressive (by using demeaning stereotypes) and transgressive (by interrogating those very stereotypes through humorous discourse)" (2004, pp. 137–138). In the case of Celes, Nelken describes the only feminine character as a subject that is able to take advantage of a suicide attempt, thereby claiming a more independent role for women, who largely encompassed an oppressed and silenced role during the first third of the twentieth century. That way, Nelken uses the humor and the car accident/suicide attempt to perform the marginality of the women. Celes is now the character that, somehow, is oppressing Juan de la Cumbre, as he wishes to get rid of her, but she would not allow so because it is her way to have a role in this dramatic scene and to belong to the intellectual circle. From oppressed to oppressor, Celes is a clear example of how female writers use humor and stereotyped discourses to perform their marginality, as stated by Gilbert.

That said, there is still one more element from the period she lives in that Nelken wants to parody and, at the same time, criticize. After the "suicide attempt" and the protection of "Duque de las Siete Partidas," Juan López y García becomes "Juan de la Cumbre." As we understand "cumbre" as the highest part of a mountain, Juan López y García has moved from the lower social groups to be considered as one of the most prestigious writers of the literary and cultural circles, as stated in one of the newspapers he reads during his stay in the hospital: "One of our young poets of greater and fairer prestige among our intellectual «elite» [...] has tried to end his life" (1924a, p. 5). The director of one of the most important print media tries to make an agreement with him in order to have him as a daily collaborator. However, Juan de la Cumbre cannot ensure it due to the high number of orders he is receiving. Paradoxically, the near end of his life has launched him to the top of the literary circles. That way, Nelken is criticizing the publishing market established during the first part of the twentieth century, which appeared at times to be more focused on making money than on creating high-quality literature. In fact, Alberto Sánchez Álvarez-Insúa and Julia María Labrador Ben point out that "*La Novela Corta* built its trajectory with important authors who do not sell: Margarita Nelken, Roso de Luna, and Cansinos [...]" (2002, p. 215). Also, many of these new publications included illustrations, worldly news, and discount vouchers or prizes in order to bring the buyer's attention. The fact that, on many occasions, these new publications were in the service of making easy money influenced this kind of literature to be considered by many critics as popular literature or sub-literature. Roselyne Mogin-Martin affirms that the readers, though they appreciated the quality of the stories, did not demand it: "These readers, both women and men, buy their magazines in kiosks, and if they appreciate the quality of the material, they do not demand it either, given the exiguity of their budget" (2000, p. 36). On the other hand, Juan de la Cumbre's fast rise to the most important intellectual circles can also be interpreted as a criticism of the advantages men have in becoming successful writers compared to women.

Nelken goes one step further if we associate her critique of the publishing market to the marginality of the women. Nelken had suffered first-hand what it meant to be a female writer and the obstacles this entailed. She is not only using the female stereotype but also the stereotype of a short novel writer, considered by many critics as a less important genre as its main consumers were women and members of a lower socioeconomic status. Therefore, through the parody of women and the literary critics, Nelken is also promoting short novels as a literary genre, as well as the role of female writers in this period. Nelken uses humor to end the stereotype of bad quality of this new literary phenomenon and to recognize the important labor women are doing during her period to produce new works that educate people somehow. As we had stated before claiming Gilbert's theory, Nelken is performing her marginality and humor in order to subvert the social status of women and the low-class population "by embodying the potential power of powerlessness" (2004, p. 137).

Conclusion

In short, Nelken uses three stereotyped characters and humor to make a realistic portrait of the society of beginning to the twentieth century in Spain where social class division, gender roles, and the publishing market are key points of her argument. In the margins of her writing, she depicts the fake suicide attempt of a low-class man, Juan de la Cumbre, and the opportunism of it for a candidate singer of zarzuela, Celes, to make readers think about the reality they live in and to call their attention to fight for social justice during one of the most turbulent ages in Spanish history. Even if, as Pedro Pascual Martínez has pointed out, the short novels were not the main literary genre for social and political claims, Nelken uses it in *Mi suicidio* as an easier way to connect with readers she was interested in, the low social class, which was the largest demographic predominant at that moment (2000). Therefore, Pilar Martínez-Quiroga's theory helps us to understand Nelken's use of well-worn topics of the popular literature, as Carmen Servén Díez had already pointed out in 1998. Nelken uses humor and parody in order to subvert the stereotypes that take place in *Mi suicidio*. Nevertheless, Martínez-Quiroga's perspective invites us to rethink and re-explore other short novels written not only by Margarita Nelken but also by other women writers that approached humor as a tool to claim a social change.

References

Barreca, R. (1988). *Last laughs. Perspectives on women and comedy*. Gordon and Breach.
Critchley, S. (2002). *On humour*. Routledge.
Gilbert, J. R. (2004). *Performing marginality, humor, gender, and cultural critique*. Wayne State University Press.
Martínez Gutiérrez, J. (1997). *Margarita Nelken (1896–1968)*. Ediciones del Orto.
Martínez-Quiroga, P. (2015). Humor, feminismo y crítica social en la novela española contemporánea. *Bull. Span. Stud., 92*(6), 931–949. https://doi.org/10.1080/14753820.2014.947854
Mogin-Martin, R. (2000). *La Novela Corta*. CSIC.
Nelken, M. (1923). La aventura de Roma. *La Novela de Hoy, 2*(40).
Nelken, M. (1924a). Mi suicidio. *La Novela Corta, 474*.
Nelken, M. (1924b). Una historia de adulterio. *La Novela Corta, 442*.
Nelken, M. (1924c). Pitimini Etoile. *La Novela Corta, 456*.
Nelken, M. (1925). El viaje a París. *La Novela de Corta, 488*.
Nelken, M. (1931). El orden. *La Novela Roja, 5*.
Nelken, M. (2013). *La condición social de la mujer en España*. Horas y Horas.
Nelken, M., & Ena Bordonada, Á. (Eds.). (2000). *La trampa del arenal (de Margarita Nelken)*. Castalia.
Pascual Martínez, P. (2000). Las escritoras de novela corta. In M. Villalba Álvarez (Ed.), *Mujeres novelistas en el panorama literario del siglo XX: I Congreso de narrativa española (en lengua castellana)* (pp. 67–94). Universidad de Castilla La Mancha.
Sánchez Álvarez-Insúa, A., & Labrador Ben, J. M. (2002). La obra periodística de Emilio Carrera (I): Sus colaboraciones en *Flirt* (1922-1925) y *La Gracia* (1923-1924). *Cuadernos para investigación de la literatura hispánica, 27*, 207–256.
Thon, S. (2010). *Una posición ante la vida. La novela corta humorística de Margarita Nelken*. Centro Superior de Investigaciones Científicas.
Verdugo Martí, V. (2012). El compromiso de Margarita Nelken. *Andalucía en la historia, 38*, 56–59.

Juan A. Godoy Peñas holds a double Ph.D. from Florida International University and the Complutense University of Madrid (Spain). He was a visiting instructor at the University of Qingdao, China, where he was also the first coordinator of the dual-degree program in Spanish between the said university and Florida International University, and teaching assistant at Harvard University. He is currently an Assistant Professor Educator at the University of Cincinnati. Godoy Peñas is interested, on the one hand, in the hybridity of literary genres, specifically of autobiographical genres, as well as in the literature of exile and the formation of identity through the concepts of nation, time, and language, and, on the other hand, in developing tasks and didactic materials that entail a greater involvement of the African-American community in the Spanish classroom.

The True Life in the False One (*Das wahre Leben im falschen*): Suicide Attempts of Literary Heroes in Eastern German Literature

Angelika Potempa

Contents

References ... 130

East Germany was one of the "world leaders" as her suicide rate is concerned. As the historian Grashoff argued, this high rate was, nevertheless, "normal" in that it followed, at least since the 1970s, West German and regional historical trends (2006). Against expectations, the majority of suicides were not related to protests against or frustrations because of the repressive political system but to utmost personal circumstances, moments of a "total personal breakdown or after a succession of painful failures or losses" (Grashoff, 2004, p. 26). Total dissatisfaction, hopelessness, broken relationships, the desire to punish others who disappointed, or to end a life that was overshadowed by extremely painful, incurable, or terminal illnesses were major motives, and often there existed a history of depression and/or other mental conditions. All this, however, the public did not know. Official policies prevented that by limiting or forbidding collection and publication of data, doing research, and to operate suicide prevention programs and use talk therapies to treat depressions (Grashoff, 2006). The questions of whether and why someone could perceive one's life as *nicht*

A. Potempa (✉)
The University of Texas Rio Grande Valley, Brownsville, TX, USA
e-mail: angelika.potempa@utrgv.edu

J. Ros Velasco (ed.), *Suicide in Modern Literature*,
https://doi.org/10.1007/978-3-030-69392-3_8

lebbar/unlivable (Fühmann with reference to Trakl, qtd. in Tate, 1995) and what it is that makes it not just bearable but dignified and happy would have opened the door to criticism on *Socialism As It Really Exists*. And the suspicion was justified. Studies by Blankenship (2011, 2017), Beutin et al. (2001), Zimmermann (2002), and Grashoff (2004, 2006) show that quite a number of literary works of the 1970s and 1980s were devoted to suicides, but not as suicide studies but discourses that subversively critiqued the political system, including its past, ineffective socioeconomic and healthcare measures, hollow and euphemistic phraseology of "official language," and, even, the official understanding of literary-cultural heritage and appropriate stylistic means. Moreover, these texts, mostly written with an audience in mind, had to offer the reader possibilities for identification (Deiritz & Krauss, 1993; Helwig, 1986) by using common cognitive schemata and emotion patterns, valuations, and symbols, as well as by providing insights into how the political and economic permeate the private and are experienced in everyday life, shape people's biographies, expectations toward life, and the scope of their ability to take control of their lives in their locale. To the audience, the ability to converse about everyday life sensibilities or the big questions in life mattered. The media were censored as were texts on the socialist way of life, coming from heavily ideologically shaped fields, such as sociology, scientific socialism/communism (according to Stalin, together with Marxist-Leninist philosophy and political economy, one of the three essential parts of Marxism-Leninism), philosophy, and ethics. Reliable data were in short supply, and topics as happiness, self-realization, love, death, suffering, failure, and injustice were not granted much space, if any at all (Herzberg, 2000; Hörz & Wilke, 1986; Mende & Mocek, 1996). The latter did not prevent critical writers from painting a picture of GDR life that could have prevented many "naïve" or inaccurate judgments by western social scientists or publicists, as the sociologist and political scientist Klaus Schroeder noted: "Hard facts provide only frameworks to understand the realities of everyday life" (1998, p. 572). Texts by Dieckmann (1999, 2000) and Engler (2002) support this insight.

Literature on (mainly) fictional suicides, because it had to take the situatedness of individuals and their personal perception of life into consideration, seems to be a treasure trough in that regard. Even texts with questionable aesthetic and/or written by authors who toed the party line or did not disavow the notion of reformability of *real* socialism can be expected to include an "excess" of reality insights that help to understand how and what value orientations and mentalities allowed for functioning and final downfall of the system and contributed to the breakdowns of individuals. Within the "Great Lie," people lived their lives in ways that they perceived as authentic: They "cursed, loved, betrayed, lied, were sad, hoped, or sank in despair," so Görlitz (1999, p. 121), one of the party loyalists. To not recognize this devalues their biographies and is based on moral absolutes and, also, ideological. Those who had left the GDR did not become *Mitläufer*/followers in this particularly oppressive system. But, if we work with absolutes, as Adorno seemed to do (1951, pp. 29, 43), does this mean that only those who lived in places that did not belong to this system could "live the truth," an undamaged life? Isn't C. Wolf's Kleist right with his, "No place on earth" (2007, p. 100)?—Even if it sounds apologetic. A wide field...

The following discussion will pursue this line of thought and fits under the umbrella term of political culture research. It will trace the imprints of two interconnected philosophical tenets of Stalinist Marxist-Leninist ideology regarding "real life" as depicted in texts by system loyalists and critics. After all, this ideology served as kind of "blueprint" for the formation of *real socialism* with its inability to democratize: (i) a teleological model of history, claiming that history worked itself toward communism, with the communist party as owner of the truth and driving force of universal human progress, and (ii) a reductionist concept of the individual, which did neither consider the individual being the owner of its own living conditions nor focus on self-determination, individuality, and embodiedness (Kolakowski, 1978; Mende & Mocek, 1996). To understand how these models influenced the literary characters' contradictory living arrangements and their reflections, a combination of an understanding and interpretative approach to literature (in Dilthey's sense of *Verstehen,* 2020) and an ideology-critical lens will be applied. The latter is, among others, shaped by Žižek's ideas of ideological disidentification, master signifiers, and the power of the fake (2002). As the former is concerned, Dilthey attested literature a "sense of reality" because it expresses lives lived by embodied individuals that are embedded in local and historic social structures. Accordingly, literature is written and read willingly and feelingly and within a broader context of interrelated meanings (Dilthey, 2020). To which Žižek (2002) might add that ideology is part of that structure:

> The future is ours... You have a goal in sight.
> (A labor movement song that was adopted by the Free German Youth).

On the side of progress, out of the dark past, forward to the ultimate goal of history, socialism/communism. The Party knows the way of history and will tell you about it. You belong to the "winners of history," since you were born in the GDR, the "first German peaceful state" and the antifascist-democratic alternative to the FDR, which is a shelter of militarism and neo-fascism....

(A brief summation of the doctrine of history for young generations).

Accordingly, the new history started with the liberation from fascism, celebrated annually on May 8, the Day of Liberation (Jarausch, 2012). As a result, history got split in a "before" that was full of hardships and an "after," that was good per se, constantly perfected, and which began with denazification and the conviction of Nazi criminals. The latter, following Dimitrov's definition of fascism (1972), was mainly done by the destruction of the fascist state and the expropriation of corporations and banks. Although antifascism was an important legitimation for the existence of and identification with the GDR, its focus on the communist resistance led to the neglect of the struggle and suffering by others, such as Jews, homosexuals, Sinti and Roma, Members of the Confessing Church and Jehova's Witnesses, and of socio-psychological reasons for the seizure of power and the ordinariness of Nazism (Jarausch, 2012; see also Brinks, 1997).

With *Horns Ende* (*Horn's Fate*) (2001), which linked this "forgetting" to another one, the one of victims and perpetrators of Stalinism, Hein did not only raise the issues of collective memory, historiography, and remembrance policies but also of historic guilt and injustice as Blankenship (2011, 2017), Zimmermann (2002), and Beutin et al. (2001) pointed out. But there is a deeper problem; it concerns the unspoken of sun around which everything rotates and in whose interest the forgetting was: The Party, with its organizing principle of democratic centralism and its myth of the "politico-moral unity of party and people" (Deutscher Bundestag, n.d.). The Party depended on strict "party discipline," according to which every member had to follow a decision once it had been made by the (top of) the party. Otherwise, the party rulership, which hid behind the ominous "the Party," could not have maintained its power. By superimposing this principle of top-down decision-making on economic and political structures, pluralism could be eliminated in the name of "the will of the people" and opponents sidelined or pushed out; fear got induced. Injustices were masqueraded as "historically necessary" (Hein, 2001, p. 83). More so, the party that portrayed itself as revolutionary reinforced thoughtless following, and subservience, and odd rituals, such as demonstrations of gratitude to the leadership or *Gegenpläne* (planned plans to surpass the planned economic headline goals). Party loyalty and the belief that history would judge the grand project "right" made even old-guard communists join the silence about the suffering under Stalinism, as H. Zinna in her novel *Katja* described (1981). The "community of the silent" of the townspeople of Bad Guldenberg was united by the power of fear, guilt, shame, cowardice, and relief to be allowed to just get on with their lives. Simultaneously, their participation in the new anti-fascist democratic state allowed them to disavow objective guilt and "enjoy the small pleasures of daily life" (Žižek, 2002, p. 91).

Thus, they gained a We-identity in the "state of the plain people"; they belonged again because of or despite their inner distance (Elias, 1994, p. 488; Žižek, 2002). By being rewarded continuity in their biographies, they became an integral part of the reproduction not just of official ideology but the system as a whole. They functioned, accepted, and indifferently complied with the decisions of "never seen authorities" (Hein, 2001, pp. 32, 186).

There was plenty of room for cynic, apolitical, indifferent, subservient, and servile behaviors; though officially deplored, they fit in. How well, Claudia, the disengaged main character of Hein's *Der Fremde Freund* (*The Distant Lover*) (1989) divulged: After having mocked traditional family roles, others' ideas of the good life, the need to push one's own life's dream on one's child, and the wish for close emotional relationships, she came to state that she had achieved what was possible for her. She was fine; her colleagues would face a riddle, if she committed suicide. As for taboo subjects, her advice was to not bring them up; these memories are embellished or contorted, nothing but "radioactive waste" (1989, p. 99). Her cynical tale was right on target: The schizophrenia that people lived in East Germany was self-made, embedded into the system. How crippling this self-destructing *Hamlet Machine* was has been expounded by the psychiatrist Hans-Joachim Maaz (1995), an Easterner himself: Having, again, settled in the "false life" came at the price of skewed needs and dammed up emotions (Maaz, 1995, p. 29; see also Barbagli, 2015, p. 126). That frustration, loneliness, depressions, and, finally, suicide of Hein's Horn character would not have been influenced by it, seems to be unthinkable. The same applies to the death of Heiduczek's Jablonski in *Tod am Meer* (*Death by the Sea*) (1999), the suicide attempt of Frank in Braun's *Unvollendete Geschichte* (*Unfinished Story*) (1989), and the suicide of the father in Krauß' *Der Dienst* (*The Service*) (1990). Conflicts between individual and state are present, as Zimmermann (2002) explained in detail, but there is a psychosocial history behind it. The state had seeped into the lives of the individuals, their value orientations, life plans and expectations, and daily emotional states and psychological conditions; it had become part of them. Also, believability and identification possibilities with regard to stories depend on showing the fictitious characters' suffering in and from life, that is, how they experience normality and abnormality of their everyday lives; suicide is a deeply individual reaction. So, some of the fictitious suicides have stronger links to the political than others, but the political played into all of them—without being necessarily dominant.

How the difficulties of life at a time when the hardships of the after-war years were in the past mixed with both the silence about Stalinism and an overabundance of talking about communist resistance and suffering in concentration camps is at the heart of H. Zinna's novel *Katja* (1981). Though including autobiographical elements, it is the fictitious story of a mother's search for the 'big Why' behind her daughter's suicide and, with it, the question of preventability. The honesty, with which the story was told, prevented it for years from being published, although Zinna belonged to the old-guard communists, was highly decorated, and did not fundamentally question the Eastern German socialism project—publication date is 1980, after Görlitz's *Eine Anzeige in der Zeitung* (*An Advertisement in the Newspaper*) (1978 [1981]). What appeared to be the tale of intergenerational conflict within a not-so-common family (communist anti-fascists) was much more than that. Though told in a much simpler and direct way than Hein's stories, it, too, provided a distressing picture of value and life-plan clashes and emotional conflicts in *real socialism* and how these contributed to Katja's suicide. Katja suffered because she could not understand the hardened attitude of her father, who, like his comrades, stayed quiet about the damage that Stalinism did unto his and many others' lives and because she was forced to live with too much of a particular history and live among the dead (Zinna, 1981). Her mother had made it her life's mission to give those a voice who had given their lives in the fight against Hitler and to tell about suffering and comradery in prisons and concentration camps. Furthermore, stories and behaviors taught Katja, like many of the younger generations, to suppress her emotions. Katja's conflicts were also shown to have been caused by a general expectation that the younger generation would be grateful for being granted to live their lives according to their parents' ideas of a good life (1981, p. 52): A little house or apartment with a garden and honest and diligent work on a job that affords a "decent" life with vacations and supports a family. What to think about this dream and how one's own life projects fit in were questions that captured the pulse of the time, as the writings of others, such as Plenzdorf (1972 [2002]), Braun (1977 [1989]), Wander (1977 [1993]), Heiduczek (1977 [1999]), and Görlitz (1978 [1999]) showed.

In this context, Zinna and Görlitz touched on the ironies of having to be grateful for something that one has not asked for and how that could happen in a 'shortage economy,' under a government that tried to dictate which needs were appropriate and, therefore, to be met. The questions, though, why "society" would expect gratitude and why this gratitude belonged to "The Party," they did not ask. If the life that's easier than the life of the parents' generation is a gift, why should one continuously feel guilty for accepting it? Refusal would have meant to have the freedom to experiment with one's life, a liberty, that Plenzdorf's literary hero in *Die neuen Leiden* (*The New Sufferings*) (2002), Edgar Wibeau, decided to take. It made him an outsider, though, and the Party had difficulties with determining the limits on what kinds of outsider existence were acceptable.... If the gift was an investment into one's future, it would require payback in form of goods and services. So, by not refusing the "gift" one was put into the position of borrower/owing without having agreed, taking from a government that, according to the Constitution, should provide. Consequently, one lost one's ability to determine one's role in the relationship, confirmed the giver's power and accepted a mission for one's life. And there was no place for failure/giving up, as Bakunin, Stalin, or Mehring had opined. Neither Görlitz nor Zinna went this route. By trying to encourage understanding for their heroes' suicide, instead of depicting them as acts of cowardice or "avoidance of life," they sided with Lafargue, Luxemburg, and Zetkin who recognized the complexities of individual life. Nevertheless, Zinna's Fini-character (Katja's mom), for instance, when revealing her fear that "the project" had not become the project of "our children" (Zinna, 1981, p. 38) offered explanations that did not go beyond official labels, such as failure to sufficiently educate, "remnants of the past," or "alien to socialism." This shows, among others, in the presentment of consumerism, black-market work, the role of "Vitamin B" (connections) in people's lives, Katja's ideas of role distribution in marriage (1981, p. 79), of love, and marital fidelity (marriage certificate as warranty), and her husband's and mother-in-law's notions of a good wife and life. How the apparently non-fit actually fit into the system, because of its economic and emotional binding power and despite its moral and emotional toll, escaped Zinna. Nevertheless, by calling attention to suppressed emotionality and the daily emotional toll of "the gap between the real and the wished for" (1981, p. 154), that is, failed or endangered life plans, disappointed expectations toward others, especially friends, family, and lovers, she grasped the "normality" of many of the suicides in Eastern Germany. People faced personal conflicts in their daily "easy life" and reacted emotionally but not irrational; they had reasoned about what to do. And suppressed past traumas were lingering, too. So, "normal suicides" were non-political but influenced by the political, not driven by endangered livelihood but galvanized by the desire to break a cycle, escape a personal situation that was perceived as intolerable, and signaled the need for help (Grashoff, 2006, pp. 13, 22–23).

The suicide of Görlitz's teacher Manfred Just in *Eine Anzeige in der Zeitung* also matches this categorization. In his case, it's a conglomeration of several factors, among them stress on the job and related to it, disappointments about friends and colleagues, the dreaded outlook on early retirement, and the collapse of his dreams for his life. The cancer diagnosis really hit him hard. Just's life centered around his profession; he was a full-blood teacher. And he desired to have a happy family life with his new love and partner. The political impacts his life especially through his clashes with Karl Strebelow, the old-guard school principle who wanted everyone to share "our" dream (Kolakowski, 1978, p. 189) of a good, peaceful life with a diligently pursed job, a little well-kept house, and a garden with orderly flower and veggie beds. By pursuing "typical" German values, such as discipline, diligence, and orderliness, Strebelow, like others, personified a mix between proletarian habitus and petty bourgeois lifestyle (Schroeder, 2000). Being in a position of power, and not sufficiently countered by the faculty, allowed him to make Just's life difficult, just because he disagreed with the less authoritarian teaching methods and the unconventional behavior of the younger, which he perceived as provocative. Lack of support by colleagues, their furtiveness, cowardice, and indifference added to the stress Just was under. Görlitz, though showing the balancing act that innovators had to perform, did not cast doubt upon Just's full-hearted affirmation of socialism. Neither did the explanatory musters he provided for Just's problems point beyond the official lines of argument in order to get to the mechanisms that made everyday life toxic. At least, the reader was offered to think about it, together with the reasons for Just's suicide. Another issue to ponder came up in connection with one of the exacerbating moments in Just's professional life, the class observation by Strebelow: Just raised the question of whether the dialogues about West German television and, in general, Eastern Germany's relationship to its alter ego, the FRG (Federal Republic of Germany), shouldn't be changed. Official propaganda was not effective, and important questions stayed unanswered. However, Görlitz stayed silent about the feeling of being walled in and the hysteria with which the state security forces tried to prevent "desertion" to the West. People were continuously trying to cross the border "illegally," despite the threat of being shot and, when caught, heavily fined and imprisoned up to 3 years (Raymond, 2000, p. 45). Just being suspected of wanting to defect created enormous stress and long-lasting difficulties, as believably shown in Braun's *Unvollendete Geschichte* (*Uncompleted Story*) (1989) and Muthesius' *Flucht in die Wolken* (*Escape with the Clouds*) (1982).

> We are young, the world is open.
> The world needs you as you need the world. The world can't be without you. (FDJ songs).

These lines really disclose the contradictoriness of different strands of the official propaganda and the wide rift between propaganda and one's life experiences. Traveling eastward was limited, even to the Soviet Union. Traveling legally westward depended on travel privileges, a passport, vetting by the state security forces, access to Devisen (foreign currency), being of retirement age, or having finally gotten approval for one's emigration permit. So, going west, be it for a short or a permanent stay, was extremely difficult. This applied specifically to younger persons with system-critical views or economic reasons (e.g., higher income, social upward mobility without having to commit to the party, professional opportunities). With the 1980s, the success of the command economy became more and more questionable, which made a growing number of people denounce the social contract that promised growing prosperity (Schroeder, 1998, pp. 554–555, 572–574, 585–586). Faced with this situation, official propaganda tried to do the impossible: Make people believe that they had to develop all their talents and creativity for the "cause" while simultaneously disowning them of their lives and talents by subordinating it to the "cause." But what was hiding behind the label "cause"?—Was it progress and a better future? What would this mean? Improvement of the living standard? Prosperity of the people? What about chances to do creative work? How do trial, error, failure, and risk fit in? What about one's interest in nature, playing soccer, or collecting stamps? More so, if it is about the cause, is it really "me" who is needed and not just a placeholder? If I am needed, why don't *you* trust me? Is something wrong with me?—which let the cat out of the bag: The "you" cannot be "the people" because the author of the questions belonged to it. What's left is the ruling political elite; nevertheless, a bit of space in the definition of the "cause" was left for people to fill in. Thereby, people got a chance to identify with the system in obviously political or apparently unpolitical ways. To overstep, and be it coincidentally, could have severe consequences.

Both Braun's sensitive Frank and Muthesius' high-strung and creative Pony got a first-hand experience of it. In the telecommunication electrician Frank's case, it was because of west contacts and the suspicion of "desertion of the republic" (Braun 1989, pp. 16, 35) and in Pony's case because of "unauthorized entering of the border zone" in East Berlin in order to "just see the West" (Muthesius, 1982, pp. 236–237). Franks' situation was complicated by his past stay at a *Jugendwerkhof* (juvenile workhouse), an institution created for the "reeducation" of youth in order to make them well-behaved good citizens (Braun, 1989, p. 30). Although the father of Frank's girlfriend Karin alleged that he had been sent there for reasons of hooliganism and petty theft, his own memory suggested that it was anti-government protests. The latter is very likely; "disciplinary problems" (Braun, 1989, p. 30) belonged to the most common reasons for committing someone to a werkhof. Many of these places used rigid systems of punishment and allowed for mistreatment and harassment, which caused traumata in their inmates (Sachse, 2011). The note about their stay that was put in their cadre dossier (portfolio) influenced their choices of professions and degrees and future treatment by the authorities. Karin got a chance to experience the latter herself; just adhering loyally to Frank, despite his west contacts and invitation to leave the country, made her suspect in the eyes of the state security, her internship supervisor, and even her father (government functionary). Promptly, she lost internship and university place and had to prove herself in a manufacturing job (Braun, 1989, p. 78). This belonged to the real-life ironies in Eastern Germany: In the state of the farmers and workers, one could be penalized with having to join the working classes.

In form of Karin's reflections about her relationship to Frank and the history of Frank's suicide attempt, Braun handed down a devastating verdict regarding the state of affairs in the GDR. There was no space for outspoken, critical people who wanted to honestly fight against exploitation; those who fell out of line got to feel the oppressive apparatus of 'the' state. This state did not need one, except for doing necessary work or serving as cautionary example to keep others in line. Life here was full of suffering and stress for both the unadjusted and the well-adjusted. The price for adaptation was to become untrue to oneself, to damage oneself by blocking one's emotionality (Braun, 1989, pp. 64, 80). This system was irreparable. The working class was alienated from power but also integrated into the state and would not revolutionize the system. Nevertheless, Frank's suicide attempt did not seem to be primarily politically motivated, despite all his suffering from the stressing and trauma-inducing political. Doubts about Karin's love, his isolation, and his prehistory were the catalysts.

In difference to Frank's, Pony's story was written, like Katja's, in search for reasons that explained a daughter's suicide. As in case of *Katja*, autobiographical elements were used. Consequently, the focus was much less on the political than on the biographical elements of the story. But it is precisely this that provided interesting insights into the penetration of private lives by the political. For Pony, a high schooler, the encounter with state security forces had tremendous consequences: In order to avoid any legal punishments, she agreed to be readmitted into a mental hospital for treatment of her depression (Muthesius, 1982). Consequently, she had to go back to a place she dreaded and had wanted to escape. Instead of restarting her life, her mental suffering and the exposure to often horrific therapies continued. Released from the institution, she was double-stigmatized—first, for having been institutionalized, which in the eyes of many people meant to be crazy, and, second, by the label of "attempted escape of the republic." Personnel managers and distributors of study slots, had to take it into account; it was in her portfolio. Ergo, she got advised to "stabilize and mature" in production (Muthesius, 1982, pp. 172–174, 236–238, 244). Not even her parents' excellent "connections" could change that, resulting in the shattering of her hopes to enter a profession that would allow her to develop and live out her enormously broad-spectrum creativity (acting, art, photography, songwriting). Her being different, an independent thinker, very sensitive, and with deep mood swings had already complicated her entrance into the work world. Considering that she was a romantic at heart and stood with both feet on the ground of (idealized) socialism, which centered life around work, that must have been devastating. Her good will to contribute to the "cause" was disregarded—as the good will of many others who were "different." The system did not offer much space for them. One of the dialogues in the book expresses this clearly by mentioning "reeducation" and asking how socialism could be built with "such" persons (Muthesius, 1982, pp. 243–244). By bringing up these questions, Muthesius touched upon a major problem of real socialism, that of failing real individuals, who are experiencing their lives, are emotional, opinionated, gendered, aged, more or less healthy, and differently talented. They all wanted to "pick up the flower of happiness," as Wolf's Kleist expressed in *Kein Ort. Nirgends* (*Not a Place. Nowhere*) (2007, p. 63). Since humans cannot be neatly divided into a feeling and a thinking part, society has to accommodate the whole and allow to live as the embodied that oneself is, that is, "authentically" (Wolf, 2007, p. 100). But none of the existing societies has granted that yet, thereby being a contributing factor to "unlivable lives" (Wolf, 2007, p. 100).

Eastern German mental health treatments attested to it, as Muthesius described. Talk therapies that took also the existential situatedness of the individual into consideration were in short supply, and many treatments were based on a reductionist biomedical picture of man, which focused on physical factors. To these belonged insulin cures and strong electroconvulsive therapies, in addition to monotonous occupational therapies. Pony endured years of these treatments. The romantic that she was, she wanted not just a livable but an enjoyable life, which had to include three things: To be unconditionally loved, to be understood, and to have the opportunity to try to make her dreams come true. Love, however, was the overarching condition (Muthesius, 1982). She gave up on it in a moment when she felt too exhausted to continue fighting.

To sum it up, the literary characters of Pony, Katja, Frank, Just, Horn, Wolf's Günderode, and Kleist shared that they were not depicted as cowards or losers but persons who were not able to live authentically; they could neither live out their emotions nor their dreams of a happy, satisfying life, personally and professionally. The affective structures of GDR society, that power relations had provided and that continued and mixed with mentalities that stemmed from the past, were a big part of what stood in the way. Mentalities have an afterlife, even after governments have changed and influence the presence. Consequently, literary suicides or attempts were also reflections of the normal in the unnormal: The trigger was deeply personal, and, in the end, those who are left behind are left with guesswork and open questions.

So, talking about suicides allowed to demonstrate how the political had become part of their literary heroes' everyday life difficulties and joys, valuations, and life plans; it showed these writers' commitment to their readers. Although the literary quality of their texts and their approaches differ, their mirror image of GDR life, lived by people who had "settled in," was in many points distressing. But it was a "microcosm" of GDR life (Blankenship, 2011, p. 133). Thereby, these writers invited their readers to participate in the precarious conversations on the guiding principles for their personal lives and whether they could live these out in real socialism, something neither official propaganda nor philosophy offered.

References

Adorno, T. W. (1951). Minima Moralia. *Theodor Adorno Archive*. http://www.efn.org/~dredmond/MinimaMoralia.html. Accessed 15 Feb 2020.

Barbagli, M. (2015). *Farewell to the world. A history of suicide*. Polity.

Beutin, W., Ehlert, K., Emmerich, W., Kanz, C., Lutz, B., Meid, V., Opitz, M., Opitz-Wiemers, C., Schnell, R., Stein, P., & Stephan, I. (2001). Die Literatur in der DDR. In W. Beutin, K. Ehlert, W. Emmerich, C. Kanz, B. Lutz, V. Meid, M. Opitz, C. Opitz-Wiemers, C. Schnell, R. Stein, & I. Stephan (Eds.), *Deutsche Literaturgeschichte* (pp. 511–579). J.B. Metzler.

Blankenship, R. (2011). *Transforming suicides: Literary heritage, intertextuality, and self-annihilation in GDR fiction of the 1970s and 1980s*. University of North Carolina at Chapel Hill.

Blankenship, R. (2017). *Suicide in east german literature: fiction, rhetoric, and the self-destruction of literary heritage*. Camden House.

Braun, V. (1989). *Unvollendete Geschichte*. Suhrkamp.

Brinks, J. H. (1997). Political anti-fascism in the German Democratic Republic. *Journal of Contemporary History, 32*(2), 207–217. https://doi.org/10.1177/002200949703200205

Deiritz, K., & Krauss, H. (Eds.). (1993). *Verrat an der Kunst? Rückblicke auf die DDR-Literatur*. Aufbau Taschenbuch Verlag.

Deutscher Bundestag. (n.d.). Deutsche Demokratische Republik (1949–1990). *Deutscher Bundestag*. https://www.bundestag.de/parlament/geschichte/parlamentarismus/ddr. Accessed 25 Jun 2020.

Dieckmann, C. (1999). *My generation. Cocker, Dylan, Honecker und die bleibende Zeit*. Christoph Links Verlag.

Dieckmann, C. (2000). *Das wahre Leben im falschen. Geschichten von ostdeutscher Identität*. Christoph Links Verlag.

Dilthey, W. (2020). *The essence of philosophy*. University of North Carolina Press.

Dimitrov, G. (1972). The fascist offensive and the tasks of the communist International in the Struggle of the working class against fascism. Main report delivered at the VII world congress of the communist international 2 August 1935. In G. Dimitrov (Ed.), *Selected Works* (Vol. 2). Sofia Press.

Elias, N. (1994). *Studien über die Deutschen. Machtkämpfe und Habitusentwicklung im 19. und 20. Jahrhundert*. Suhrkamp.

Engler, W. (2002). *Die Ostdeutschen als Avantgarde*. Aufbau Verlag.

Görlitz, G. (1981). *Eine Anzeige in der Zeitung*. Verlag Neues Leben.

Görlitz, G. (1999). *Keine Anzeige in der Zeitung: Erinnerungen*. Karl Dietz Verlag.

Grashoff, U. (2004). *Let me finish*. Headline Publishing Group.

Grashoff, U. (2006). *"In einem Anfall von Depression..." Selbsttötungen in der DDR*. Ch.Links Verlag.

Heiduczek, W. (1999). *Tod am Meer*. Aufbau Verlag.

Hein, C. (1989). *The distant lover*. Panth eon.

Hein, C. (2001). *Horns Ende*. Aufbau Verlag.

Helwig, G. (Ed.). (1986). *Die DDR-Gesellschaft im Spiegel ihrer Literatur*. Verlag Wissenschaft und Politik.

Herzberg, G. (2000). *Aufbruch und Abwicklung. Neue Studien zur Philosophie in der DDR*. Ch.Links Verlag.

Hörz, H. E., & Wilke, U. (Eds.). (1986). *Ethik*. VEB Deutscher Verlag der Wissenschaften.

Jarausch, K. (2012). The failure of east German antifascism: Some ironies of history as politics. *Historical Social Research / Historische Sozialforschung, 24*, 212–228.

Kolakowski, L. (1978). The breakdown. In *Main currents of Marxism* (Vol. 3). Oxford University Press.

Krauß, A. (1990). *Der Dienst*. Suhrkamp.

Maaz, H. J. (1995). *Behind the wall. The inner life of communist east Germany*. W.W. Norton.

Mende, H. J., & Mocek, R. (Eds.). (1996). *Gestörte Vernunft? Gedanken zu einer Standortbestimmung der DDR-Philosophie*. Edition Luisenstadt.

Muthesius, S. (1982). *Flucht in die Wolken*. Fischer Verlag.

Plenzdorf, U. (2002). *Die neuen Leiden des jungen W. und andere Stücke: Stücke und Materialien*. Suhrkamp.

Sachse, C. (2011). *Der letzte Schliff. Jugendhilfe/Heimerziehung in der DDR als Instrument der Disziplinierung (1945–1989).* Die Landesbeauftragte für Mecklenburg-Vorpommern für die Unterlagen des Staatssicherheitsdienstes der ehemaligen DDR.

Schroeder, K. (1998). *Der SED-Staat. Geschichte und Strukturen der DDR.* Bayerische Landeszentrale für politische Bildung.

Schroeder, K. (2000). *Der Preis der Einheit. Eine Bilanz.* Carl Hanser Verlag.

Tate, D. (1995). *Franz Fühmann, innovation and authenticity: A study of his Prose-writing.* Editions Rodopi E. V.

Wander, M. (1993). *Guten Morgen, du Schöne.* Deutscher Taschenbuch Verlag.

Wolf, C. (2007). *Kein Ort. Nirgends.* Suhrkamp.

Zimmermann, M. D. S. (2002). *Suicide in the German novel, 1945–89.* Peter Lang.

Zinna, H. (1981). *Katja.* Fischer Verlag.

Žižek, S. (2002). *Did somebody say totalitarianism? Five interventions in the (mis)use of a notion.* Verso.

Angelika Potempa is a Professor of Philosophy at the University of Texas Rio Grande Valley. She is originally from Germany, where she has also taught and published on ethics, political philosophy, and political humor. Her degrees are from Humboldt University Berlin (M.A., Ph.D.) and Martin Luther University Halle-Wittenberg (Ph.D.) in Germany.

The Life of Others: Marx and Durkheim on Suicide and Social Good(s)

Ricardo Gutiérrez Aguilar

Contents

Introduction: The Great Chain of Goods—Sharing and the Economic Life of the Community 134
Life and the City: Advantages and Disadvantages of Modern Collective Maladies 139
Our Life for Others: Altruism, Real Socialism, and Suicide 145
References 151

> They always met for a special purpose of religious, festal or martial kind; and this purpose seemed to sanctify their state. A man attending a sermon honestly believed that it was the sermon which mattered to him, and he would have felt astonished or even indignant had it been explained to him that the large number of listeners present gave him more satisfaction than the sermon itself. All ceremonies and rules pertaining to such institutions are basically intent on capturing the crowd: they prefer a church-full secure to the whole world insecure. [Canetti, *Crowds and Power* (1978)]

R. Gutiérrez Aguilar (✉)
Universidad de Alcalá de Henares (UAH), Madrid, Spain
e-mail: ricardo.gutierrez@uah.es

J. Ros Velasco (ed.), *Suicide in Modern Literature*,
https://doi.org/10.1007/978-3-030-69392-3_9

Introduction: *The Great Chain of Goods*—Sharing and the Economic Life of the Community

Let's talk about the nature of sharing. Maybe is against our prompt first well-meant judgment that not all malaises are to be held in contempt. If we are right in this, there are malaises and *there are* malaises consequently: The usual and the special occasion, so to speak. But usually to be sick, to be threatened by an ailment, is not a motive for joy. It is rather a matter of concern for everyone. In these very days, contagion is not among the words to tread on even lightly either. Notwithstanding:

> Some readers [maybe the boldest ones] may wonder if the term 'contagion' [can be] meant in [other] than a derogatory way. [And the response to them is that it can be. In fact,] [...] laughter and joy can be contagious, and even beneficial microbes are still contagious. (Lynch, 1996, p. viii)

First things first, it seems like we are facing a matter of character for the very illness. And we were only—and sadly—aware of one of its species. The good or ill character of the contagion obviously determines its lenient spread, as it is in the case of laughter and joy. They are welcome. As for the Holy Mass in a church-full, it depends eminently on our judgment of what is made to circulate. Thus, laughter and joy merit with no doubt for social goods: Goods deeply appreciated. And their dissemination would end in a community afflicted by happiness. A sermon is intended apparently to be of the same kind of goods and to have an akin nature with laughter and joy regarding social esteem and social expectancy. It is possible to have the sermon itself as that which truly matters. All of them—laughter, joy, and sermons—are goods deemed welcome to be distributed with good reason. But when a man attending a sermon honestly believes that it is only the sermon which matters to him, he is mistaken: Honestly but wrongly mistaken—Canetti *dixit.* If festooned—secondly—with the mark and sign of the ritual, the ceremony, and some customary rule or norm that vindicates social frequencies, there is though a main concern on the question of solidarity, on the large number of those present, on who shares what, for ritual, ceremony, and rule are—of course—the public and physical marks that lead the tempo of the distribution. But there has to be a paired tempo for the acquisition too. The positive moment of religion, the material public aspects in the rite, within the relic, should be supported in the same representative move by highlighting the trait of its transitive and communicative nature. The last, not being a material aspect in reality at all. That is the real measure of goods in question here. At the end, it boils down to their commonality value. Astonishment and indignation would make their entrance then just in the fashion of a symbolic knot between the disputed value of the goods themselves involved and the yet unnoticed added value of the community of stakeholders to the equation. What really matters to the pious sermon listener is to be sharing the experience, the shared presence of his fellows within the symbol the summoning words of the homily embody. To discuss heresy in the indignant movement of the zealot is to project reversely the real standard of value. Not the sermon but the faithful assembly is what matters to him. And so concealed, the treasured value of the homily hides its character as a mere symbolic substitute. Had it been explained to them that the satisfaction felt was due to the crowds and not to the words themselves, they would have been astonished or even indignant. The argument on solidarity turns surprisingly into one on desacralization: The attempt against the sanctity bestowed onto the community. It is to coin an absolute standard of value for the special occasions in which we live with others. And the suspected ripping off of all sanctity can be understood as the negative vicarious representation of a total judgment, a judgment on the real value of the dissolution of the social bond, and as non-recognized standard where it is not the honest belief that it is the item shared which matters but having something to share at all. Under this logic, *is all sharing to be judged as* good?

Like joy and laughter, festal, religious, and martial spirits are highly regarded contagions. Spirits are transported and stitched together with ease. Community sprouts. Lord Shaftesbury knew it already better there in the far 1707:

> One may with good reason call every passion 'panic' which is raised in a multitude and conveyed by aspect or, as it were, by contact or sympathy. Thus, popular fury may be called 'panic' when the rage of the people, as we have sometimes known, has put them beyond themselves, especially where religion has had to do. And in this state their very looks are infectious. The fury flies from face to face, and the disease is no sooner seen than caught [...] Such force has society in ill as well as in good passions, and so much stronger any affection is for being social and communicative. (2000, p. 10)

Pan's influence flies on the wings of the conspicuous representation. Present to everyone and partaken by everyone. The emblem, the sign, must be shown as much as it must be shared. We are told the concrete aspect of this special Eucharist involves some sort of contact. Of passing from hand to hand or from face to face. The public mark presented by Shaftesbury bonds all those present capturing them physically by means of its circulation. It is a matter of ascription by appropriation, no sooner seen than caught. The aspect and the looks work in the manner a catalyst would do toward the constitution of an assembly. Looks are infectious. But the alleged multiplier effect of passion—the threat of the large numbers, the pathological aspect of the disease—is not such a threat. It is a production, the production of an increased meaning. The numbers do not grow merely in quantity but in quality as well. The threat is nothing more and nothing less than the astonishment felt after the constitution of a shared newly emergent dimension accessible to the crowd who built it: A state, a communication structure, an in-between, and a network ultimately.

Some "theories of social psychology [...] view social structure as a distribution system. Network approaches, for instance, see actors in a network as possessing varying amounts of valued resources that, in turn, set into motion a variety of exchange processes" (Turner, 2006, p. 356). This approach in social psychology is fond of establishing four main principles in regard to social interactions: (i) actors are basically agents. They put themselves beyond their own actions. So, their role is encrypted in their behavior. That is the piece of evidence we have to pay attention to. And behavior is stubbornly object-oriented. In attending to the object, the agent honestly believes that it is what really matters to him. Items work more like nodes, crossroads of facilitated interactions, though. They redirect and expand the reach and sense of the agent's action in a feedback. Following this, it can be said that we are bound to a *representational realism*, an onto-epistemological position that states all interactions are accomplished only with the due intervention of such objects. (ii) Metaphorically, these items give shelter to meanings. More properly said, it can be held that they are in fact vicarious meanings, sense-laden icons. They take in certain representational content as the item flies from hand to hand or face to face, within the distribution system. The object is a focus for meaning and is thickened by it in the procedure. It is not just something in the place of something—*presentational*—but the ontological chance to tell the story of a process, *representational*. A process of gaining value. It is a fetish in relation to value, in short. This value stems from a chain of *symbolic interactions*, a chain in which distribution, administration, and appropriation occur in due time around the related item, promoting its meaning. Be it laughter, joy, ceremony, or ritual, there is an *economy of the symbol* in the works in which (iii) actors develop their own social identities as necessary—or complimentary—cooperators in the dynamic distribution of the system. They do it in the growing of the symbolic capital within the network. If representational items and actors are structural parts of the system, then it is only in the fashion of agents that are capable of starting a process and, with this move, they engage at the same time in constructing their own role within the system as the system acquires a new dynamic dimension giving rise to new possible nodes; (iv) actors entangled in this activity come to share a common reality: A common life or life in common. Contentwise, it is obviously an artificial one, elaborated, manufactured by them. That is a possible definition of goods, the economic one. Goods are non-natural resources in the context of a planned distribution chain. And under these circumstances, these goods should be called accordingly social goods. Regarding its relative character, it is a decentered reality, a social realism sustained by the intersubjective character of the exchange in which actors trade meanings—i.e., representations (McCall, 2006).

Deepening our inquiry into social goods, it seems like *s*olidarity, property, and satisfaction are social lines of force—or tension—we should count in. They bring us inadvertently near the territory of a most interesting three-way dialectics:

> Individuals as responding to the distribution of goods, bads, and other valued or devalued resources in terms of their perceived fairness or justness [...] [concoct] a comparison theory. Expectation-states theorizing and related approaches such as status characteristic and status construction theories all conceptualize status structures as both an effect and cause of the differential distribution of prestige, power, and evaluations; moreover, status itself is conceptualized as a distributional process whereby power and prestige are unequally distributed across a set of interacting individuals. (Turner, 2006, p. 356)

Individuals perceive their relative position in the chain of representational distribution, the distribution of representational goods and bads and its fairness or not, and have therefore the need to respond to it. And not all exchanges preserve the equity momentum of the process. Their would-be response is a claim within rights for the fair share, because some exchanges are deemed unequal by its very nature and meaning, i.e., status. In its balance, this explains partly the problem with dialectics as well, for if it is inherent to the idea of prestige or power as a resource that we would face an unequally distributed network position, it is no less evident that as communicative forces can have natural inertia toward solidarity, they can indulge in forgetting the subjective counterparts of the equilibrium. Is all sharing to be judged as good? Are we correspondingly bound to share in an absolute sense? Some exchanges are deemed unequal, but not all. Nonetheless, it is not a moral claim, at least in principle. It is just a matter of discussed proportions. Sometimes the structure simply fails to balance adequately its distributive tensions. However, in the representational realm, justice does not have to be commutative nor symmetric. An incipient theory of justice is so born, and its regulative criterion is but comparison: First, a comparison of course with the fellow with whom we share. The subject of evaluation in the case referred—as an illustration for the argument—is the status perceived. Status is in itself an effective representation, definitely not a structurally neutral one—if unequal—part of the goods and bads and other valued or devalued resources. It is something worth trading then, item and node at the same time once in the administration system. Thus, in the same move, any effective structure can officiate as both an effect and cause of the network differentials. Furthermore, symbolic resources administration is made dependent on the weighing of a perception. Status is constructed, built out of a combined representation: What we can expect in the sharing. Status, prestige, power, and authority would join the cause with joy and laughter concerning goods farmed in common. Conveyed into the multitude, they have put it beyond itself. Such performative force has a society. But the possibility of an argument on a just and fair distribution—as with the one presented above on the offense of desacralization—warns us about considering the restitution of the classical economic categorization between economic and free goods. If the judgment of value—or disvalue—is able to engender indignation, then a measure to it is possible and a criterion for valid (non)distribution conceptually achievable. Some goods are off the system and should remain like that. There is no positive evaluation for sharing in an absolute sense. It is then understood that not all sharing has to be good—or that sharing in a restricted sense implies distribution of a limited resource and the expected threat of dissatisfaction in deprivation. Goods sharing is now morally sensitive to the nature of the goods.

Free goods are intended to be off the economic system. For example, we are prone to think better under this light both of laughter and of joy, not disputed or scarce goods, but will find difficulties with the dialectics of status, prestige, and power which is always controversial. Laughter and joy would be candidates for a type of free goods, not overseen ones. In conclusion, is there any good that individuals should and could not share at all in accordance, a special one that we would unrelentingly avoid to cash out as common property?

Let's move forward to the special case at issue. Allow us at this point to give Émile Durkheim space, enough to make his proper entrance once the conversation is already that advanced: Talking about goods and bads:

> Among the different species of death, some have the special quality of being the deed of the victim himself, resulting from an act whose author is also the sufferer; and this same characteristic, on the other hand, is certainly fundamental

> to the usual idea of suicide [...] The intrinsic nature of the acts so resulting is unimportant. Though suicide is commonly conceived as a positive, violent action involving some muscular energy, it may happen that a purely negative attitude or mere abstention will have the same consequence. Refusal to take food is as suicidal as self-destruction by a dagger or firearm [...] The causes of [such] deaths are outside rather than within us, and are effective only if we venture into their sphere of activity [...] Of course, in common terms, suicide is pre-eminently the desperate act of one who does not care to live. But actually life is none the less abandoned because one desires it at the moment of renouncing it; and there are common traits clearly essential to all acts by which a living being thus renounces the possession presumably most precious of all. (2005, pp. xl–xlii)

Life and the City: Advantages and Disadvantages of Modern Collective *Maladies*

Talking about goods and bads, valued and devalued resources, life should be presumably the possession most precious of all. But is it a possession at all? It is 1897 and Durkheim publishes the capital classical study on suicide—*Le Suicide: Étude de Sociologie*. Conceptualized there as a possession, one more property, the theorizing Durkheim points out at the negative dialectics brought by the inclusion of it without due care into the chain of distribution and exchange. Life is, at times, also ruled by the social regularities of trade and administration. *Possession* is *economic goods*. And economic goods are to be distributed, partaken, since only in the act of management and administration of them—the act of making them circulate—can the value and disvalue of goods change. Same with life if it is going to be so categorized by the indignant response of the suicidal. The differential distribution is both cause and effect of an act; the deed of the agent shows a plausible representational connection between active—violent—and passive acts. There is an absolute structural difference—a relational one—between including or removing an item off the chain of distribution. But its removal if noticed can be measured in comparison with the effect of its former presence in the chain alone.

Supposing that life has some sort of representational status—and according to Durkheim it does—we could presume it has necessarily among other structural goods. Hierarchy of value is the result of a distributive process. It is in relation to other structural goods that life would reap its worth. It has it back again once into a communicative network. Durkheim underlines a contradiction in the dialectics just to enlighten and strengthen the underlying economic logic and does it not with one but with two intertwined paradoxical cases which support each other: The first one presents the desperate act of one who does not care to live, a case in which he assigns apparently zero value to the goods in dispute, but referring suicide the deed of the victim himself is an act whose author is also the sufferer: Cause and effect. And the suffering in question is but the deprivation of the most precious possession, something of worth, an absolute value, on the other hand. The value perceived of the supposed item should be off charts then and should be not tradable, zero value versus absolute value. A necessary connection in meaning comes in handy here to help us disentangle the connection between contradictions. Because in the second one, renouncing life and desiring it, renouncing the most precious possession of all and appreciating it as it is, is solved in a comparison as soon as we realize that mirroring it, both the action and the omission—deed and abstention—of disposing of one's life, has the same absolute differential value within the network. It is a conceptual equivalent, as happens with life and death, appreciation and renounce, in the first contradiction. When value is unequally distributed across a set of symbolically interacting goods, a claim to fairness must be represented inevitably by a renewed exchange. In the case of the most valued goods along the distribution chain, presence and absence should matter the same and amount to the same regarding structure differentials. In the same sense, deed and omission are equals.

This is rounded up in one of the most insightful commentaries Durkheim displays in his monography on suicide: The Alsacian author has come at the last part of his work, the development of a succinct taxonomy for suicidals exclusively dependent of institutional factors. The taxonomy abounds in details of the social and communicative connections across multiple sets of interacting individuals and groups. Each group and each dynamic system of social interactions or network puts into circulation its own set of symbolic goods, of valued and devalued items, and these create consequently what we could call a *symbolic niche*. An environment in which—in Durkheim's words (2005)—a *temperament* or representational and emotional profile is constituted for the group: A moral constitution or fluid identity that differs from group to group, from time to time. Unfortunately, identities are usually inclined to collide, either in between or against groups. Drawing in part on Spencer's writings influence, the so-called *egoistic suicide* (*le suicide égoïste*) and the *anomic suicide* (*le suicide anomique*) are the assumed individual's response to the (im)possible social economy of his own symbolic capital within the network. That is, being the distribution equally unsatisfactory for types of suicidal, their position pushes to the limit the dialectics of solidarity and *property—intégration and régulation* according to Durkheim. In fact, their position challenges it. They are dependent on their perception of the fairness of the distribution structure—or on the presence of a distribution structure at all—dependent on the compatibility or non-compatibility within the system of their own particular expectations-states. The egoistic expects too much, the anomic too little. The relation of ideas that binds an administered chain and the lot we can expect of its trade of goods is easily brought into the argument. Expectation-state is property prediction. Bargaining over deserved property:

> Anomy indeed springs from the lack of collective forces [from the lack of expectations-states satisfied, of administration of any possible goods] at certain points in society; that is, of groups established for the regulation of social life [and its representational economy]. Anomy therefore partially results from the same state of disaggregation [or lack of symbolic economy] from which the egoistic current also springs. But this identical cause produces different effects. (Durkheim, 2005, p. 263)

The lack of any valuable exchange and the lack of any possible exchange at all are obviously tantamount. And they presumably have identical cause. It equates to the absence of any expectation-state satisfaction. These expectations of validity would be off charts by definition, not classifiable inside the scope of what should merit as exchange in that group, one of them by falling short and the other by not finding any criterion. Suicide is a claim against the current evaluation of goods. Durkheim's arguments trying to correct the utilitarian position on suicide tend to highlight this conclusion. To judge of the deed or the omission thereof in the manner of a projected benefit—the case of the suicidal that renounces to life as it was not the value he expects—is to surrender to the symbolic economic logic at stake here; maybe it could help at least to explain the cases of *partial* and *attempted suicide* (Fenichel, 1945, p. 401). For Durkheim, the suicidal recognizes the logic but rejects it. Symbolically, it is a transcendental act—an act on the verge of the group's limit—that confronts the group's value frame in that case. It is a good moment to recall that there is a temperament profile for each group. Is there any social interaction and distribution system that fosters more than others that extreme act of self-destruction?

> The fact that suicide, like insanity, is commoner in cities than in the country [...] [seems to indicate that] the social causes of suicide are, as we shall see, themselves closely related to urban civilization and are most intense in these great centers. (Durkheim, 2005, p. 16)

Cities promote the tendency, but why is it so?

For each group, a temperament. These temperaments present themselves in the form of tendencies. Urban civilization is depicted along the lines traced by industrialization and centralization. The city is the big industrial center of life. There is an urban life running through the processes of modern civilization harbors. Quantitatively, it is obvious that in urban life, the city dwellers are freely exposed to a myriad of unexpected encounters in comparison with the countrymen. It is a matter of large numbers, and an ever-growing population is the mark *par excellence* of the big city. Mobility and travels broaden the city's horizon. Citizens are open to a myriad of exchange opportunities with their fellows. Either desired or not, the social frequencies escalate. The chance? The nodes of interaction that public spaces like squares, main streets, avenues, theaters, *cafés*, and markets provide, making social and communicative passions more easily infectious. They are modern mediation spots, hubs of transition, and places to confront the difference in the encounter with others. To confront the difference and to allow it to pass the barrier of our privacy to intimacy. The history of Paris—biographical base camp of Durkheim—would never be the same without the *Palais-Royal*, *le Temple*, or the revolutionary *Place Vendôme*, where Jacobin assemblies took place. Interactions qualitatively multiply too with a multifarious new universe of enticements and expectations due to new goods and roles, roles amplified by the nodes and tendencies in the distribution of the very symbolic goods. It is a complex system. Goods as status, prestige, authority, and power, let alone the new ceremonies, rituals, or rules, accumulate with cultural products that expand expectations furthermost: Cause and effect in the same move. Simultaneously, material abundance brought by the endless repetition praxis of industrialization indulges in conspicuous consumption (Sennett, 2003; Veblen, 2007). Merchandise is born. The distribution network is hypertrophied: More interactions around more goods. And so an exchange should be made efficiently, easier and faster. Acceleration in life occurs, more quantity to juggle with. The city is the place for a new extended cosmos. Durkheim talks about the profound representational change—a new *Weltanschauung*, a brand new intuition of the World—that modern centralization played erasing administrative boundaries and frontiers. He calls it *hypercivilization* (Durkheim, 2005). In good positivist spirit, the analysis of the facts appears to indicate a place and a time for the start of such unintended sociological experiment: The 1789 Revolution and the bureaucratic compulsion that followed it through. Just to make things happen easier and faster, *provinces*, *départements*, and *quartiers* were legally recomposed, at the end of the cosmic chain, *l'État* (*the State*), its dweller, a troubled cosmopolitan. The global new dimension of facts puts into tension once more the old equation between expectations-states, satisfaction, and solidarity.

L'étranger (*the stranger*), *l'immigré* (*the immigrant*), *le dilettante* (*the dilettante*), or *le flâneur* (*the wanderer*) along with the shiny figure of the *dandy* illustrate perfectly the city's general character, its emotional and representational profile, what is of worth, valued, and devalued to it. They are characters without roots, endlessly mobile but without certain direction nor expectation, void both in desires and vocation, although involved in the exchange chain, narcissists in short (Sennett, 1980)—free and autonomous individuals, open to the adventure of writing for themselves the most interesting autobiography, but who are wary enough of possibilities as to avoid decidedly to begin the enterprise. Anomy and egoism are the *élan vital* of urban melancholy. *Le suicidaire* is another character in this civilized *Comédie Humaine*. Playing the antagonist role, those who are naturals to the environment, the equivalent figures of the *bureaucrat* and the *bourgeois*:

> For a whole century, economic progress has mainly consisted of freeing industrial relations from all regulation. Until very recently, it was the function of a whole system of moral [and institutional] forces to exert this discipline [...] Nations are declared to have the single or chief purpose of achieving industrial prosperity; such is the implication of the dogma of economic materialism, the basis of both apparently opposed systems [that is, freeing industrial and personal relations and exert at the same time the necessary discipline to achieve it in prosperity]. And as these theories merely express the state of opinion, *industry, instead of being still regarded as a means to an end transcending itself, has become the supreme end of individuals and societies alike.* (Durkheim, 2005, pp. 215–216)

It is institutions that give society its characteristic demeanor. Institutions are social devices that administer and discipline needs, a perfect example of a network or chain of distribution. In this sense, so the institutions, so the society. They are signs of expectations-states to be satisfied. Tendencies climb back to their cause. For Durkheim, these causes crystallize in social facts susceptible to be measured, to be compared. It is social facts and not individual tendencies what should be traced back to their origins. The rest of the figures are but symptoms for a social etiology. There are constant collective inclinations in each society and group, the temperaments of which are a subject for social physics. The data multiply and either collected in repositories, archives, or public governmental statistics departments they are for sure the materials to the successful correlation of social concomitants. Sociology should concern itself exclusively with structural considerations and should concern itself with a comparative and quantitative history of institutions, not with the motives and desires of particular individuals. If the trigger for suicide is mental illness, climate, race, heredity, or imitation, the intrinsic value of the acts so resulting is unimportant at the level we consider.[1] It is strongly recommended not to put the cart before the horse. Moral and personal concerns come after, they are *extra-social*, microcauses—emergent traits in putting together the sketch of the semblance of society. It is the network and its differential distribution what really has importance sociologically speaking. And suicide rates are a constant social fact defining the character of a society. For Durkheim, there is not enough emphasis put in the term *constant*. As society springs out of eased tensions between solidarity, property, and expectations-satisfaction, suicidal tendencies are a trait intrinsic to all societies. There is no one without the tendency:

> When we forgot the individual [...] [We] sought the causes of the suicidal aptitude of each society in the nature of the societies themselves. The relations of suicide to certain states of social environment are as direct and constant as its relations to facts of a biological and physical character were seen to be uncertain and ambiguous. Here at last we are face to face with real laws, allowing us to attempt a methodical classification. (Durkheim, 2005, p. 263)

Real laws for a real society. Laws that assembled will help to devise a portrait of the particular group and its special dynamics. Of what to expect—and predict—of it. Durkheim is optimistic regarding the possibilities of a social realism. Advances in statistics methodology in France made him hope for the best, even when we know that it was rudimentary progress in the field. But, is it true that there are social inclinations that threaten constantly the existence of society? Is the very concept of society the shared common paths of distribution in its nature, doomed to produce frictions? If talking about idealism against realism, is there a social structure that could honor the idea of an eternal motion machine for goods and expectations-states?

[1] Durkheim had a direct addressee of his work in the figure of Gabriel Tarde (Jean-Gabriel De Tarde, 1843–1904), whose own work on imitation (*Les lois de l'imitation*, 1890 [2009]) confronted some of Durkheim's thesis abounding in the mimetic element: There is a strong subjective cause comparably to social tendencies. It is in acquaintance and emulation that we can find an inner flow of worth which triggers comparison (see Abrutyn & Mueller, 2014; Niezen, 2015).

Our Life for Others: Altruism, Real Socialism, and Suicide

Das Leben der Anderen (*The Life of Others*), by Florian Henckel von Donnersmarck, premiered in March 2006 in Berlin with great public acclaim (n-tv.de, 2006). The *Filmbuch* depicted on detail what could be called one of this social contradictions we are talking about: The intricacies and stern duties in which *living under* the surveillance of the State Apparatus—and the political police in GDR (German Democratic Republic), the *Stasi*—in the East Berlin 1980s consisted of and what living could amount to once time, body, thought, and feelings (all elements that surely should be counted with when it comes to evaluating what life is made of) have to cope with those imposed social conditions, once they have to enter the endless chain of social goods, the conditions of the so-called real socialism. Life under or according to something, though legitimized, should be of a different species than life itself or so it seems, a second-hand something. Social realism and *real socialism* double in structure. There is an inner logic all through the *Filmbuch* that confronts devotion and passion, altruism and egoism, with its relative weight in the service (or not) to the common good. The common good is represented obviously by the Party—that is, the SED, *Sozialistische Einheitspartei Deutschlands* (*Socialist Unity Party of Germany*). Rephrasing again our fundamental question, *is it* life—*each one's life—the lives of others*, as the translation to English of the title of the film states, *some kind of goods we actually possess, an amenity?* Is it sort of merchandise that we can rearrange in order to cope with a fair and just distribution? At the end, would be fair to rate it—in time, body, thought, and feelings—as other commonality to be shared, as an issue of social duty?

In January 1846, a young Karl Marx was *avant la lettre* more than sure of the truth of Durkheim's approach to society, not, though, with the scope of the elements to be counted in. It is true that there are measurable social facts, and that they are descriptive of social life, but we have to decide well which ones are decisive enough to pick and important enough to decipher. These facts cannot be circumscribed to social concomitants alone. If social life is to be properly depicted, it has to include *naturally* the intimate response of the interacting individuals to structural differentials: The subjective point of view as cause and effect of the structure's recurrent dynamics. Between the pages 14 and 26 of the second volume of an obscure monthly gazette edited by a friend, the *Gesellschaftsspiegel* (*Mirror of Society*), Marx published a concise excerpt of social analysis on a statistical study about suicides in France parting from the beginning of the eighteenth century. *Peuchet: vom Selbstmord* (*Peuchet: On*

Suicide) is a unique piece of evidence on the intellectual development of Karl Marx (1971). Since his prior French stay in Paris, influenced by Engels, Marx had made good use of the terms *Klasse* (*class*) and *Stand* (*estate*). They were inherited as conceptual synonyms and structural categories. Understood as a node of social worth, a point of convergence, a class is for actors always a constant focus of distribution tendencies for goods. A place for a certain crystallization. Individuals within the scope of a node have certain particular representational landscapes of their own in comparison to other *Klassen*. The estate-expectations is the *class consciousness* (*Klassenbewußtsein*). The gazette was intended precisely to be *the organ for the representation of the dispossessed popular classes* (*zur Vertretung des besitzlosen Volksklassen*), but not only. Those classes that had a fair and just claim referring to the (un)equal distribution of goods were more in numbers. A consciousness of the distribution differential regarding social goods, suicide is one of these types of claims in the same spirit as Durkheim defended. A claim essentially addressed to the nature of one special type of distribution and structure. Barely a brief account of the *memoirs* of a first-tier bureaucrat of the Restauration with Louis XVIII—Jacques Peuchet, Royal Archivist for the *Préfecture* of the Paris Police—the text on suicide is for Marx the occasion to show:

> The contradictory and unnatural [*Unnatur*, monstrous] character of modern life –not only in regard to the reciprocal relations amongst particular classes, but in all circuits and figures of the common everyday exchange. By the way, they are characterizations with the vital warmth of immediacy. (Marx, 1971, p. 14)

To directly reach the pulse of those intimate social frequencies, we should seek for evidence in:

> All sickness present to the social body; [the gazette] will publish general descriptions, monographs, statistical items and particular typical cases [...] [It] shall include within the scope of its research the spiritual conditions of workers, moral and intellectual alike, and not only the physical ones. (Heß, 1971, p. 1)

Characterizations that have to summon us as affected. The *maladie* permeates modern society in its entirety, and then the scope should be the whole of it. It goes through all estates, situations, and material circumstances. Statistics are essential to the task, but bones have to be covered by flesh to move. Macrocauses need to add up microcauses, and the particular example serves very well too to build on the tendency. If not, "critique of property relations [that leads to the major division in society between *possessed* and *dispossessed individuals*, apart from the critique] of familial relations, of the rest of private relations, in short" would be an incomplete and biased exercise in its aim (Marx, 1971, p. 14). The end station of the critique of representational goods in circulation goes as deep as the sphere of social life reaches, goes deep into every nook and cranny of community. Justness and fairness determine the reach. Social goods will include exchanges within the niche of private life, open to an economy of symbolic interactions as well. For if not, do we dare to assert that:

> The only ones in bearing the present social conditions [of Modernity and industrialization] would be the workers [the *dispossessed classes*], as if in respect of the rest of society, the outer [and inner] standing reality was [judged] the best of all possible worlds? (Marx, 1971, p. 14)

Real laws for real societies.

In accordance with Durkheim's statistical narrative, the apple does not fall here far from the tree. In the inner *sanctum* of private life, children and women are most eminent signs and figures and the final proof for the sad argument:

> Suicide is extremely rare among children [...] [None the less] the child too is influenced by social causes which may drive him to suicide. Even in this case their influence appears in the variations of child-suicide according to social environment. They are most numerous in large cities. Nowhere else does social life commence so early for the child, as is shown by the precocity of the little city-dweller. Introduced earlier and more completely than others to the current of civilization, he undergoes its effects more completely and earlier. This also causes the number of child-suicides to grow with pitiful regularity in civilized lands. (2005, p. 49)

As for the women "with assistance of the *Code Civil* and property rights [...] *Women are part of the inventory*" (Marx, 1971, p. 20). They are *Sklaven.* They are *the proletariat of the proletariat*, surrounded by a double standard of social duties —demands on social goods. Inner and outer in relation to the core the family would be, it comes not as a surprise then that the leading role in the *Filmbuch Das Leben der Anderen* is and should be the one played in the film by Christa-Maria Sieland (Martina Gedeck). Taking on the role of an actress in the film, she gathers around all the implications of the abovementioned *comédie humaine* traits plus the one just referred: An actress is a character who makes a profession out of not having roots, of being endlessly mobile in the chain of representations; her expectations are not really of her own, but those determined by the role, void both of her own desires and vocation—duly deprived of them—although totally involved in the exchange chain of communal possibilities. Each position of the chain could be hers in an eventual moment like a possession. She is bestowed with all possessions and yet dispossessed. But what social goods are here in trade? As in the case of the poet, actors are *soul engineers*—states in a celebration party the despiteful Bruno Hempf (Thomas Thieme), Minister of Culture and former Minister of National Security, quoting Stalin— and technicians of feelings, but technicians who have the duty to correct the possible tensions of those emotional goods within the distribution chain. Furthermore, Christa-Marie Sieland is the pearl of the GDR in his own words, a worth to protect, a worth to keep, a significant metaphor when we come to terms with it. A woman, Christa-Maria, represents the paradigmatic case of someone who is the representative organ of the allowed and forbidden transitions between inner and outer world, public, private, and intimate spheres of existence. The boundaries between home—family—and labor—State—blur. "It is *natural to our present society* to produce a lot of suicidals [...] but not all societies have the same products, though," affirms Marx no matter what Durkheim says (1971, p. 15). A well-designed society—by engineers of all sorts that could even indulge themselves in counting not only with the physical conditions but with the moral, intellectual, and spiritual ones of interacting individuals in the community of sharing—would solve rapidly without a doubt this urgent problem, or so we think. Does not the unity in sharing of the socialist community produce voluntary deaths?

At the peak of the *Filmbuch*, suicide makes its entrance into the plot of the film in the form of a symbol: A place of passage, a crossing point. The omnipresence of the possibility of an all-goods porose chain of distribution is overwhelming. All is in all. There is no right to keep anything out of the distribution cycle. There should not be an interest in an *outer* world. In that case, it would be pointless. GDR is *the best country in the world*, comprehends all fulfillment possibilities at hand. Living in another one would be foolish, not an option—never a competing value. And yet, the references to trespassing the limits of the democratic republic in idea or in reality multiply. Becoming an obsession sanctifying a most desired rite of passage, references crystallize in the very physical act of an escapee concealed in the backseat of a golden Mercedes that reaches West Berlin through the customs in Heinrich-Heine Straße (!), through the idea of indulging in reading western literature as a moral weakness to stronger ones including the reference to the *otherness* as a passing by, a transition and a disappearance, the radical symbolism of detaching oneself of the system at all, in the flesh, not being at all in the GDR, not in body, not in thoughts. Under a rattling floorboard, the typewriter with which the secret *manifesto—on someone that left to the other side*—on suicides in the GDR has been written in red ink is hidden at plain sight, precisely on the threshold between apartment environments, a forbidden secret. Albert Jerska (Volkmar Kleinert), a good-old friend and stage director commits suicide as he can no longer bear the thought of not directing anymore, inducted as he is in a—allegedly—nonexistent blacklist. It is just an advance of the ending of the film, in which Christa-Maria redoubles the thesis with her own *self-assassination* (*Selbstmord*). Both are pushed to this tragic end, more to the argument as she cannot even salvage her own intimacy—thoughts, feelings, etc.—from the lewd interests of Minister Hempf, who takes Sieland for his private possession... as he represents the almighty State. Sieland and Jerska take maybe *(un) justly* their lives then.

Suicide represents all of these relations to life in their complex structure: Vocation as property, the dispossession of expectations and aim, the presence and absence of one's own name in Party's Providence, the gratuitous character of this whimsical distribution... The concept of suicide officiates as a dialectical reminder of the tensions among private and public solidarity, property, and fulfillment, the functional substitute of satisfaction when in a socialist paradise:

> At Athens a man who had killed himself was punished with 'atimia' for having committed an injustice to the city; the honors of regular burial were denied him [...] these punishments were applicable only when the person had killed himself without having previously asked permission of the proper authorities. At Athens, if he asked authority of the Senate before killing himself, stating the reasons which made life intolerable to him, and if his request was regularly granted, suicide was considered a legitimate act. (Durkheim, 2005, p. 295)

Life is a social good, not entirely of our own under this light. Only *if... if... if... is a right to life considered as legitimate.* Loss of intimacy in relation to public and private property is to keep at least the right to detach oneself of the sharing within the unending distributional chain of social concomitance (Foessel, 2008). *ἀτιμία* is the deprivation of honor. It is a total judgment on the value of life: In comparison with status, prestige, power, and all social goods depending on structural differences of exchange. Life is of social value under this logic. This special occasion for the exercise of underworld ostracism points to a social humiliation that would explain why the term for suicide in German is so descriptive in the movie. *Selbstmord—Suizid* is an alternative nowadays—is the illicit act of assassination turn onto oneself. One can only unjustly take his own life. As it is a social good, the rest of society is the harmed party. It is the society that is forced to renounce to a possession to which is somehow entitled.

Concluding our argument here, it would be helpful to add a corollary question to the ones already presented above. Each suicide is a direct accusation against the public sanity of a society. Is Marx right over Durkheim with respect to the possible absence of this social product once the correct material and representational sharing conditions for the social structure would be achieved? A plausible response extracted from an article by Udo Grashoff:

> Except for the period between 1956 and 1962 suicide statistics were not published in the statistical yearbooks [in the GDR]. However, the 'State Central Bureau for Statistics' recorded suicides with Prussian accuracy, but kept them a state secret […] Although there was no public discussion of suicide, there was a limited, if diminishing, coverage of the issue in professional journals. From 1977, even specialists could not access data. [It is surprising though that] suicide rate of East Germany was, indeed, consistently 50 percent higher than in West Germany (about 6,000 suicide cases were registered every year in the GDR until the fall of the Wall). But East German suicide rates have to be viewed in a broader comparative context. European states like Austria, Czechoslovakia, Denmark, Hungary, and Finland also had high suicide rates, despite variations in their political systems. (Young, 2014)[2]

Probably the majority of the film's audience, along with our own reading of Durkheim and Marx, could be tempted to make a fine correlation too between confinement, repression, and suicide but, according to what just have been stated, maybe is more of a matter of concealment, of the bare negation of one social product whose existence could rise fair moral claims against just one more society among others.[3]

---

[2] See the outcome of the revolution of 1989 for GDR-public servants (Appelius, 2010).

[3] This essay is a direct result and should be understood on the basis of its relationship to the individual research project *On the Letter and Spirit of Imitation: Exemplum and Exemplarity* (2017–2020), a project ascribed to the Department of Logic and Theoretical Philosophy (Faculty of Philosophy, Complutense University of Madrid) and under the tutelage and endorsement of Prof. Dr. Ricardo Parellada. Its academic outcomes are research additions to the scientific results already published in several formats in collaboration with two other national projects: *PAIDESOC – El desván de la razón: cultivo de las pasiones, identidades éticas y sociedades digitales* (FFI2017–82535-P), with Prof. Concha Roldán Panadero (Institute of Philosophy, CSIC) as a PI; and a second one, *Proyecto de INNOVA-Docente. Precariedad, exclusión y diversidad funcional (discapacidad) (II): lógicas y efectos subjetivos del sufrimiento social contemporáneo* (PIMCD-84), led as a PI by Prof. Nuria Sánchez Madrid (Complutense University of Madrid).

References

Abrutyn, S., & Mueller, A. S. (2014). Reconsidering Durkheim's assessment of tarde: Formalizing a tardian theory of imitation, contagion, and suicide suggestion. *Sociol. Forum, 29*(3), 698–719. https://doi.org/10.1111/socf.12110

Appelius, S. (2010). Die Toten der friedlichen Revolution. *Spiegel Geschichte.* https://www.spiegel.de/geschichte/selbstmorde-nach-der-wende-a-946683.html. Accessed 4 Aug 2020.

Canetti, E. (1978). *Crowds and power.* Continuum.

Durkheim, É. (2005). *Suicide: A study in sociology.* Routledge.

Fenichel, O. (1945). *The psychoanalytic theory of neurosis.* W.W. Norton.

Foessel, M. (2008). *La privation de l'intime. Mises en scènes politiques des sentiments.* SEUIL.

Heß, M. (1971). *Gesellschaftsspiegel. Organ zur Vertretung der besitzlosen Volksklassen und zur Beleuchtung der gesellschaftlichen Zustände der Gegenwart* (Vol. 2). Glashütten im Taunus.

Lynch, A. (1996). *Thought contagion: How belief spreads through society.* Basic Books.

Marx, K. (1971). Peuchet: vom Selbstmord. In M. Heß (Ed.), *Gesellschaftsspiegel. Organ zur Vertretung der besitzlosen Volksklassen und zur Beleuchtung der gesellschaftlichen Zustände der Gegenwart* (Vol. 2, pp. 14–26). Verlag Detlev Averman KG.

McCall, G. J. (2006). Symbolic interaction. In P. J. Burke (Ed.), *Contemporary social psychological theories* (pp. 1–23). Stanford University Press.

Niezen, R. (2015). The Durkheim-tarde debate and the social study of aboriginal youth suicide. *Transcult. Psychiatry, 52*(1), 96–114. https://doi.org/10.1177/1363461514557560

n-tv.de. (2006). "Das Leben der Anderen" Bejubelte Premiere in Berlin. *n-tv.de.* https://www.n-tv.de/archiv/Bejubelte-Premiere-in-Berlin-article175178.html. Accessed 4 Aug 2020.

Sennett, R. (1980). *Authority.* Penguin Random House.

Sennett, R. (2003). *The fall of public man.* W.W. Norton.

Shaftesbury, A. A. C. (2000). *Characteristics of men, manners, opinions, times.* Cambridge University Press.

Tarde, G. (2009). *Les lois de l'imitation.* BiblioBazaar.

Turner, J. H. (2006). The state of theorizing in sociological social psychology: A grand theorist's view. In P. J. Burke (Ed.), *Contemporary social psychological theories* (pp. 353–374). Stanford University Press.

Veblen, T. (2007). *The theory of the leisure class: An economic study of institutions.* Oxford University Press.

Young, S. J. (2014). 'The death of others': The myth and reality of suicide in the German Democratic Republic. *UCL – SSEES Research Blog.* https://blogs.ucl.ac.uk/ssees/2014/11/27/the-death-of-others-the-myth-and-reality-of-suicide-in-the-german-democratic-republic/#:~:text=The%20suicide%20rate%20of%20East,the%20fall%20of%20the%20Wall. Accessed 1 Aug 2020.

Ricardo Gutiérrez Aguilar (MA in Philosophy, 2006; National Prize in Philosophy, 2008; MA in Teachers Training, 2008) is an Assistant Professor and Researcher in Philosophy in the History and Philosophy Department at Universidad de Alcalá de Henares (UAH). He holds a Ph.D. (2014) with a European Mention awarded by the UNED. He is Doktor der Philosophie by the Technische Universität zu Berlin (Germany, 2014). Predoctoral fellow in the National Spanish Research Council (CSIC) and a *Marie Curie* Early Stage Researcher in *TU Berlin* (Project *ENGLOBE. Enlightenment and Global* History, 2010–2013), Dr. Gutiérrez Aguilar research interests are Analytical Philosophy of History and Philosophy of Mind. Dr. Gutiérrez Aguilar's most recent publications are *Virtud y Sistema. Juicio moral y filosofía de la Historia en Kant* (Alamanda, 2018), *Deuda y legado en la filosofía de la Historia de Schiller* (Herder, 2018), *Empathy: Emotional, Ethical and Epistemological Narratives* (Brill, 2019), and *The Philosophy of Kant* (Nova Publishers, 2019).

Part II

Existential and Psychological Reasons for Suicide in Modern Fictional Literature

Desire of Death, Suicide, and Salvation: Problems with Eternity in Miguel de Unamuno

Rodolfo Gutiérrez Simón

Contents

Suicides in Unamunian Narrative: A Selection 156
Premeditation: Regretful Agony 156
Death as an Escape from Hopeless Solitude 159
Hope, Hopelessness, and the Others: From the Desire for Immortality to the Difference Between the Hero and the Suicide 160
Life as a Novel 163
References 168

Suicide, although it has not been highlighted in his most recent interpretations (Orringer, 2020), is a recurring element in the work of Miguel de Unamuno (1864–1936). This persistence, united with a tragic vision of human existence, has brought him on occasion, to be considered the "suicide inducer" (Unamuno, 1995a, p. 302, 1995b, p. 416). However, despite being an exit that the author portrays for many characters from his narrative—like other contemporaries such as Baroja (2005)—the self-inducement of death should be understood as an antagonist figure from the "hero" category in Unamunian thought. Thus, while heroism is a reappearing theme in several of his texts, suicide will be its non-categorized counterpart. The following pages

R. Gutiérrez Simón (✉)
Complutense University of Madrid, Madrid, Spain
e-mail: rodolfo.gutierrez@ucm.es

J. Ros Velasco (ed.), *Suicide in Modern Literature*,
https://doi.org/10.1007/978-3-030-69392-3_10

will be dedicated to analyzing suicide in the Basque author's literary works, by highlighting his specificity and binding it to the author's general philosophy by contrast to the heroic figure.

Suicides in Unamunian Narrative: A Selection

Although on some occasions Unamuno has considered suicide and other evil as an escape from apathy (Unamuno, 1984)—including before the crisis he suffered from in 1897, embodied in *Nicodemus the Pharisee* (1974)—he always foresaw that he would quickly regret it, because he would always be followed by a terrible panic of the "experience" of ceasing to exist (1974, p. 56). In this way, suicide had a definite presence in his life, especially if we consider the tragic passing of Ángel Ganivet, with whom Unamuno maintained an acquaintanceship and whose death poses a thought-provoking issue, although not very noticeable in the Basque author's work: That being, how an author's suicide can determine the interpretation of his or her work (Álvarez Castro, 2018).

In Unamunian literature, nonetheless, suicides seem to appear as a central theme/concept. These suicides are explicit or uncertain (in the case of Augusto Sánchez) and include the possibility of "suicide of another" (Unamuno, 1995b, pp. 17, 554). They are presented in literary works responding to the idea that these compositions and their characters allow the exposure of problematic ideas that the philosophical essay cannot always adequately express (Unamuno, 1995a). However, the philosophical depth is clear: Unamunian understanding of suicide starts from the conception of man as a mortal and contradictory being. But let us start from the beginning.

Premeditation: Regretful Agony

The first thing that draws attention in the suicides in Unamuno's work is that in no case is it something angry, sudden, or impulsive. Premeditation of the act is always present[1]: At a given moment, the subject decides to kill himself. The suicide, then, deliberately chooses death, but normally does not carry out

[1] Regarding the suddenness or not of the decision to commit suicide, it is interesting to bring to light a parallelism between what Unamuno highlights about such a decision and some theses of an author who influenced him notoriously, William James: For both, although a radical decision (like a conversion) whether it is apparent or externally sudden, actually respond to a succession of previous situations, which makes it possible to postpone the suicidal act (Unamuno, 2005; see also James, 1920).

the act at that very moment (Unamuno, 1995b). The clearest example is found in *Love and Pedagogy*. In this novel, Apolodoro—a young man whose positivist father hoped he would become a genius inspired by the education received by J. S. Mill (1981)—chooses to hang himself by adding to the paternal coldness, the loss of a desired woman. However, his suicide is not instantaneous, instead he will wait for two events to occur: The foreseeable death of his sister Rosa and making a woman pregnant by force (Unamuno, 1995a), thus allowing him to eternalize himself. The situation is similar in the case of Augusto Sánchez, protagonist of *Mist*: His suicide—deliberately questioned in the prologue (Unamuno, 1976a)—occurs after going too far with Unamuno(1976a).

All of this is particularly meaningful because in Unamunian work, there exists a relationship between suicide and regret in itself, but this only takes place when it has been performed and it becomes irreversible. It remains to be seen, then, what class of regret this is.

It has already been indicated, alluding to the examples of Apolodoro and Augusto, how there can be a guilt that precipitates events in Unamuno's work. This kind of guilt is not coincidental, given the religious undertone of Unamunian thought (Baker, 1990); it acquires lustful tones—relating to those generated by another capital sin, envy—central passion in *Abel Sánchez* (Unamuno, 1976a)—as both implicate a feeling of persecutory mania: The culprits detect an accusation in every look, even if it is not real, according to a psychological complex that sums up well the protagonist of *Saint Manuel Bueno, Martyr* (Unamuno, 1976b). However, it is not this guilt that generates the regret analyzed here.

There are two excerpts that will clarify what regret means in the case of suicide. First of all, there is the case of the already mentioned Apolodoro in *Love and Pedagogy*, whom after hanging himself tries to grab hold of the rope, unsuccessfully (1995a). Ergo, the author puts his character in a situation of immediate regret which he foresaw would overcome him if he committed suicide, as shown above.

The second exemplary excerpt is perhaps even more revealing. It appears in *Saint Manuel Bueno, Martyr*:

> "A stillborn child, or one who dies soon after birth are, like suicides, the most terrible mystery to me," I once heard him say. "Like a child crucified!"
>
> And once, when a man had taken his own life and the father of the suicide, an outsider asked Don Manuel if his son could be buried in consecrated ground, the priest answered:

> "Most certainly, for at the last moment, in the very last throes, he must surely have repented. There is no doubt of it whatsoever in my mind."
> (Unamuno, 1976b, p. 144)

In addition to the classification of suicide as a mystery, two other issues stand out. The first has to do with the fact that Saint Manuel refers to the exact instant in that one passes from life to death—Unamuno establishes an analogy with the passage from wakefulness to sleep, impossible to consciously perceive (1995b)—like *agony*. This concept acquires an explicit technical and philological character in Unamuno's work: Agony (*ἀγωνία*) is *struggle*, further pointing out that "He who lives in the throes of struggle, struggling against life itself, lives in agony, agonizes. And he struggles against death as well" (1974, p. 5). It should be noted that this struggle between opposites, this inherent contradiction to human existence (1976a), is in a certain way typical to the sensibility of this time period and of the generation of 98—still with romantic reminiscences (Scari, 1984)—that the Basque author leads on (Tomás, 2007). Thus, Antonio Machado also points out that "Man is by nature the paradoxical beast, / An absurd animal that needs logic" (1974, p. 155).

But let us take back up the quote of *Saint Manuel Bueno, Martyr*. The suicide's father's concern is, naturally, the salvation or not of his son, considering that suicides suffer Catholic condemnation (Durkheim, 2005; see also Díaz, 1973; Jiménez Lozano, 2002). And the priest, having the ability to act in another way, decides to bestow something that will be crucial to understanding Unamuno: Hope. With it, Saint Manuel adopts a given trait of heroism in the Unamunian sense of the term: Beyond his absence of faith (the plot of this short novel), he dedicates his life to the people, to the others, over his life, constructing them in his own mission. This contrast will be critical later; for the moment noting how we have passed from regret with respect to the enabling guilt of self-induced death to a regret of the desire to die: The suicide, at the final moment, believes in something that he did not believe in, and this leads to his belated regret. Death can then be considered as the key to a purifying regret, whose maximum exponent—especially in several of Unamuno's writings—would be Saint Dimas, counterpart to suicidal Judas (Unamuno, 1974, 1976b, 1984).

However, this purifying element of death is not the crucial point of the Unamunian theses on suicide. Thus, there are two other important aspects that must be considered before getting to the core of the issue: Death as an escape and the relationship between suicide and solitude.

Death as an Escape from Hopeless Solitude

Unamuno repeatedly relates the idea of death with escape (1976a, 2004), and the cases mentioned so far would be paradigmatic in this regard. Apolodoro and Augusto Sánchez see a way of fleeing from their drama by ending their existence: They escape from time, space, and even logic, being the most radical way of fleeing and moving themselves—paradoxically—to safety (1995a). This also happens with Enrique in "The Godfather Antonio" (Unamuno, 1995b, p. 572).

The mentioned texts are linked to underlying philosophical ideas. In *How to Make a Novel* (which mixes fictional, explanatory, and autobiographical), Unamuno presents us with the creation of a novel and its parallelism with life. The protagonist, "U. Jugo de la Raza," finds a book whose reading catches his interest but promises him that he will die when he finishes it (1976a, p. 427). Although later on it will be necessary to return to the Unamunian understanding of life as a novel, it is now interesting to recover an idea from this text: Sometimes, leaving is the victorious exit in the game, in politics... and in life (1976a). Here we have a clue that the suicide narrative of Unamuno is based on an intellectual construction of greater depth than that merely adequate to the development of his stories. And in this way, although he did not get to do it, in his most relevant philosophical work (*The Tragic Sense of Life*) he talks about killing oneself as a way out in the face of drama that affects us all because we are human: That of reaching *the depths of the abyss* (Unamuno, 1921).

Now, for "death-as-escape" to make sense, it is necessary that that of which one is fleeing from is considered less valuable than the possibility of condemnation or even ceasing to exist altogether. It will therefore be necessary for the suicide to perceive as a central aspect of their existence, an unbearable pain[2] that turns death, even if it means nothing, into something desirable (Unamuno, 1976a); and this pain is particularly reflected in a peculiar feeling of solitude—different from the solitude of the hero.

There are many things that the human being does in that strict solitude which is "the marrow of our essence" (Unamuno, 1976a, p. 397), especially dying. And Unamuno, who relies on an increase in communicability through the love of seemingly individual aspects such as dreams (1976a), cannot share death (1995b, 1984). The peculiar thing about suicide is that his feeling of solitude is before he dies: He does not die alone but he is alone and then commits suicide.

[2] Pain is an essential theme in Unamuno's literary and philosophical work (1995a, b, 1976a, 1921; etc.).

Although it appears in other places (Unamuno, 1995b, pp. 551–554), the characteristic loneliness or solitude prior to committing suicide is shown especially clearly in the story "Ramón Nonnato, Suicide." The remarkable thing about this story is that in it exists two lonely characters: Ramón and his mother, who passes away just before giving birth to him. Both one and the other are neglected—when not mistreated—by Ramón's father; however, while the protagonist commits suicide, his mother endures. In the difference between their loneliness lies the core of the Unamunian theory of suicide: Ramón's loneliness is hopeless, while the mother does not reach that point as she puts her hope in her son's arrival to the world and the changes that this may generate in the behavior of the abuser (1995b). The key is this central concept of hope (and its counterpart, hopelessness), which contains important technical nuances.

Hope, Hopelessness, and the Others: From the Desire for Immortality to the Difference Between the Hero and the Suicide

The relationship between hopeless radical solitude and suicide is clarified in *Saint Manuel Bueno, Martyr*. There we find its protagonist in constant activity, fleeing his solitude toward the only place he can do so to escape the suicidal idea (Putnam, 1935): Toward others, dedicating his life to his community (Unamuno, 1976b). And it is only by establishing a certain relationship with others that we can escape a loneliness that goes far beyond physical distance: Mere loneliness is not enough to explain the suicide's behavior because the hero is also—as it will be seen later—a loner.

The role of others regarding the suicide is heightened at the moment in which it is suspected (with or without basis) that native incommunicability exists with the otherness. Apolodoro, a future suicide, begins his fall to radical negative solitude when he begins to think that what he thinks he says and does is different from what he says and does, believing that the others take him for mad and there being no possible mediation between one another (Unamuno, 1995a).

That of which makes any aspect of human interiority transmissible and communicable (breaking solitude) is what Unamuno considers "reason" in broad terms (1921, p. 113); however, it can be sensed that an unavoidable and very human part of our interiority is "irrational" in part because of what is incommunicable: Here you find a range of passions, among which solitude is found. Man, essentially solitary, cannot fully rationalize nor communicate to others his state of being; he may not even be able to explain it rationally to himself. Hence, the passionate and the rational collide, which we can clarify with the clash between "truth" and "religion" according to *The Agony of Christianity*: If truth is collective, religion is individual and incommunicable (Unamuno, 1974, p. 5). This struggle between religion and communicative reason tries to be remedied through writing, ritual, etc. At its very root, however, religious passion is essentially solitary and incommunicable depending on grace. Undoubtedly, although Unamuno points out—like William James (1920)—that man is more passion than reason (1921, 1984, 2014), a specific point should be made: man is above all the struggle between both extremes, and Unamuno already recognizes this in his first novel *Peace in War* (1983; Ouimette, 1987).

The struggle as an essential element to human life (Unamuno, 1976a, 1984, 1995b; etc.) will be that which allows one to speak about the tragic sense of life. Ultimately, that struggle (agony) between passion and reason, between faith and rationality (1995a, 1984), is a classic argument which confronts the knowledge of our mortality with our inherent desire for immortality and eternity. Such eternity, to top it all, is in the case of extreme Unamuno: It is not only a matter of lasting, but doing it exactly as we are, without relinquishing the body which gives us *unity*—to which a *principle of continuity* can be added (1921). Thus, "In a word, be it with reason or without reason or against reason, I am resolved not to die" (Unamuno, 1921, p. 130), not wanting to die is closely linked to Spinoza and his conception of the *conatus*. So far, we have faced a trite problem; Unamuno's singularity will lie in making this intimate contradiction, of this unsolvable struggle, the starting point of hope: Contradiction, far from being a destructive element, becomes a generating element. The characteristic of suicide from this point of view would be the incapacity to find hope, while his counterpart (the hero) would be one who finds hope even if it may be absurd.

Although it involves summarizing a complex and extremely counterintuitive doctrine, it is necessary to state the argument of *The Tragic Sense of Life*. This book is, in itself, pure deliberate contradiction (Fraser, 2010): Unamuno attempts to show formally and physically, that the human being is a contradictory animal (remember the "paradoxical beast" to which Machado alluded, indicated above), far from the rationalist ideal. Thus, it will explicitly indicate that the first six chapters clash with the last six. Therefore, if in the first half of the book he attempts to approach with reason a series of passions which are impossible to completely translate to logical reasoning, in the second half, he tries to predominate the passionate part by using only the minimal essential reasoning, trying to verbalize and convey what cannot be rationalized in itself.

Regarding the content of the text, the main concept is found in the first half of the book. There Unamuno gathers what he has been anticipated here: Man is an animal that is in permanent conflict between reason and passion, between his longing for immortality and his finitude. In this regard, mere reasoning inevitably leads us to a dramatic dissolution in which truth and solace divide, which gives place to "skepticism of reason encounters the despair of the heart" (Unamuno, 1921, p. 105). Thus we arrive at the aforementioned *depths of the abyss*; and it is at this point, in this extreme contradiction, where Unamuno inserts his proposal, critical for understanding suicide in his work: What must be achieved is "to accept the conflict as such and to live by it," by attaining that "this despair may be the basis of a vigorous life" (1921, p. 124).

This is how the contradiction converts itself into a generatrix, a concept that Unamuno does not use but is underlying in many passages of his work (1921, 1984, 1974, 1995a; etc.): Tension allows creation, pro-creation,[3] and the possibility of hope (which only makes sense in uncertainty).

That contradiction is the basis for hope that is attested in various places (Unamuno, 1976a, 1984). However, less attention is given to the fact that hope is a concept with a certain technical nuance that should be clarified to the extent that the suicide's given trait will be to have lost it completely. In this context, it is appropriate to note that Unamuno differentiates hope from faith, because the latter arises from the former and is subordinate to it (1921). And adds something very meaningful:

> Love hopes, hope ever (always) and never wearies of hoping [...] And if faith is the substance of hope, hope in turn is the form of faith. Until it gives us hope, our faith is a formless faith, vague, chaotic, potential; it is but the possibility of believing, the longing to believe. But we must need to believe in something, and we believe in what we hope for, we believe in hope. (1921, p. 200)

Now, as well, Unamuno gives us something close to a definition of hope:

> [...] faith is to believe in what we did not see. To believe in what we see—and what we do not see also—is reason, science; and to believe in what we shall see—or shall not see—is hope. (1974, p. 11)

[3] The contrast between "matter" and "form" which refers to Marina and Avito, Apolodoro's parents in *Love and Pedagogy* (Unamuno, 1995a, p. 320).

The relationship of these passages and concepts with suicide is noted by perceiving that suicide is, precisely, one who lacks hope: A hopeless person. Unamuno is not going to confuse two similar terms in Castilian, but which have quite different consequences for the argument presented here: Hopelessness and despair. While the person who definitely lacks hope remains passive, the desperate person is capable, through despair itself, of denying, affirming, or refraining from denying or affirming (1921). In this respect, the desperate person can carry out a desperate action; the hopeless person, on the other hand, tries nothing but, at best, to bring an end to his hopelessness (committing suicide). In other words, "many of the greatest heroes, perhaps the greatest of all, have been men of despair and that by despair they have accomplished their mighty works" (Unamuno, 1921, p. 130) but no suicide in Unamuno's narrative is desperate (remember what was indicated above: Suicides in his literature are not sudden, but are postponed if necessary). Despair is not, therefore, disconnected from hope: A desperate person can believe in something (1921) and go from despair to hope. And if reason does not allow them to illuminate any hope, it will be achieved against reason. That is the characteristic of the hero: Believing in something although it may be absurd (1921). And thus, the suicide acquires his condition, opposite to the hero: He is not capable of giving way to hope from his peculiar solitude. Now, on the contrary, it is the hero's relationship with others that allows him to escape from the real or figurative suicidal temptation, because it is them who allow him to avoid the induction of his own death (1976a).

Life as a Novel

The differentiation between the hero and the suicide, as I have indicated at the beginning, is not carried out by Unamuno to the extent that he does not expressively use a categorization of suicide; however, it is evident that the suicide is the counterpart of the heroic figure. In this sense, several passages in *Love and Pedagogy* that implicitly differentiate the hero from the suicide (1995a) are suggested in that they are traversed by the intimately linked Unamunian conception of life and the novel.

Anticipating later philosophies, Unamuno will consider life as a novel in numerous passages of his work, although the most characteristic approach in this regard is found in his complex and strange literary piece *How to Make a Novel*, which in reality is a common theme in the author's philosophy and narratives (1976a, 1995a, etc.). This allows him to make himself a character in various literary works and explicitly allude to the novel's fictional character, things from his own life (Unamuno, 1995a): Men are just, as much, characters as those in a novel (1976a, 1995a). This analogy between creator and creation, between author and characters, is possible first of all, because the theory of Unamuno's novel dictates that, as with human life, the novel properly lacks a plot beyond its own making (1995a, b, 1976a).

Here we have an essential problematic point: The understanding of an individual as a suicide since birth (1995b, 1976a). If life is a novel and its fate all the same is inevitably death, the life-novel will be the story of one's ongoing death, of an unborn or dis-born, and of the unraveling of the path that goes from cradle to grave (1984, 1976b, 1974). In this context, the Unamunian approach to suicide acquires a noticeably clear identification that can be attributed only to some individuals. And it is not accidental that the verb "attribute" is used here: In Unamuno's approach, the reader is given the authority, at the time of interpreting the true actions of the characters, over the author.

Since the prologue of *Mist*, as noted from the beginning, we are faced with a debate between Unamuno and his characters with respect to whether Augusto Sánchez commits suicide or not. Leaving the content of the text open to the reader's interpretation is the consequence of the Unamunian conception of the novel: Something without a plot, or whose only plot is its development. It is the literary works' reader, therefore, who is as much as their creator and that of their characters as the author (1976a): The relationship between the one who reads, the one who writes, and the characters becomes something profound, determining each other just as in the "real" world we make one another… and just as characters in a novel make each other (1976a, pp. 63, 154–155). Although there are many examples, it is especially clear in the story, "The Reason of Being":

> They say that in a certain place in Guadiana River its course is hidden below the sand and only a few sections appear to you mixed in it. This is the life of the teacher… Did he marry? Did he not marry? As the reader likes, as I am indifferent. (Unamuno, 1995b, p. 682)

This relationship between the reader and the writer maintains the same approach that Unamuno uses when he elaborates *The Life of Don Quixote and Sancho* and offers us the interpretation of the thoughts that these characters "really" had—those of which had been resurrected (1976a, p. 16)—facing the mistakes of Quixote's "historian": Cervantes (Unamuno, 1967, p. 26). Thus, the readers that follow revive the story and, through it, the author… so they can feel it and not only understand (1974). Thus, two pending themes reappear: The desire for survival and the superiority of passion in the face of reason. The first failed in the suicide case, the hero triumphs by the second. It is time to address the difference between the two notable figures in order to gather what has been said here and bring it to full clarity.

Although Unamuno dismisses the greatest names in history, a coherent approach can be found in his vision of a hero aside from the fact that in Spain's history, no one meets that description. Actually, exactly as it has been pointed out in *On Casticism* (*En torno al casticismo*), Spain would have lacked what Carlyle called heroism of the people: Perhaps there have been heroes, but they have not been recognized (Unamuno, 2007). Therefore, Unamuno's main heroic literary referent would be Don Quixote (González Vicen, 1943). The Quixotic figure brings together the traits characteristic to a hero, highlighting that he endures new degrees of contradiction (e.g., between different duties) and the split duality of his being (Unamuno, 2007). And, as always in the Unamunian approach, the split between reason and passion will appear in an especially dramatic way in the hero to the extent that we can call his heroic wisdom a kind of non-intellectual but sentimental knowledge—which allows him to do (out of despair) things that I characterized as absurd, above. The hero knows that God—at least in the example of Don Quixote—had chosen him to do something and that the rest will not believe him, just as what happened to Apolodoro while believing that everyone saw him as crazy to the point of hindering his destiny. Therefore, the heroic mission is a matter of fundamental willpower: The desire to do what that strange non-intellectual wisdom dictates.

When characterizing this non-scientific knowledge—with the ultimate purpose in disputing dominance of the prevailing positivism in the era, *Love and Pedagogy*'s theme—Unamuno is inspired by the Quixotic passage of the fulling mills (Cervantes, 1998, I, XVIII-XX): Upon hearing an unknown sound at night, Don Quixote wants to set out on an adventure while Sancho is frightened; at sunrise, discovering that the pounding came from the fuller of a mill, Sancho laughs superbly with the consequent reprimand from his master. Unamuno points out:

> In order to right wrongs and resurrect chivalry and establish the kingdom of good on the earth, it is not needful to distinguish sounds, and be able to tell which are fulling hammers and which are not. Such a distinction has nothing to do with heroism, nor do the numerous other disciplines acquired by learning add one whit to the total sum of good in the world. A knight has more than enough to do with listening attentively to the sound of his own heart and distinguishing the sounds it makes.

> This quixotic doctrine must be preached all the more nowadays, when Sanchopanzism ceaselessly repeats to us that the essential thing is to distinguish between sounds and be able to tell which are made by fulling mills and which are not, regardless of the fact that as long as it is night time and fear lingers in us, even Sancho cannot tell the difference, despite his hearing them clearly, and even though they really need not be seen. But Sancho needs to see them; in order to be sure and to dare make mock, he needs to see the cause of the noise. Sancho, who by night dares not leave his master's side for fear of the terrible sounds, and who fails to distinguish them because of fright, mocks Don Quixote when he sees the object which produces them. Thus, it is with Sanchopanzism, now called positivism, now naturalism, now empiricism; once cured of fright, it mocks the quixotic ideal. (1967, pp. 94–95)

The opposition to this mockery of quixotic idealism, to Sanchopanzism, will be the hero himself, who neither fully knows what he is doing nor is able to explain it (or explain it to himself) rationally: His knowledge is not scientific (1967). This act, guided by irrational knowledge, and therefore of a passionate character, allows us to bring up another hero-propitiated characteristic caused by his passion: That of being a *sinner by ambition*, in the manner of Adan and unlike the devil (1967). The Quixotic hero is not content with the way he is; he will always want to be more, "extracting strength from weakness and turning degradation into glory and forcing sin to serve as the groundwork for his redemption" (1967, p. 51). And how does one pass from degradation to glory, but through hope?

Some loose ends from above are in need of being tied, mentioned earlier in the text. This *sinner by ambition*, whom is the hero, is in no way a Herostratus (1967): He does not do things for fame, but for glory. Hence, in *The Life of Don Quixote and Sancho*, it has been recorded that Alonso Quijano praises Dulcinea with the robes of glory, the context in which an essential statement makes sense: The love for women is where all heroism arises; the hero wants to perpetuate himself with her and forever be in her memories rather than conserve himself to preserve oneself (the Spinozian instinct of perpetuation and the desire to eternalize oneself, by not dying, has already been alluded to above). Of course, what the hero intends to do is to produce spiritual children, not of the flesh: Don Quixote does not win the heart of Dulcinea, to the Glory, and he does not need to conceive children with her: His adventures and his works are for her; he realizes them to put them at her feet without waiting to be recognized or rewarded (1967). This prevents them from entering in the hero category like Joaquin Monegro, from *Abel Sánchez*, or suicides as Apolodoro, who aims to leave *earthly children*.

The hero, that is not Herostratus, is not selfish either: He is not a vigilante who moves at his own risk or expense, but one that lives for his followers. This is the case of Saint Manuel Bueno, as seen above. The hero needs the faith of his followers, he is fed by it, while these followers, perhaps, do not need him. It is the hero who is the one that cannot be left alone: Don Quixote needs Sancho—who personifies humanity in its entirety—more than Sancho needs him (1967, 1921).

This fits with other elements that characterized the suicide: The true feeling of solitude. But if the solitude of the hero ends up accepting the presence of others, in the suicide's case, this does not occur. The relationship with others is what ultimately determines the eagerness of the suicide: Desperate hope may be directed toward them. Unamuno is, therefore, an heir in a certain way to Durkheim and points to the community as an essential preventative element to the suicide. Thus, the pessimist that plays the lead in "See with your Eyes" ("Ver con los ojos") does not kill himself: By crying, he shares his pain with the others, conveying it (1995b).

Consequently, the hero and the suicide share, through their humanity, the extreme, dramatic situation of the tragic sense of life: This is portrayed in what Unamuno characterizes as *depths of the abyss*. Furthermore, they are cases in which radically a particular sense of solitude is noted. If the suicide is the counterpart of the heroic figure, it is because in him reason prevails over passion, which explains his vital failure: Giving in to hopelessness. In this way, in despair at *the depths of the abyss*, the hero is capable of guiding himself with an irrational hope, including contrary to reason and of which can provide him with eternity; the suicide is not capable of taking such a step, remaining rationally in a despair that becomes hopelessness (a rational coldness that allows the character very little choleric and nothing rash of the suicides that appear in Unamunian narrative). And perhaps the most important part will be the best closing: The hero and the suicide are still two extreme cases that Unamuno's work exaggerates, with the intention that we see that we are all between both poles depending on whether we experience the appropriate transformation which allows for hope—like Sancho with the death of Don Quixote (Unamuno, 1967)—or not—that of which happens to the suicide. Therefore, all of us have or can have something heroic... and something as suicide has, beyond turning pages in the novel of life.[4]

[4] I want to thank Shannon Emery for her help in translating this text into English. This chapter was founded by the "Biblioteca Digital de Pensamiento Político Hispánico Saavedra Fajardo (BSF) - Ayudas Fundación BBVA a Equipos de Investigación Científica 2018."

References

Álvarez-Castro, L. (2018). Ángel Ganivet (1865–1898) ante la crítica: el suicidio del escritor como negación de la "muerte del autor". *Revista Canadiense de Estudios Hispánicos, 42*(2), 225–248. https://doi.org/10.18192/rceh.v42i2.3113

Baker, A. F. (1990). Unamuno and the religion of uncertainty. *Hispanic Review, 58*(1), 37–56. https://doi.org/10.2307/473157

Baroja, P. (2005). *El árbol de la ciencia*. Alianza.

de Cervantes, M. (1998). *Don Quixote*. Wordsworth Editions.

de Unamuno, M. (1921). *The tragic sense of life in men and in peoples*. MacMillan and Co..

de Unamuno, M. (1967). *Selected works of Miguel de Unamuno, vol. 3. Our lord Don Quixote. The life of Don Quixote and Sancho with related essays*. Princeton University Press.

de Unamuno, M. (1974). *Selected works of Miguel de Unamuno, vol. 5. The agony of Christianity and essays on faith*. Princeton University Press.

de Unamuno, M. (1976a). *Selected works of Miguel de Unamuno, vol. 6. Novela/Nivola*. Princeton University Press.

de Unamuno, M. (1976b). *Selected works of Miguel de Unamuno, vol. 7. Ficciones. Four stories and a play*. Princeton University Press.

de Unamuno, M. (1983). *Selected works of Miguel de Unamuno, vol. 1. Peace in war. A novel*. Princeton University Press.

de Unamuno, M. (1984). *Selected works of Miguel de Unamuno, vol. 2. The private world. Selections from the Diario Íntimo and selected letters 1890–1936*. Princeton University Press.

de Unamuno, M. (1995a). *Obras completas I*. Fundación José Antonio de Castro.

de Unamuno, M. (1995b). *Obras completas II*. Fundación José Antonio de Castro.

de Unamuno, M. (2004). *Obras completas VI*. Fundación José Antonio de Castro.

de Unamuno, M. (2005). *Obras completas VII*. Fundación José Antonio de Castro.

de Unamuno, M. (2007). *Obras completas VIII*. Fundación José Antonio de Castro.

de Unamuno, M. (2014). *Abel Sánchez*. Alianza.

Díaz, J. W. (1973). Socio-religious context for a poem of Unamuno. *Romance Notes, 15*(1), 18–24.

Durkheim, É. (2005). *Suicide: A study in sociology*. Routledge.

Fraser, B. (2010). *Encounters with Bergson(ism) in Spain. Reconciling philosophy, literature, film and urban space*. University of North Carolina Press.

González Vicen, F. (1943). La figura de Don Quijote y el donquijotismo en el pensamiento de Miguel de Unamuno. *Romanische Forschungen, 57*(2/3), 192–227.

James, W. (1920). *The varieties of religious experience. A study on human nature*. Longmans, Green & Co.

Jiménez Lozano, J. (2002). *Ni venta, ni alquilaje*. Huerga y Fierro.

Machado, A. (1974). *Poesías completas*. Espasa-Calpe.

Mill, J. S. (1981). Autobiography. In J. S. Mill (Ed.), *Collected works of John Stuart Mill* (Vol. 1). University of Toronto Press.

Orringer, N. R. (2020). Dinámica de la otra vida en la filosofía de Unamuno. *Claridades. Revista de filosofía, 12*(1), 11–34. https://doi.org/10.24310/Claridadescrf.v12i1.5449

Ouimette, V. (1987). Paz en la guerra y los límites de la ideología. *Revista Canadiense de Estudios Hispánicos, 11*(2), 355–376.

Putnam, S. (1935). Unamuno y el problema de la personalidad. *Revista Hispánica Moderna, 2*, 103–110.

Scari, R. M. (1984). Unamuno: fruto tardío del romanticismo español. *Hispanófila, 81*, 51–70.

Tomás, F. (2007). La invención estética de España. *Journal of Iberian and Latin American Studies, 13*(2/3), 149–167. https://doi.org/10.1080/14701840701776223

Gutiérrez Simón is Ph.D. in Philosophy at Universidad Complutense de Madrid (Spain) with the thesis *Ortega y Gasset and North American Pragmatism*. He is a Professor of Contemporary Spanish Philosophy, History of Aesthetical Ideas, and History of Modern and Contemporary Philosophy. He is a member of the editorial board of *Revista de Hispanismo Filosófico* and the author of several papers in scientific journals on Spanish Philosophy in the twentieth century and winner of the IV Philosophical Essay Contest "María Zambrano" (2014). In 2019, he published his first book, entitled *Devenires de un acontecimiento. Mayo del 68 cincuenta años después* (Cenaltes).

"The End of the World? Let Me Die": Guido Morselli's *Dissipatio H. G.* Between Suicide and Mankind's Dissolution

Roberto Risso

Contents

"An Event (Unimaginable)": Morselli's Movement Toward the Cave 171
In the Cave: Suicide in Morselli's Dissipatio H. G 173
After the Cave: Dissipatio Humani Generis 178
References 182

"An Event (Unimaginable)": Morselli's Movement Toward the Cave

Guido Morselli's novel *Dissipatio H. G.* was written during the early 1970s, not long before the author's suicide. However, it was not published until 1977, after his death in 1973. It is tempting to trace the cause of his suicide to the many publication attempts of his works and his frustration toward the cultural and literary establishment that kept refusing them; critics have too often traced easy parallels, but the case of Morselli's unsuccessful publication

R. Risso (✉)
Clemson University, Clemson, SC, USA
e-mail: rrisso@clemson.edu

J. Ros Velasco (ed.), *Suicide in Modern Literature*,
https://doi.org/10.1007/978-3-030-69392-3_11

attempts and his suicide must be kept separate and not strictly consequential.[1] The choice is too simplistic and leaves out the fundamental natures of his works: The philosophical reflections on the existence of man, its relationships with the world of ideas, and the very concept of otherness. These are crucially intersected with narrations of events that have happened, could have happened in the past, could happen in the future, and, more importantly, have never happened, the extreme modernity and sophistication of Morselli's prose consist of a linear and clear description, in a rather neat and common language, of very plausible events that did not actually occur in history. Take, for example, his work of the year 2000 in *Rome with no Pope* (*Roma senza Papa*) (1974), of Germany winning World War I thanks to a secret tunnel in the Alps—*Contro-passato prossimo* (*Next Counter-Past*) (1975a)—and more interestingly of the Italian King Umbert I's secret vacation on the Alps, which is plausible but never documented—*Divertimento 1889* (*Fun 1889*) (1975b). All these novels, written with wit and thorough documentation of places, dynamics, and people, clearly refuse two of the prerequisites of Italian literature of the 1960s: *Impegno*, or "engagement with society," and on the other side, the neo-avant-garde's formal and content experimentation. If Morselli's works were to have been published before his death, they would have created an entirely new canon, and he would have had a substantial impact on the 1960s and 1970s.

During his life, Morselli had two book-length essays published: One on Marcel Proust and the other on philosophy. Included with these are numerous short stories and articles that were published during his lifetime, both in local Lombard and national magazines.[2] He lived the life of an intellectual

[1] Critics have found the equation quite easily: Frustration and refusal plus isolation and disappointment equal the desire to die and disappear from the world. One example is a book written by Marina Lessona Fasano, *Guido Morselli. Un inspiegabile caso letterario* (*Guido Morselli. An Inexplicable Literary Case*) (2003). In her perspective, *Dissipatio H. G.* is Morselli's "last" novel and understandably becomes his "literary testament" (2003, p. 159). It is the final artistic document of a troubled and disappointed intellectual who revolted against the society that never accepted him and his works, as well as pushed him to the border. Although the aforementioned factors may have played a role in his state of mind and choice, it is important to stress the fact that *Dissipatio H. G.* was *not* truly the last work by Morselli, as shown by other scholars; the collection of essays by Valentina Fortichiari (1994) spanning over more than four decades can contribute to this. Another important thing to note is that suicide is an element of deep reflection in his *Journal* (*Diario*) (1988) since his youth, and it is a choice that many of his fictional characters make to opt out from reality, one with such complexity and troubling dimensions that had already been explored by the author.

[2] Morselli also had published an excerpt from his first novel, *Uomini e amori* (*Of Men and Loves*) (1948 [1998]). According to archive materials, another novel, *Il Comunista* (*The Communist*) (1976 [2017]), was in the advanced stage of publication—proofs already corrected—with the prestigious publisher Rizzoli, but due to economic and internal problems with the publisher, it was aborted. However, Morselli's short works—essays, book reviews, journalistic reports, and opinion-based writings—were published all throughout his life, many in culturally relevant newspapers and magazines, such as the *Corriere Della Sera* and *La Cultura* (*The Culture*).

profoundly dedicated to the *otium litterarum*. Coming from a wealthy family, he managed to avoid working and substituted the *negotium* with a rigorous *otium* that consisted of writing, reading, studying, and attempting to be in epistolary contact with an amazing array of theologians, scholars, professors, and experts in all fields. He also lived a healthy life following strict nutritional and hygienic routines, distancing himself from the pollution and chaos of urban living, and committing himself to agriculture (possibly taking to heart Voltaire's famous sentence, "*Il faut cultivar son jardin*," as well as the humanistic concept of balance between studying and physical activity). He additionally went horseback riding and took excursions on the mountains, since he lived most of his life tucked away in a private villa, immersed in nature at the feet of the Lombard Alps.

After having been provided insight into this peculiar and mighty author's life and themes of his works, it is important in this essay to focus on the two major themes of *Dissipatio H. G.*: Suicide—better yet, the *attempt* of suicide—and the vanishing of humanity. The novel begins in medias res, with the unnamed protagonist narrating in first person of his new "normal" life near the fictitious city of Crisopoli (*City of Gold*, possibly embodying Zurich), located between Lombardy and Switzerland. All animals and objects still exist and function, but all humanity has disappeared. The protagonist thinks back to the time *it* happened—more than a month prior—and coincidentally it was when he was hiding in a cave in the mountains, acting on an elaborate plan to kill himself and disappear from the world.

In the Cave: Suicide in Morselli's *Dissipatio H. G.*

The cave in which the protagonist intends to commit suicide is not a metaphorical space but a real cave, where he will disappear during the night between the first and second day of June; "That night, it was decided, I would kill myself. Why? Because of the prevalence of the negative over the positive. In my ratio. A prevalence of 70%. A *cliché* reason, all too common? I am not so sure" (1977a, p. 18).[3] He describes himself as unhappy, a trait common with so many other characters of Morselli's novels and short stories. In a work of nonfiction significantly titled *Happiness Is Not a Luxury* (1994)—published by Fortichiari in a 1994 anthology of the same title, also including both of the two short essays Morselli dedicated to suicide—he writes, "Happiness is not something unnecessary. It is not a luxury, and it is for this simple reason that

[3] All quotations from *Dissipatio H. G.* are taken from the Adelphi Edition of 1977 reprinted in 2012, and all translations from Italian to English are written by the author.

it is a necessity of life" (1994, p. 94). He additionally notes, "Suffering is a symptom of the isolation, the recession of life from within us, and at the limit arrives the impossibility, either physical or psychological, of surviving" (1994, p. 94). For Morselli, happiness coincides with life itself, in the very possibility of living; therefore, the impossibility of reaching happiness leads inevitably to death. The man who is completely alive, according to Morselli within the same essay, is able to live his own life in harmony with all the other men of society; he is not separated from the community of individuals who constitute reality and the present society. He writes, "The single man who lives in full the life he's destined to and is happy about it is an active, useful, open individual and largely resourceful to himself, as well as directly or indirectly useful to others around him" (1977a, p. 109).

The narrator of *Dissipatio H. G.* is openly disgusted by his contemporary society which he describes as sold-to-profit, one-dimensional, and obsessed with money and materialism. Ironically quoting Durkheim (1951), of whom Morselli states "was not without wit" (1977a, p. 20),[4] the author adds the technical term on suicide, "To put it in Durkheim terms, here was the primer" (1977a, p. 21), the primer of his suicidal decision being the construction project of a highway close to his home. The building of a highway that is very close to his quiet home makes him literally sick with fever; he describes the project in these terms: "A heinous 'Euro-Autoroute', a company famously owned by two very relevant and mighty local businessmen, was working on a continental artery Le Havre-Athens" (1977a, p. 21).[5] This triggers his

[4] For the Italian reader, this sentence also closely recalls a similar expression about Shakespeare used ironically in the novel *The Betrothed* (*I promessi sposi*) (1830, p. 152) by the father of the modern Italian novel Alessandro Manzoni: "a barbarian who was not without wit." In *Dissipatio H. G.*, Morselli seems to enjoy inserting hidden quotations, for at page 18, he names depression "*mali oscuri*"—meaning "dark pains"—quoting Giuseppe Berto's famous novel *Il male oscuro* (1964), which deals with depression.

[5] Morselli had always been very close to nature and its preservation, especially during the 1950s and 1960s, when in Italy the environmental conscience was almost nonexistent. He not only had chosen to live immersed in nature in a countryside home, but he also had been writing extensively in favor of the preservation of the local fauna and of the beauty of the city near where he lived, Varese in Lombardy. Some of these essays which appeared in local newspapers are collected in a 2012 anthology of Morselli's nonfiction, titled *Una rivolta e altri scritti (1932–1966)* (*A Riot and Other Writings (1932–1966)*). Among those essays, "Le case di sette piani e la difesa delle bellezze naturali" ("Seven Floor High Rises and the Conservation of Nature," pp. 89–91) is significant for its environmental engagement and clear consciousness of the damage men inflicted upon it; there is another essay dedicated entirely to the city of Varese, "Vecchi e nuovi temi d'interesse cittadino" ("Old and New Topics About Our City," pp. 123–126) though the most explicit one on this issue is "La difesa del verde è una necessità sociale" ("The Defense of the Environment is a Social Necessity," pp. 143–146). He writes, "In Italy everyone always agrees when it comes to wage war on nature" (2012, p. 144), which is exactly what triggers the protagonist of *Dissipatio H. G.* In the novel, the building of the artery would in fact destroy the whole valley, since it would come as a complex of interconnected constructions; "It provided: a huge tunnel in the high part of the valley and many other projects including a viaduct in concrete on the Zemmi brook and many junctions and ramps. And a Motel" (1977a, p. 21).

decision to die and disappear, to dissolve from society, "without leaving any trace" (1977a, p. 21). In Morselli's first essay on suicide, dated 1949 and published in the Milanese magazine *Il Tempo* (*The Time*), he strictly connects the choice of suicide to the others within society, being men strictly "dependent on others and on nature at large" (2004, p. 32). Suicide then becomes the rebellion of a man who is not like the others, the ones who "do not live if not as an element of the crowd, of the 'tribe': the men of the mass" (2004, p. 32). Referring to the Italian society still traumatized by the horrors of the civil war and World War II, he claims that people react in two very different ways: By way of procreation and, on the opposing side, isolation and "the supreme negation of the self" (2004, p. 34), that is, suicide itself as an open act of rebellion. In 1956, seven years later, he writes the *Brief Chapter on Suicide* (2004), an essay to be published posthumous—which is less tied to the Italian historical situation and is more sophisticated in both language and content. In these pages of pain and suffering, Morselli adds solitude to the causes of suicide, which heightens suffering itself. This is a crucial moment to better understand the author's poetics, especially *Dissipatio H. G.* as a novel of failing and solitude. In a note on the text of the *Brief Chapter on Suicide*, Morselli mentions the possibility of self-reclusion, engaging first the possibility of segregation in a home, then into a cave (*grotta* or *cava* in Italian). Both elements are well present in the novel but ordered differently since the cave comes first, then the protagonist barricades himself at home for some time, traumatized by the *dissolution* of mankind (1977a). Although the allegory of the cave in Plato's *Republic* (2012) may be recalled, more present in Morselli's mind is that of Mary Shelley's *The Last Man* (1826 [2004]) of which a cave in the Neapolitan region of Italy is the beginning of the long narration of a plague that depopulates the entire earth. Morselli's protagonist is drawn to the cave with the exact intent of committing suicide, as mentioned before, after hiking up to a mountain, entering the cave, reaching a pit full of water in which he intends to fall and die and disappear forever from mankind. He describes the place in a precise and fascinating manner: "The pit is a natural siphon, where water collects" (1977a, p. 23). However, a rather comical accident occurs; he falls against a rock head-first, and the pain itself seems to recall him back to life since he exits the cave. Trying to go back home, he mistakes the path and becomes lost. I argue that this ironical element—also rendered by an acute series of reflections on fermented liquor wines when he was still in the cave—serves the author to render not only the importance of chance (in Italian, *caso* or *fatalità*), once more evident in his work as in so many of his novels, but also the very essence of suicide, according to the reflections of *Brief Chapter on Suicide* mentioned:

> Despair, for instance, is not necessarily glamorous or loud as people imagine it. It is often dumb squalor of the soul; it is silent and dark inertia [...] We feel so alone with such pain that even annihilates vision, not to mention the consideration for other beings although related to us. (2004, pp. 120, 125)

The protagonist of *Dissipatio H. G.* is desperately alone both before and after his first suicide attempt in the cave. Before, he was living alone close to a city he calls Crisopoli, or *City of Gold*, a place where banks and tourist attractions rule, for which he has no sympathy or love. It is the quintessential human creation with the most artificial and complex systems where history, technology, humanism, and progress coexist. Cities' familiar though ever-changing shape is the ideal setting for, among other things, narration. The word *civis*, derived from its Latin origin of *civitāte*, still carries the Indo-European stem meaning to "settle" or to "found." All this does not apply to Morselli's character who feels alienated by the city and all his inhabitants, feeling alone in the crowd, not connected to anyone, completely and hopelessly isolated. The environment was at risk, and Italian political and social reality was anything but safe. All those de-stabilizing elements must have played a role in the atmosphere in which Morselli wrote this novel of suicide and annihilation. The year 1968 with all its rebellion and protest was over, but not the years of inner terrorism that gave almost two decades of homicide, bloodshed, attacks, and death. The late 1960s and 1970s were the epicenter of the "Years of Lead" (*anni di piombo*) and the infamous strategy of tension, orchestrated by extra-parliamentary right-wings together with sections of state agencies and the P2 deviated Masonry.[6] From the year 1968 onward, even from a legal and parliamentary point of view, scholars argue that a long legal and administrative crisis began, destined to last for the rest of the First Republic (that is until 1993–1994). It was called the "constitutional crisis," and it was due to the failure of the reforms proposed by the center-left parties, triggering a long cycle of short-lived governments and party alliances (Paladin, 2004).

It was in this complex setting that *Dissipatio H. G.* was written, and its protagonist feels what a scholar of suicide has called the "disorientation"

[6] For the cultural and literary context in general, see Tellini (1998). For *Dissipatio H. G.* in particular, see Rinaldi (1996), D'Arienzo (1998), Mari (1998), Pischedda (2000), Mussgnug (2003), and Bertelli (2013). A very good and useful essay on Morselli is the *Introduzione* (*Introduction*) by Valentina Fortichiari to the first volume (2002) of Morselli, *Romanzi* (pp. IX-LXIII), and the *Cronologia* (*Chronology*) (pp. LXVII-CVXII) by the same scholar.

(Barbagli, 2009, p. 239) of not knowing how to cope with reality. Morselli's character finds himself twice in that discouraging condition: First in the chaotic consumerist society and then after the event of humanity vanishing. At this point, he considers committing suicide again, like many other characters in Morselli's narrations,[7] now with a gun that he jokingly calls with black humor "my black-eyed girlfriend" (1977a, p. 26). He eventually decides for the second time to live, perhaps mindful of a famous verse of the poem "I Am a Creature" (1916 [1997, p. 68]) by the poet Giuseppe Ungaretti: "*La morte / Si sconta / Vivendo*," or in English, "We pay for death by living." Also, by nullifying both suicide attempts and quickly adapting to the new reality as a lone survivor, Morselli kindly ironizes with Durkheim, jokingly quoted together with Freud and many other authors. He does this by recreating two cases of suicide analyzed by sociologists of the past: The anomic suicide—consequent to inadaptability to a disaggregated but prosperous and dynamic society—and suicide of despair after a catastrophe. Both cases are related to society and the others in relation to the self. It is a self that in *Dissipatio H. G.*, after the cave and the house, is now left alone to roam free in a solitary world with no

[7] Morselli had not only theorized in his nonfiction on suicide but had often depicted suicide as a narrative element in his novels. After editing a small book collecting the two essays on suicide, scholar Valentina Fortichiari has written an essay at the end titled "Note to the Text" (1984, pp. 23–29), where she reconstructs all references to suicide done by Morselli, from his *Journal* to the novels. I do not want to repeat her words, but I directly refer the reader to her volume *Guido Morselli, Il Suicidio e Capitolo breve sul suicidio* (*Suicide and Brief Chapter on Suicide*) (2004). For my essay on suicide and human dissolution in *Dissipatio H. G.*, it suffices to say that in no other work of fiction has the author given any reason for the characters' suicides or attempted suicides. In *Un dramma borghese* (*A Bourgeois Tragedy*) (1980), the daughter of the protagonist possibly attempts to commit suicide at the end, or it is an accident with her father's gun; the author voluntarily leaves the question open-ended, just as he leaves to question the survival of the girl, and the reader will never know if she is dead or alive. Same goes for *Il Comunista*, where the protagonist's estranged ex-wife is hospitalized for an "accident" that could suggest a suicide attempt, but the ambiguity is left unsolved. In *Disspatio H. G.*, maybe not coincidentally, the narration is in the first person, unlike the third person of the other novels, and reflections on suicide are relevant, insisted, and developed with a clear and focused aim. Even though both suicide attempts are not successful, there is no chance of mistaking them as accidents. This peculiarity has led scholars to interpret the whole book as a great and witty suicide note of the author. Although I do not completely agree with this interpretation, it surely is appealing; there are many autobiographical elements in the novel—the isolated villa threatened by the construction of a highway and the protagonist being a writer who deeply feels unsatisfied with society and life in general—that directly recall Morselli's last years, not to mention that *Dissipatio H. G.* is his last finished novel. Despite all that, I am convinced that a work of art must be read and studied without exaggerating its relations with the biography of its author.

people, but it remains full of animals, objects, machines, and all the remnants of society.[8]

After the Cave: Dissipatio Humani Generis

It is relevant that in the whole book—a rather short novel of roughly 130 pages—there is neither an explanation, theory, nor reflection of the disappearance of mankind. People just vanish with no exceptions other than the protagonist; this is unlike the novels that surely had an impact on Morselli, such as Shelley's work, but even more so M. P. Shiel's *The Purple Cloud* (2012), a peculiar 1901 novel translated into Italian by Rodolfo Wilcock in 1967, just years prior *Dissipatio H. G.* Unlike the mysterious cloud of poison that kills humanity leaving but two human beings alive, a man and woman—in Shiel's novel—the protagonist in *Dissipatio H. G.* is the only one left, and he questions neither the reason nor the dynamics of the event. What he does is use quotations from Iamblichus, a Neoplatonic thinker from present-day Syria who lived between the third and fourth centuries AD. The three Latin words—two of them abbreviated in the title—are presented as a quotation from this author. Critics have often overlooked or neglected researching this element, and it has been qualified as a fake quotation. I argue that, although the three words do not appear in that order in Iamblichus' work, Morselli had his reasons to mention this author, since the concept of *dissipatio* comes down to the relations among men and deities. In an 1821 English translation of Iamblichus' major work on divination and prayer, it is possible to find many aspects that lean toward isolation, caves, and even dissolution. The author mentions the importance of a cave, making it possible to get closer to the

[8] In a short essay published in 1964 in the local publication *Questo e altro* (*This and More*), Morselli had given a short and poignant description of his contemporary society, one that completely fits the novel *Dissipatio H. G.*; "If we keep our eyes open we cannot but see that we are at the mercy of things – machines, goods, money – a society in which the laborer is enslaved and dehumanized by labor itself, and the rulers themselves are enslaved to the cult of richness" ("L'ideologia, un tramite" ["Ideology, a Means"], 2012, p. 196). In an original short story published in the magazine *La Prealpina* in 1950 and significantly titled "Una rivolta" ("A Revolt"), Morselli imagines that society collapses due to *the revolt* of everyday tools such as screwdrivers, can openers, etc., that after a plague of the metal become soft and unable to function. Toward the end of the short story, the narrator ironically affirms, "Triumphant of the most hazardous deeds in every field, sociological, moral, speculative, man had to realize he was powerless in front of the necessity of rolling a bolt" (2012, p. 113). In *Dissipatio H. G.*, objects do survive; only mankind disappeared, not animals, plants, or objects. However, tools and machines became unused, immobile, and deprived of their meaning and function. For this reason, the protagonist collects some on them in a grotesque, open-air museum. The city itself, untouched and completely empty thanks to all the objects left behind, immediately becomes archeology: "The city is intact, just abandoned. It is already archeology" (1977a, p. 35).

gods, hence worshipping in isolation, "by being seated at the mouth of a cavern, as those who prophesy at Delphi" (1821, p. 5). Later in his work, he will elaborate on the oracle of Delphi, adding something that would be very close to what Morselli's protagonist finds in his cave. Iamblichus writes, "It is acknowledged then by all men, that the oracle in Colophon gives answers through the medium of water, for there is a fountain in a subterranean dwelling from which the prophetess drinks" (1821, p. 141). Morselli's character goes into the cave and drinks liquor wine in front of the water siphon in which he is planning on committing suicide by drowning. Although already quite a strong ironical subversion, he goes further, engaging the modern "medium" par excellence of the press. After going back to the journal he worked for, traveling around the city, and to the now empty and inactive airport, he reflects (almost paraphrasing the ancient oracles and, of course, Marshall McLuhan's book), "The medium is the message. With its indisputable consequence, no medium means no message at all" (1977a, p. 52).

After a thorough investigation and description of the beliefs and religious practices of the Egyptians, Chaldeans, and Assyrians, Iamblichus approaches some very important thoughts on the possibility of the *dissolution* of men, after having mentioned multiple times "the indefiniteness and instability of the human condition" (1821, p. 24) and "corporeal dissolution" (1821, p. 177). He finally mentions the possible source of Morselli's words when discussing people's abstinence from animal meat for spiritual clarity and religious practices; he writes, "Nor is it the power of the Gods only that abolishes all bodies, and causes them to vanish, without any approximation to them" (1821, pp. 228–229). This is the most the author says about what Morselli calls *dissipatio humani generis*, but in an entirely different context. It is more a description of the humans-Gods relationship, technical instruction on liturgies, and sophisticated descriptions of ancient cults and beliefs. Morselli's "quotation" is hence more a transliteration and adaptation than a real quotation, but it is not at all fake, being the element of human (body) dissolution mentioned and described by the ancient Iamblichus. Morselli's collective vanishing is a more philosophical and ironical realization of what he had been theorizing and describing during his speculations; it is also a reflection on the thinking self and otherness, particularly on the theme of solitude and solipsism to which must be added his extensive reflections on religion and the crucial problem of evil.

The overnight vanishing of all men and women, the only exception being the narrator, does not constitute an "apocalypse," not even a secular one as many scholars have written. Still, using Slavoy Žižek's term (2014), it constitutes an event, a moment of change from the before and the after. There is no revelation during or after it, nor tribulation as expressed in the Gospels or in the Book of Revelation. Morselli uses the post-disaster form—although the "post-event" narration would be a more accurate definition by all means—only to transcend it and use it to ironically express with deep wit many of his religious, philosophical, and moral reflections. The novel *Dissipatio H. G.* has nothing in common with novels or novellas like *Earth Abides* (1949), *The Purple Cloud* (2012), *The Last Man* (2004), or *The Scarlet Plague* (2019); it is closer to Voltaire's *contes philosophiques* such as *Candide* (2011) and Giacomo Leopardi's *Operette Morali* (*Moral Operettas*) (1827) and especially *Storia del genere umano* (2015) which could be seen as good starting points to understanding Morselli's novel. Morselli himself poses the basis of this interpretation of his novel by making his protagonist reflect with candid irony on the wake of the event:

> I used to play my usual game, putting on hold the existence of all my peer human beings, envisioning myself as the only thinking of being in a completely deserted creation. Deserted by men, of course. In this case, my inner thought can be depicted as pedantry. As Hegel has dreamt of a reality in itself by itself, I was dreaming of a reality with me and for me. Because the others simply were not there. (1977a, p. 29)

Morselli, who had conducted lifelong intense studies on religion and philosophy alongside his literary works, was deep into the problem of the presence of evil in the world, as well as a profound criticism of the neo-idealist philosophy. This philosophy was represented in Italy by two major thinkers with whom Morselli, ideologically, had an intense though problematic fascination: Benedetto Croce and Giovanni Gentile. Both were quoted and discussed numerous times throughout Morselli's works together with philosopher Giuseppe Rensi, particularly the most speculative ones. An important statement about philosophy and its unavoidable conjunction with theology is made by Morselli in 1964, in a book review published in the popular cultural magazine *La Cultura.* Reviewing C.B. Offner and H. van Strafelen's *Modern Japanese Religions* (1963, reviewed in 1964, and later collected in the 2012 volume *Una rivolta e altri scritti*), Morselli argues that philosophy itself is inspired by what he calls "the mystery of evil" (2012, p. 207), or evil in its real substantial reality, which is for him in the "suffering of souls and bodies" (2012, p. 207). This is the same powerful source of evil that brings the protagonist of *Dissipatio H. G.* twice on the verge of suicide, before and after mankind's vanishing. It is no coincidence that a major work of Morselli's philosophy, a collection of essays published in 1977b meaningfully titled

Faith and Criticism (*Fede e critica*), contains at the very beginning two essays completely dedicated to the themes of suffering, evil, and the relationship between God and man: "Why Do People Suffer" and "The Book of Job." However, in the third essay of the book titled "An Easy Criticism," Morselli describes the biblical narration as a kind of a "transfiguration, rather than fiction, allegorical allusion rather than mythical and incise adherence" (1977b, p. 80). Keeping this in mind, I argue, is crucial to understanding the allegory of the vanishing of mankind in front of the protagonist; this is especially so when it is known how deeply Morselli's thoughts were influenced by the philosopher Giuseppe Rensi, whose major work on religion and philosophy dealt with the "vanishing of religion" (*Le aporie della religione* [*The Aporias of Religion*], 2017).[9]

In *Dissipatio H. G.*, Morselli imagines the dissipation of all men and women except for one, who he calls "intellectual monad" (1977a, p. 28). This intellectual monad survives the "mysterious annihilation, a vanishing onto nothingness" (1977a, p. 21), just to progressively lose contact with the new state of things. He then wanders to all the places he used to know, searching for traces of the past and his friends, the woman, and the doctor. He is aware of his condition as the last member of society, which he becomes the society itself: "I am yet Humanity, I am Society" (1977a, p. 31),[10] which ironically stresses the capitalization of the initials. He adds, "There is nothing left but the self, and the self is only mine. It is me" (1977a, p. 31). This condition of the self is the allegory of solitude and suffering that grips every human being, as Morselli depicted in a short essay on blasphemy. In this essay, the desolation and solitude of men and the image of the cave are so striking, and it recalls the novel with a clarity that is beyond doubt; "The world is a cave in which echoes, empty, a silence that possesses the dimension of our being, horribly enlarged"

[9] Morselli himself wrote a theological essay that has only recently been published as an appendix of a broader work by scholar Paola Villani, *Un mistico ribelle. A-teologia e scrittura in Guido Morselli. Con l'inedito* Teologia in crisi (*A Rebel Mystic. A-theology and Writing in Guido Morselli. With the Unpublished* Theology in crisis) (2012). The essay *Teologia in crisi* is found on pages 233–287. Explaining Rensi's approach to theology, Morselli writes, "[Rensi's] assumption, 'God's volatilization' as he incisively calls it, does ignore (or fights against) atheistic positions of idealistic subjectivism, and so it should be, since it moves on the grounds of negative theology" (2012, p. 249). In *Dissipatio H. G.*, Morselli significantly ironizes against subjectivism by imagining one subject left completely alone on earth and by depicting the series of his actions and reflections in the wake of the vanishing of all referents.

[10] Another possible element of parody, although it is not certain that Morselli read the book, could be Richard Matheson's *I Am Legend* (2007), which was published in America in 1954 and in an Italian translation three years later, by the title *I Vampiri* (*The Vampires*) (1957). It is the story of a lone survivor after an event that caused humanity to transform into vampires, ending with the protagonist calling himself legend. Morselli, whose English was very proficient, could have read the book in the original language. In *Dissipatio H. G.*, the lone-surviving protagonist ironically calls himself 'society,' possibly paraphrasing Matheson's book into *I Am Society*.

(1977b, p. 221). In *Dissipatio H. G.*, the self comes into the cave as enlarged, and when it comes out, nobody is there to see or challenge it. The hellish experience of the self becomes the impossibility to have any relationship with other human beings, since hell can be both the others and the complete absence of them, as Morselli seems to suggest.

Haunted by these reflections and by the difficulties of a peculiar life, during the night of July 31, 1973, Guido Morselli himself commits suicide. Since then, most of his work has been published; however, there are some that remain untouched. It is now the scholars' duty to finish publishing his works and to popularize them globally, for only writing may defeat death, and the only way life wins over suicide is through art.

References

Barbagli, M. (2009). *Congedarsi dal mondo. Il suicidio in Occidente e in Oriente.* il Mulino.

Bertelli, D. (2013). Morselli, Rensi, Leopardi and the suicide philosophy. *La Rassegna della letteratura italiana, 117*(2), 471–484.

Berto, G. (1964). *Il male oscuro.* Rizzoli.

D'Arienzo, S. (1998). Il cantiere della *Dissipatio H. G.*: Ipotesi di lettura degli appunti preparatorî. *Autografo, 14*(37), 9–21. https://doi.org/10.1400/157923

Durkheim, É. (1951). *Suicide: A study in sociology.* The Free Press.

Fortichiari, V. (1994). *Invito alla lettura di Morselli.* Mursia.

Iamblichus. (1821). *On the mysteries of the Egyptians, Chaldeans, and Syrians.* C. Whittingham.

Leopardi, G. (1827). *Operette morali.* Stella.

Leopardi, G. (2015). *Storia del genere umano.* Zona.

Lessona Fasano, M. (2003). *Guido Morselli. Un inspiegabile caso letterario.* Liguori.

London, J. (2019). *The scarlet plague.* Read & Co. Books.

Manzoni, A. (1830). *I promessi sposi* (Vol. 1). Baudry.

Mari, M. (1998). Estraneo agli angeli e alle bestie (Lettura di *Dissipatio H. G.*). *Autografo, 14*(37), 49–58. https://doi.org/10.1400/157925

Matheson, R. (1957). *I Vampiri.* Longanesi.

Matheson, R. (2007). *I am a legend.* Tor Books.

Morselli, G. (1974). *Roma senza Papa.* Adelphi.

Morselli, G. (1975a). *Contro-passato prossimo. Un'ipotesi retrospettiva.* Adelphi.

Morselli, G. (1975b). *Divertimento 1889.* Adelphi.

Morselli, G. (1977a). *Dissipatio H. G.* Adelphi.

Morselli, G. (1977b). *Fede e critica.* Adelphi.

Morselli, G. (1980). *Un dramma borghese.* Adelphi.

Morselli, G. (1988). *Diario.* Adelphi.

Morselli, G. (1994). *La felicità non è un lusso*. Ed. Fortichiari Adelphi.
Morselli, G. (1998). *Uomini e amori*. Adelphi.
Morselli, G. (2002). *I romanzi* (Vol. 1). Adelphi.
Morselli, G. (2004). *Il suicidio e Capitolo breve sul suicidio*. Edizioni Via Del Vento.
Morselli, G. (2012). *Una rivolta e altri scritti (1932–1966)*. Milan.
Morselli, G. (2017). *The communist*. New York Review of Books.
Mussgnug, F. (2003). Finire il mondo. Per un'analisi del romanzo apocalittico italiano degli anni Settanta. *Contemporanea, 1*, 19–32. https://doi.org/10.1400/20367
Offner, C. B., & Van Strafelen, H. (1963). *Modern Japanese religions*. Brill.
Paladin, L. (2004). *Per una storia costituzionale dell'Italia repubblicana*. il Mulino.
Pischedda, B. (2000). Morselli: una *Dissipatio* molto postmoderna. *Filologia antica e moderna, 19*, 163–189.
Plato. (2012). *The republic*. Penguin.
Rensi, G. (2017). *Le aporie della religione*. La scuola di Pitagora.
Rinaldi, R. (1996). I romanzi a una dimensione di Guido Morselli. *Critica letteraria, 24*(91–92), 667–691.
Shelley, M. (2004). *The last man*. Wordsworth Classics. (Original work published in 1826).
Shiel, M. P. (2012). *The purple cloud*. Penguin. (Original work published in 1901).
Stewart, G. R. (1949). *Earth abides*. Ballantine Books.
Tellini, G. (1998). *Il romanzo italiano dell'Ottocento e Novecento*. Bruno Mondadori.
Ungaretti, G. (1997). I am a creature. In G. Ungaretti (Ed.), *A major selection of the poetry of Giuseppe Ungaretti* (p. 68). Exile Editions. (Original work published in 1916).
Villani, P. (2012). *Un mistico ribelle. A-teologia e scrittura in Guido Morselli, con l'inedito Teologia in crisi*. Grauseditore.
Voltaire. (2011). *Candide*. Gallimard.
Žižek, S. (2014). *Event: A philosophical journey through a concept*. Melville.

Roberto Risso holds a Doctorate in Italian Literature from the University of Turin, Italy, and a Ph.D. in the same field from the University of Wisconsin-Madison. From Fall 2015, he is an Assistant Professor of Italian Studies at Clemson University (USA). His field of research is the Italian Narrative Prose of the Modern and Pre-modern periods, with a particular focus on the interconnections between literature, cinema, and art. He has published 3 monographs and 45 peer-reviewed essays in journals and books both in English and Italian.

The Existential and Suicidal Crisis in the Work of Walker Percy

Barbara Hawellek

Contents

Introduction 185
Phenomena of the Existential Crisis in Selected Novels 188
Origin Models of the Existential Crisis 196
Summary 200
References 201

Introduction

The phenomenon of existential and suicidal crisis is becoming a central challenge for a modern human, especially in an age when death is increasingly becoming a taboo on the one hand and suicide rates are rising steadily on the other. Historically, suicidal behavior has gone through different evaluations, from suicide as an expression of free will to a maximum restriction of the will in the form of mental illness. Among the scientific theories, that of Émile Durkheim (1951), who sees suicide as a symptom of social grievances

B. Hawellek (✉)
Beta Clinic Bonn, Bonn, Germany
e-mail: barbara.hawellek@betaklinik.de

J. Ros Velasco (ed.), *Suicide in Modern Literature*,
https://doi.org/10.1007/978-3-030-69392-3_12

which can be solved restructuring the society, had a lasting effect at the beginning of the last century. Later, the representatives of psychoanalysis (Freud, 1961, 1953; Klein, 1972; Menninger, 1956) emphasized the importance of the unconscious by introducing the concepts of the "death instinct," "primary aggression," and its psychological defense mechanisms. The definition of suicidality, which is based on Haenel and Pöldinger (1986), regards suicidal tendencies as the sum of all mental forces that tend toward self-destruction. In this context, the phenomenon is almost always understood as an expression of subjective constriction without the possibility of unimpaired choice. When looking at the suicidal spectrum from a psychiatric-psychosocial point of view, however, the impression of a continuum rather emerges, ranging from the interactional subject-object relationship crisis based on Wolfersdorf (1994a, 1994b, 1995) to psychopathological abnormality in the sense of a mental illness. Within this continuum, suicidality is conceived not only as an illness in the sense of a medical entity but as a generally possible way of thinking and acting. A comprehensive analysis of this meaning spectrum can only be adequately met by interdisciplinary perspectives, in this article based on the literary work of Walker Percy.

The Person of Walker Percy (1916–1990)

Percy, who is an American author from Louisiana, adopted after the early death of his parents, studied medicine at Columbia University in New York, yet, quit the medical profession in 1944 due to his pulmonary tuberculosis. Pursuing a medical career, Percy was greatly influenced by his time spent at the National Institute of Mental Health (NIMH), where he got actively involved in numerous psychiatric projects. After leaving the medical field, he devoted himself with great energy to European literature and philosophy. The author comes from an educated family, which left a deep mark of melancholy on his character, with multiple suicides among the family members, including the author's father and grandfather. Affected by this experience, he was concerned with this issue in his life and writing. Percy converted to Catholicism in 1947 and was intensely committed to the field of faith and religion until his late creative years (Tolston, 1992).

Percy's Phenomenology of Suicide

In his literature, Percy uses a philosophical, psychological, and neuroscientific approach to the existential issues of life and death. Using the method of the *empathic horizontal and vertical "unrolling,"* the author conducts a multidimensional situation and a personality analysis of his characters, which at the same time contains a deep philosophical reflection. For Percy, a discourse on yearning for death and suicide emerges where traditional suicidology ends. He creates a phenomenology of suicide whose uniqueness lies in the change of perspective from the outside to the suicide victim's inner world.

With a considerable amount of psychological expertise and philosophical reflection, the author makes up a profile of the human being, who is "sick to death" in an empty and artificial world. Far from creating an apologia of suicide, he is rather concerned with relativizing an exclusively psychopathological model and, beyond the traditional research, finding an understanding approach to the process of despair and longing for death, especially on the background of the prevailing *Zeitgeist*, which is largely exposed as the bearer of the "moribund." In the style of Pascal, he shows a portrait of a restless modern human thrown into the chaos of the world, driven by escapism, who is more capable of destroying himself instead of facing the true self.

Literary Works

Percy's literary work experienced an existentialist interpretation early on. In reference to Kierkegaard's *The Sickness unto Death* (2013, p. 322), he defines as the motto of his work: The special thing about despair is that "it is despair but does not know it" and thus shows the depth and intensity pervasive in his work in the consideration of the problem of meaning.

As a modern realist, Percy is anchored in the philosophical tradition of the nineteenth century. He also refers to Charles S. Peirce (1998), an American language theorists, and creates his own theory of the "essentially human." The reflection of the language, understood as a process of liberation, has a close relationship to Peter Handke and thus to the German-language literature of the 1960s, which was influenced by naive linguistic realism. Anchored in existentialism, both authors attempt a new orientation in a meaningless world without real values and ideals. The German translation of Percy's first novel *The Moviegoer* (1961) by Peter Handke is an expression of spiritual closeness of both authors.

The initially secular orientation of Percy's work changes later into a clearly religious one. Undoubtedly, the mythologizing of the past of the American South is a significant element in Percy's work, whereby he almost always writes from the standpoint of the already lost, without excessive sentimentality and with a strong degree of irony. A central role is played by certain main issues that run through his entire oeuvre, such as the omnipresent states of the continuous *search*, the *banality of everyday life*, the situation of the *outsider*, and the *experience of catastrophe*.

For Percy, the disintegration of tradition results in the loss of identity: At the end of the world oriented toward progress with an extreme desire for self-realization, especially in the areas of science and sexuality, for him, the individual is degraded to an abstract mind with an attached sexual organ.

The Existential Conflict: Loss and Transmission of Meaning

The central topics in Percy's work capture mainly the omnipresent search for identity, rootlessness, the right to exist, and a sustainable reference to the question of meaning. His protagonists are people who are well anchored in the bourgeois world, but inwardly uprooted, searching for content and meaning, to whom social and family structures cannot provide the necessary basis for existence. Increasingly, individuals experience an existential loss in space with a feeling of inner emptiness and at the same time of being trapped in the repetition of patterns. The escapism and growing alienation that often result from this lead to existentially borderline situations of a catastrophic character and allow through this the only true confrontation with one's own deeper self. Based on the interpretation of various extreme situations, Percy puts the central question of the suicidal crisis not only in terms of self-destruction but also in terms of its cathartic, identity- and meaning-transmitting character.

Phenomena of the Existential Crisis in Selected Novels

With his first novel *The Moviegoer* (1961), which encountered an existential interpretation at a very early stage, Percy made his first significant impact on American literature. A central subject of the novel is the protagonist's *search*, which constantly leads him, a young, quite successful American businessman, rooted in the bourgeois milieu, to existential border situations. The author calls this state of mind, which usually occurs at the experience of a standardized, predetermined, and secure life, the *malaise*. For the young Binx Bolling, all seemingly routine situations are images of horror.

These kinds of feelings take him unaware when a condensed banality of life suddenly hurts, e.g., during Sunday afternoon excursions, business consideration on the subject of cars or almost routinely performed erotic efforts and sexual activities:

> Everydayness life is the enemy. No search is possible. Perhaps there was a time when everydayness was not too strong and one could break its grip by brute strength. Now nothing breaks it—but disaster. (1961, pp. 117–118)

The real experience of catastrophe is underlying for the protagonist, who experienced a traumatic life event: The story of his father, who voluntarily moved and fell in the World War II, and his sister, who attempted suicide in order to escape the unbearable for a while: "I took six or eight capsules altogether. I knew that wouldn't kill me. My Lord, I didn't want to die—not at that moment. I only wanted to—break out, or off, off dead center" (1961, p. 145). And he points out the meaning of a catastrophe as an authentic experience: "Have you noticed that only in time of illness or disaster or death are people real?" (1961, p. 69).

The protagonist discovers an opportunity to escape from the real world into the world of movies. There's no denying, it is a kind of relocation into a personal virtual reality, in which Binx is able to experience feelings in a kind of distance, more detached from the self and thus less fearful.

Percy assumes that a human being is able to find out the trail to the essential, but only with a deeper and global approach:

> He was actually like one of those scientists in the movies who don't care about anything but the problem in their heads—now here is a fellow who does have a "flair for research" and will be heard from. Yet I do not envy him. I would not change places with him if he discovered the cause and cure of cancer. For he is no more aware of the mystery which surrounds him than a fish is aware of the water it swims in. (1961, p. 47)

The author implies an individual freedom and responsibility of the human: "I had discovered that a person does not have to *be* this or *be* that or to be anything, not even oneself. One is free" (1961, p. 94). Free also in the sense of choosing a very personal way of looking at life; hence, it becomes clear again for Percy; the mature and deep experience goes hand in hand with his relation to the inner and outer evil:

> In the thirty-first year of my dark pilgrimage on this earth and knowing less than I ever knew before, having learned only to recognize merde when I see it, having inherited no more from my father than a good nose for merde, for every species of shit that flies—my only talent—smelling merde from every quarter, living in fact in the very century of merde, the great shithouse of scientific humanism where needs are satisfied, everyone becomes an anyone, a warm and creative person, and prospers like a dung beetle, and one hundred percent of people are humanists and ninety-eight percent believe in God, and men are dead, dead, dead; and the malaise has settled like a fall-out, and what people really fear is not that the bomb will fall but that the bomb will not fall. (1961, p. 180)

In his social satire *Love in the Ruins* (1971), subtitled *The Adventures of a Bad Catholic Shortly Before the End of the World*, Percy describes the decline of basic structures of social order, with a critical analysis of American politics and customs, sexual therapy, euthanasia, racism, and religious fundamentalism. The main protagonist of the novel, a psychiatrist Dr. More, himself depressed and suicidal in the past, makes a great discovery of a device for detecting mind disorders, so-called qualitative-quantitative ontological lapsometer. This "stethoscope of the spirit" (1971, p. 60) is able to measure quantitative correlations in the individual Brodmann regions of the cerebral cortex and to influence them:

> The Heavy Sodium ions hit his pineal body, seat of self, like a guillotine, sundering self from self forever, that ordinary self, the restless aching everyday self, from the secret self which happens on in dreams, in poetry, during ordeals, on happy trips. (1971, p. 351)

In psychiatry, the lapsometer is celebrated as the scientific breakthrough par excellence, since it finally creates the possibility of recognizing states of depression and suicidality and treating them by means of brain stimulation.

Dr. More himself also suffers from a deep crisis of meaning with a suicide attempt. Through this experience he finds back to life again: "One morning [...] my wrists were cut and bleeding. Seeing the blood, I came to myself, saw myself as itself and the world for what it is, and began to love life" (1971, p. 92). As a counterpart to his "lapsometer" (1971, p. 88), his individual way to overcome the crisis and redefine the ego was to experience his own existential pain. The author criticizes here the reductionist neuroscience approach to explore and influence the human self and shows that a simplified causality and one-dimensionality is unable to recognize the essential issues.

Subjective failure, low self-esteem, and emotional instability are the central factors, which can lead by Percy to existential crisis. In his last outstanding work, *The Thanatos Syndrome* (1987), he is concerned with the questions of living or dying. In this context, Percy deals with the problem of failure, its individually different definitions and coping strategies, and consequently brings to mind the phenomenon of one's own sense of values, which can only arise meaningfully from a mature, individual self-perception:

> Life doesn't have to stop with failure. Not only do you have to in the creek, you can even take pleasure in the general fecklessness of life, as I do, a doctor without patients sailing paper P-51s at a martin house. I am a failed but not unhappy doctor. (1987, p. 75)

Here it becomes clear that a failure that comes up in Percy's work is a very relative, individual term, usually based on the external criteria of a civically defined achievement in society. It is up to the individual to internalize these criteria and accept them as the basis for one's own behavioral imperative or to create his own value system. All things considered, Percy acknowledges two important aspects leading to mental crisis and life weariness: an excessive hedonistic lifestyle and an inability to deal with own aggressive instincts.

In the autobiographically influenced novel *The Last Gentleman* (1966), his own family is a driving factor for the protagonist to a lifelong reflection and a border walk on the edge of the abyss with recurring images of his father's suicide. He works as a technician in a New York department store, lives completely uprooted, homeless, roaming aimlessly through the countryside and observing the events of life with a telescope. The role of the *observer* defines most clearly the bizarre figure of William Barrett, who, suffering from epilepsy, permanently experiences *déjà vu*, as well as depersonalization and derealization, with the special gift of a childlike, simple-minded view. A close parallel to Dostoyevsky's *The Idiot* (2017), who portrays a seemingly naive person, unfit to live, yet inwardly rich and still unspoiled by the progress of civilization, becomes all too clear. Almost throughout his life, accompanied by the ambivalence between life and death, he is repeatedly caught up in self-destructive memories of his father's suicide:

> The father went on without saying anything: went into the house, [...] opened the country food press which had been converted to a gun cabinet, took down the double-barrel twelve-gauge Greener, loaded it, went up the back stairs into

> the attic, and, fitting the muzzle of the Greener into the notch of his breastbone, could still reach both triggers with his thumbs. (1966, p. 261)

His father's fatal solution to the existential dilemma makes Barrett feel an immanent familiarity with the nihilistic mindset.

In his scientific paper, Dr. Sutter (main protagonist in *The Last Gentleman*) raises the issue of sexuality as a solution to overcoming the existential loneliness. For the protagonists, however, the area of sexuality, which is related to hopes of transcendence and essence, seems at the same time to be a source of deep disillusionment. It is clear that eroticism, as an everyday occurrence, has become just as obvious as all the other areas of civilized life, cannot put life on a higher level. The existential basic need for transcendence cannot be realized in this field and, in consequence, mostly leads to a deep frustration.

In *The Second Coming* (1981), motivated by a deep feeling for a woman, Barrett succeeds in overcoming a crisis of meaning that has been continuously pushed ahead in *The Last Gentleman*. It resulted in ending an existential loneliness and spiritual homelessness that he had felt permanently until then. On his inner journey to this point, Barrett repeatedly reaches the borders of his own existence and reflects on the despair. On the one hand, he admits that his feeling of absurdity stems from his depressive state, but at the same time he realizes that the world is indeed absurd—which again underlines his basic conviction that the world itself is illogical and meaningless, and particularly sensitive people tend to grasp it and despair of it. Suicide appears to be a method to escape the absurdity of the world on one's own initiative. In the confrontation with the father figure, he becomes aware of the aggressive component of the suicidal act in which a violent aggression toward the world finally turns against himself. Throughout his entire life, Barrett takes laborious pains to distance himself from the paternalistic solution of the life-death paradigm and to find a less destructive path of his own. The painful way of life-affirming self-discovery is accompanied by serious mental crises. His whole life condenses into a struggle for meaning and a possibility to overcome the world of absurdity. Beyond the catastrophic life story, the epileptic disease with depressive feelings, and the experience of alienation, Barrett represents the contemporary man par excellence, who is thrown into the world without being asked and, deprived of the power of his own individual decision, forced to live according to the principles of the generally prevailing *Zeitgeist*. In the figure of Bill Barrett, Percy portrays an extraordinarily sensitive human being, in whom civic security and prosperity fail to make him blind to the essential:

> There at any rate stands Will Barrett on the edge of a gorge in old Carolina, a talented agreeable wealthy man living in as pleasant an environment as one can imagine and yet who is thinking of putting a bullet in his brain. (1981, p. 16)

Percy also deplores the increasing distortion of interpersonal relationships and the lack of authenticity in the society: "[...] people [...] were never a hundred percent themselves. They occupied a place uneasily and more or less successfully" (1981, p. 18).

In this novel, the significance of the catastrophe as a kind of existential awakening and impulse for action becomes clear: "Disaster gave me leave to act. Between times I didn't know what to do. Now I know" (1981, p. 142). Particularly in the area of interpersonal relationships, the experience of illness and disaster, as Percy correctly recognizes, plays a significant role in creating real closeness:

> People notice very little indeed, ghost-ridden as they are by themselves. You have to be bleeding from the mouth or throwing a fit for them to take notice. Otherwise, anything you do is no more or less than another part of the world they have to deal with, poor souls. (1981, p. 201)

And further he asks himself: "Is it possible for people to miss their lives in the same way one misses a plane? And how is it that death, the nearness of death, can restore a missed life?" (1981, p. 144).

In Percy's novels, death emerges as the most intensive form of border experience and allows his protagonists to deal with the meaning of life against the background of limitation and transience. The actual catastrophe, however, is rather to be presumed in the fact that only the experience of the own abyss enables the feeling of depth and meaning. Thus, the experience of being close to death, whether voluntarily in the form of a suicide attempt or involuntarily in the form of a serious illness, is of main importance. In this sense, Percy also raises a question: "Why is it that without death one misses his life?" (1981, p. 144). Most people perceive death as the greatest tragedy of all; however, for Percy, there is a far greater tragedy in the pitifulness of a life plan that lacks depth and reflection: "Life is better than death but there are worse things than death" (1981, p. 147).

One of the protagonists' strategies is no longer to take life seriously, not to get involved in anything properly, not to recognize moral values, and, on the whole, to play a game in which life exists only in the dimension of an experiment, outside of ourselves: "You might call the ultimate scientific experiment in contrast to dreary age-old philosophical and religious disputations which have no resolution" (1981, p. 216).

In Percy's contemplation of striving for death, a closely related love and death instinct gets a central meaning in the context of Freud's psychoanalysis. Life is understood as a struggle to maintain a balance between these two instincts, with the consequence of shifting to the one side or the other:

> Did you not believe, old mole, that these two things alone are real, loving and dying, and since one is so much like the other and there is so little of the one, in the end there remained only the other? (1981, pp. 187–188)

By the example of Bill Barrett, Percy created a kind of higher human being, in his own way a sighted person "but there is a difference between feeling dead and not knowing it, and feeling dead and knowing it" (1981, p. 371) who feels like an outsider and spectator:

> It was his, Will Barrett's, own sly way of "being smart," that is, of standing aside and keeping quiet, looking on, observing commonplace disaster which everyone else accepts as a matter of course, then figuring something out which converts a necessary evil to an ingenious good. (1981, pp. 211–212)

The fact that Barrett gains an opportunity to make something meaningful out of his own life, paradoxically in a way that is completely misunderstood by others, is of particular importance. In the end, he clearly distances himself from his father's life-rejecting attitude and thereby gives a clear sign of hope for the survival:

> It dawned on him that his father's suicide was *wasted*. It availed nothing, proved nothing, solved nothing, posed no questions let alone answered questions, did nobody good. It was no more than an exit, a getting up and going out, a closing of a door. (1981, p. 211)

At no point does Percy distance himself so clearly from suicide as a solution to the existential dilemma by emphasizing the senselessness and absurdity of the act.

The main protagonist in *Lancelot* (1977) shows many parallels to the character of Bill Barrett: An outsider, a mature person, thinking differently, outwardly apparently conformist, but inwardly a brooding person suffering from feelings of alienation, who rebels against the decadence and hedonistic immorality of his family and the American society. In a paradoxical way, he tries to destroy the immorality with an immoral act, narrowly escaping death himself, finally losing his own connection to reality and spending the rest of his life in a mental asylum. In this novel, Percy deals with the American South more strongly than in his earlier works, approaching conservative-cultural-restoration tendencies and identifying with a violent unambiguity of the ailing forces decomposing the individual in the sick *Zeitgeist* of modern civilization.

Specific Coping Mechanisms for the Meaning Crisis

Even beyond the acute existential, depressive, and destructive distress in form of suicidal crisis, Percy's protagonists develop various milder, less harmful mechanisms to feel and relativize their own existential pain. The concepts of *rotation* and *repetition*, which are closely related to *malaise*, have a particular significance. Rotation describes a constant search for exciting events and sensations, repetition the analysis of the past with a focus on one's own failures. In both cases, these are dysfunctional strategies, and the escape from the current life only deepens the self-alienation.

In *The Moviegoer*, the defense mechanism of *dissociation*, especially *derealization* and *depersonalization* emerge, allowing the protagonist to move into another world, who eventually discovers a chance to abandon the real world for the world of movies. Undeniably, it is a kind of escape into a virtual reality. Binx is able to undergo important experiences in the virtual reality from a distance, detached from the self, and thus less fearful, in terms of *reality transfer*.

Overcoming the existential meaninglessness and loneliness allows Barret in *The Second Coming* to fundamentally *relativize* his own existence by shifting his own actions to an imaginary level and hence to see everything as a game and experiment.

In *The Last Gentleman*, the protagonist successfully keeps his own feelings of concern and danger at a distance through a scientific approach to the subject of suicide. Treating and healing patients, he indirectly helps himself, in a psychoanalytical sense of *rationalization* and *projective identification*.

Origin Models of the Existential Crisis

The existential roots of Percy's work emphasize a personal responsibility for creating an individual life concept: "I had discovered that a person does not have to *be* this or *be* that or to be anything, not even oneself. One is free" (1961, p. 94). Free also in the sense of choosing a very personal way of looking at life, whereby it again becomes clear that, for the author, a deeper and mature experience goes hand in hand with getting in touch with one's own unconscious world.

The ambivalence conflict arises from the fact that at the same time a human being gets exhausted by that freedom since he cannot find an absolute reference to meaning in such a world. The absurdity of existence is a central element for Percy, in which he remains in close ideological connection with Camus, who in *The Myth of Sisyphus* (1991, p. 40) describes suicide as "the absurd, which is the metaphysical state of the conscious man." A further painful ambivalence conflict comprises longing for the meaning contents, on the one hand, and intolerability of the established patterns, on the other. The confrontation with the unconscious and the experienced despair is an essential part of life and most particularly this can open up new ways and perspectives on life and induce authentic self-reflection.

From a psychoanalytical point of view, in Percy's work, a special role is played by the primary aggression and the death wish. The primary aggressive potential, triggered by subjective experiences of hurt and frustration, often leads to autoaggression and self-destruction (Freud, 1961). The difficult balancing act between the confrontation with one's own desperation, which does not lead to self-destruction but to a new perspective on life, seems to be the key challenge.

With reference to relationships, Percy identifies the difficulty of establishing and experiencing true interpersonal closeness. In this way, he makes a reference to Leibniz's "soul monads," which are self-contained entities with certain commonalities, but without any real possibility of influencing each other (1989). In his analysis of social structures, Percy particularly criticizes the disintegration and dying of fundamental values of the social order in America in the 1960s, especially American customs and politics shaped by religious fundamentalism.

Connections to Modern Neuroscience

The principles that are currently applied in neurosciences originate from the nineteenth-century neuro-anatomy, especially with regard to the localization brain theory with a brain mapping of numerous neurological functions. In the meantime, it was possible to assign a corresponding brain area to almost every function in the field of behavior and emotions. In the last decade, localization diagnostics experienced a huge upswing, in particular, due to the extended possibilities of imaging techniques such as PET (positron emission tomography) or fMRI (functional magnetic resonance imaging). This tendency is likely to continue, and certainly it will be possible at some point not only to localize a functional area anatomically but to follow every single thought and feeling on its track through brain areas.

With the possibility of technical advancement to allocate structurally and functionally numerous behavioral, cognitive, and emotional elements to specific brain regions and, at the same time, with still very limited possibility of adequate intervention, Percy is radically questioning the scientific world view as a dominant form of knowledge. As follows, Walker Percy addresses the question of progress in neurosciences and its significance in relation to the essential questions of existence. Currently, being aware of where our thoughts come from and how information is transmitted between neurons, do we really know much more about ourselves? The representatives of the reductionist tendencies among the localizationists are severely criticized. For Percy, such an approach is not only useless but also harmful, as it degrades the human being to a functioning machine according to complex cause-and-effect principles. In the form of the "ontological lapsometer," the author creates an ironic warning against a simple reductionist mind model. Although Percy largely accepts the principles of neuroscience for himself, he resolutely distances himself from the arrogant presumption of science to be considered as a basis of social value systems and judgments. He stresses that individual and social values cannot be developed exclusively through science and the change in values anchored in the idea of progress necessarily requires a multidimensional perspective.

Modern biopsychology, deriving from the post-Darwinian continuity hypothesis of basically quantitative graduations between individual beings, offers Percy an actual target for criticism. According to the author, modern science represents a very incoherent and deficient area in terms of essential questions, which is unable to understand fundamental existential issues, creating a deep epistemological dichotomy between the field of science and being in the world.

Relations to Philosophical Systems

In his novels, Percy tries to establish a critical reflection of the predominant *Zeitgeist* in neurosciences, which are based on the philosophical concept of interactional dualism. In his literary work, analogies can be found, in particular, to the elements of Descartes (2013), Leibniz (1989), and, as a modern representative, Popper and Eccles (2012).

Percy's most important ambition is an attempt to overcome classical Cartesian duality by creating a completely new existential dimension. The origins of Descartes' philosophy, like Percy's approaches, are rooted in the disappointment with the questionability and uncertainty of the sciences. The main subject of Cartesian metaphysics is the difference between the material and immaterial existence. Percy's main aim is to fill this fundamentally existential gap in between with a new content.

In his *Meditations on First Philosophy*, Descartes considers the difference in essence between mind and body, ultimately concluding that each body is essentially divisible, whereas consciousness is completely indivisible. The experience of the uniqueness of consciousness forms an important ground for the experience of freedom to act independently and responsibly. A being that is exclusively determined by natural laws, which apply, above all, in the area of material things, could not make a free decision in the true sense of the word. According to Descartes, only the experience of freedom confirms the spirituality of its subject and the essential difference between spirit and matter. In the sense of the Cartesian *res cogitans*, the conscious individual substance, the concept of "individual consciousness" and "personal freedom," is also defined. Descartes emphasizes the importance of a human being's inner freedom, which can be realized by taking responsibility for own actions. From Percy's point of view, certain conditions, such as special personal courage and inner maturity, are required to recognize and realize this thinking and acting ability.

Furthermore, both authors are concerned with the aspect of knowledge criteria in terms of the neurosciences. For Descartes, there are first of all "degrees of being" or "stages of perfection" in the realm of objective reality; for him, the idea of a substance contains more reality than one of its modes. Descartes developed the ontology of ideas according to the definitions of the pre-nominalist scholasticism; for the process of cognition, he suggests a distinction between the consciousness-dependent conceptions of things and the consciousness-independent things as such. The connection between the things existing in objective reality and our consciousness-dependent conceptions of them is thus seen as a process that can only be carried out on an individual level. From the fact of doubting and thinking, the fact of the existence of a thinking subject can certainly be deduced, in the sense of the famous "cogito ergo sum". In parallel to this, Percy states the awareness process of the individual who goes through extreme and painful experiences, which only allows reality to be clearly felt. Here one might postulate that Percy formulates his first principle of life in the style of Descartes as *Doleo ergo sum.*

In this context, the theories of science in the epistemology of Popper and Eccles are particularly relevant. Within the framework of interactionist dualism, they create the so-called three worlds doctrine, in which the objects of world III (mental objects) can have effects on the objects of world I (physical objects). World II (consciousness) is the place where the "mental objects" of world III can only be received and communicated. Percy's concepts are most likely to find expression in this system of thought, with special attention paid to the objects of the world II, which for him represent the individual, *actually and essentially human* element.

Due to the uncertain condition of an objective reality, Percy is strongly guided by a very questionable image of the world, the good reflection of which is Plato's parable of the cave (2012), where people merely perceive shadows of the objects thrown against the wall and, for lack of other reference systems, consider them to be the real things. The author's greatest ambition is to find an anthropology of man free of the positivistic presuppositions of scientism.

Concerning the issues of the search, meaninglessness of the world, and the despair of existence, the early work of Percy is anchored in the existentialist tradition, with close connections to Kierkegaard (2013), Sartre (1992), and Heidegger's existential ontology (1982; 2010). The absurdity of existence is a central element for Percy, in which he remains in close ideological connection with Camus, who in *The Myth of Sisyphus* describes suicide as a metaphysical problem of necessarily absurd logic.

According to J. Améry's philosophical essay *On Suicide: A Discourse on Voluntary Death* (1999), Percy is discussing the act of self-inflicted death as a supposed attempt to overcome one's own despair and imprisonment. For Percy, a suicide discourse is interspersed with strong aspirations for self-determination, overcoming the meaninglessness in the violent universe, against the background of the inclusions in the bourgeois and religious life of America in the 1960s. Understandably, the author's desire for liberation arises from the everyday constriction. In this spirit, he developed the idea of an authentic confrontation with one's own self and the world until desperation and emotional pain. Only in conquering this extreme experience a deep and life-affirming relationship with the world can develop.

In his analysis of interpersonal relationships, Percy illustrates that human beings cannot create real closeness resulting in loneliness and sorrow. A good reflection on this point could be the concept of Leibniz (1989), the founder of monadology. People are thereby regarded as "soul monads" equipped with the ability of a conscious and clear perception. Since the monads cannot exert any real effect on each other, they have only a kind of a slight communicative connection among each other. Percy's protagonists are usually at the level of Leibniz's monads, which appear completely sealed and closed in their core, with only a very reduced possibility of real communication and connection.

And finally, following Kierkegaard (2013), Percy considers language to be the basis of human alienation and despair, whose deep ontological and epistemological roots are defined by man's ability to name all things except himself, the one who names them. According to Wittgenstein (2010), he follows the hypothesis that limits of language are the limits of our cognitive knowledge. In this context, the human ability to symbolize seems to Percy an important way to overcome the boundaries of language (and knowledge). Following the philosophy of language of Cassirer (1992) and Langer (1990), there are symbolic forms of world perception that can grasp the *unsayable* in form of a visual and presentational symbolization.

The ability to symbolize represents for Percy the highest stage of development in the ontogenetic and phylogenetic context. In this regard, para suicidal behavior and an approach to the aggressive and catastrophic factors in one's own self can be understood as a symbolic act, transcending the limits of existence.

Summary

The Cartesian dualistic division of the traditional neurosciences is criticized in its deficient character with regard to the actual comprehension of psychologically essential phenomena. In this context, the broad spectrum of suicidal tendencies, which can experience the most diverse attributions against the background of personal intra- and interpersonal relationships, is seen as a fundamental possibility of thinking and acting. For people in crises who undergo psychiatric treatment, this results in a holistic imperative for action, which can only be meaningful if all aspects of the individual's being are considered. Percy's suicide and crisis discourse appears stimulating above all thanks to the author's broad perspective, based on his psychiatric, psychological, and philosophical experiences. The resulting interdisciplinary approach enables relativizing systemic thinking and recognizing the limits of neuroscientific and medical progress.

References

Améry, J. (1999). *On suicide: A discourse on voluntary death*. Indiana University Press.
Camus, A. (1991). *The myth of Sisyphus*. Vintage International Editions.
Cassirer, E. (1992). *An essay on man: An introduction to a philosophy of human culture*. Yale University Press.
Descartes, R. (2013). *Meditations on first philosophy*. Broadview Press.
Dostoyevsky, F. (2017). *The idiot*. Palmyra.
Durkheim, É. (1951). *Suicide: A study in sociology*. The Free Press.
Freud, S. (1953). Mourning and melancholy. In S. Freud (Ed.), *Collected papers* (pp. 152–170). Hogarth Press.
Freud, S. (1961). *Beyond the pleasure principle*. W.W. Norton.
Haenel, T., & Pöldinger, W. (1986). Erkennen und Beurteilen der Suizidalität. In K. P. Kisker, H. Lauter, J. E. Meyer, C. Müller, & E. Strömgren (Eds.), *Psychiatrie der Gegenwart II* (pp. 107–132). Springer.
Heidegger, M. (1982). *On the way to language*. Harper Collins.
Heidegger, M. (2010). *Being and time*. State University of New York Press.
Kierkegaard, S. (2013). *Fear and trembling and the sickness unto death*. Princeton University Press.
Klein, M. (1972). *Das Seelenleben des Kleinkindes und andere Beiträge zur Psychoanalyse*. Rowohlt.
Langer, S. (1990). *Philosophy in a new key: A study in the symbolism of reason, rite, and art*. Harvard University Press.
Leibniz, G. W. (1989). The principles of nature and of grace, based on reason. In L. E. Loemker (Ed.), *Philosophical papers and letters* (Vol. 2, pp. 636–642). Springer.
Menninger, K. (1956). *Man against himself*. Harcourt Brace.
Peirce, C. S. (1998). *Phänomen und Logik der Zeichen*. Suhrkamp.
Percy, W. (1961). *The moviegoer*. Avon Books.
Percy, W. (1966). *The last gentleman*. Ivi Books.
Percy, W. (1971). *Love in the ruins*. Dell.
Percy, W. (1977). *Lancelot*. Farrar, Straus & Giroux.
Percy, W. (1981). *The second coming*. Pocket Books.
Percy, W. (1987). *The Thanatos syndrome*. Farrar, Straus & Giroux.
Plato. (2012). *The republic*. Penguin.
Popper, K., & Eccles, J. (2012). *The self and its brain*. Springer Science & Business.
Sartre, J.-P. (1992). *Being and nothingness*. Washington Square Press.
Tolson, J. (1992). *Pilgrim in the ruins. A life of Walker Percy*. Simon & Schuster.
Wittgenstein, L. (2010). *Philosophical investigations*. John Wiley & Sons.

Wolfersdorf, M. (1994a). Suizidologie als moderne Wissenschaft. *Suizidprophylaxe, 2*, 47–53.
Wolfersdorf, M. (1994b). *Der suizidgefährdete Mensch. Zur Diagnostik und Therapie bei Suizidgefährdung-eine Einführung*. Van den Hoeck & Ruprecht.
Wolfersdorf, M. (1995). Begriffsbestimmung und Entwicklungsmodelle suizidalen Verhaltens. In M. Wolfersdorf & W. Kaschka (Eds.), *Suizidalität* (pp. 1–16). Springer.

Dr. Barbara Hawellek is specialized in psychiatry and psychotherapy and has completed training in psychoanalytical therapy and applied philosophy. Therapeutically, Dr. Hawellek focuses on psychotherapeutical, psychopharmacological and "Deep Brain Stimulation" treatment of people in existential crises and patients with affective (e.g., depressive, anxiety), obsessive-compulsive, and personality disorders. She has written several academic papers on suicidal ideation and the prevention of suicidal behavior.

What *Darkness* Reveals: A Look at Depression and Suicide in the Works of William Styron

Robyn R. Gaier

Contents

Suicide and Moral Agency 204
Styron and the Self as Other 207
Compassion in Place of Judgment 211
Conclusion 212
References 213

Albert Camus claimed that "there is but one truly serious philosophical problem, and that is suicide. Judging whether life is or is not worth living amounts to answering the fundamental question of philosophy" (1955, p. 495). In this chapter, I take a philosophical approach toward understanding suicide by focusing upon William Styron's account of depression. In doing so, however, I am neither claiming that depression is a necessary precursor in suicide nor am I claiming that Styron's account of depression is representative of other accounts of depression. Instead, I believe that Styron's account of depression offers insight regarding the social stigma against suicide which, in part, appears to rest upon a moral ambiguity as expressed in the following paradox. On the one hand, suicide is an intentional—not an accidental—action, and persons

R. R. Gaier (✉)
Youngstown State University, Youngstown, OH, USA
e-mail: rgaier@ysu.edu

J. Ros Velasco (ed.), *Suicide in Modern Literature*,
https://doi.org/10.1007/978-3-030-69392-3_13

are typically held morally accountable for what they intend to do. On the other hand, however, depression as a mental illness can compromise a person's intentions and, consequently, their actions, such that it is inappropriate to hold such persons morally accountable even for what they appear to intend. The moral ambiguity of claiming that persons somehow can be both accountable and not accountable for the same action perpetuates misunderstanding and fuels social stigma with respect to suicide. Styron wrote: "[...] the sufferer – whether he has actually killed himself or attempted to do so, or merely expressed threats – is often [...] unjustly made to appear a wrongdoer" (1990, p. 30).

Finding this social stigma unacceptable, Styron wrote that "the stigma of self-inflicted death is for some people a hateful blot that demands erasure at all costs" (1990, p. 31). Toward that end, I believe that debunking the aforementioned paradox is a necessary step in chipping away at the social stigma against suicide. Specifically, I believe that Styron's account of depression as expressed in his memoir *Darkness Visible* is particularly helpful in understanding how, in the grip of depression, moral agency can become fragmented. In sum, I believe that one way to debunk the paradox is by recognizing that even intentional actions, or choices, can be unfree in a profound way. Before turning to Styron's account of depression, however, I must first address both the concepts of suicide and moral accountability as a feature of moral agency.

Suicide and Moral Agency

It is surprisingly difficult to define suicide. One reason for this difficulty appears to be that suicide is an umbrella concept under which various types are to be distinguished. Another reason for this difficulty concerns the need to define suicide in a morally neutral way that nevertheless entails its various types. Several authors writing for the *Oxford Handbook of Suicide and Self-Injury* provide the following definition: "suicide is defined as death resulting from intentional self-injurious behavior, associated with any intent to die as a result of the behavior" (Posner et al., 2014, p. 11). Clearly, intention is a key component here if an individual must both intend the behavior that results in their death and intend death as the outcome of the behavior. In other words, suicide ideation accompanied with reckless behavior that happens to result in death would not count as suicide if death is unintentional. The authors further complicate their claim by adding that "importantly intent can either be stated explicitly by the individual (as in a suicide note or report of communication to someone) or inferred" (2014, p. 11).

An intention, however, can be surprisingly difficult to identify and to grasp. It might be that intentions can only be known from a first-person perspective. Yet even a first-person perspective does not ensure transparency. The possibility of self-deception and a lack of introspection, for example, might keep one's intentions hidden even from oneself, especially since intentions can be rather complex and multifaceted. Even if one's intentions are clear, further complications arise. For example, a person might foresee their death through a particular action, *intend* to do that action, but somehow *not intend* their death (as, for instance, sacrificing oneself for another). Or, alternatively, a person might intend death not for its own sake, but to end their pain. Such deaths would not satisfy the definition of suicide noted above. It is important, therefore, to gain clarity with respect to a person's intentions.

One way to gain some clarity with respect to the elements of intentionality in suicide is to consider a person's agency, which is foundational to the formation of intentions. Therefore, I will follow the observation of Igor Galynker, author of *The Suicidal Crisis*, who proposes that the "possibility of suicide begins with agency" (2017, p. xiii). At minimum, agency entails having reasons for acting. These reasons might come from beliefs or desires, and they might be either conscious or unconscious. But since I am focusing upon *moral* agency here, a more precise understanding of agency is in order. Specifically, philosopher Harry Frankfurt (1971) claims that only persons can have moral responsibility because only persons are able to reflect upon and to evaluate their reasons for acting. Therefore, only persons can be moral agents even though nonhuman animals, for instance, can appear to act for various reasons.[1] Moral agency entails the ability to recognize a moral situation as a moral situation, as well as the cognitive ability to evaluate alternative courses of action. Additionally, moral agency is thought to be a threshold concept, which means that persons develop a capacity for moral agency, and then, at a particular stage of development, they are held morally responsible for their actions. A child, for example, may exercise agency insofar as having reasons for acting in certain ways while still developing their moral agency. Since the idea that suicide is morally wrong rests upon the general assumption that suicide is an action of a moral agent—or of a person who is able to reflect upon and to evaluate their reasons for acting—my focus here will be on moral agency rather than simply agency. In sum, suicide as an intentional action entails agency. The question then remains as to whether suicide also entails, or

[1] For a position that calls for an extension of Frankfurt's scope of responsible agency, please see Marina Oshana (1998).

presupposes, a person's moral agency. Those who attribute moral wrongdoing to persons who die by suicide, attempt suicide, or who struggle with suicide ideation are assuming moral agency. Following Styron, however, I believe that their assumption is mistaken.

To be sure, philosopher Michael Cholbi emphasizes a person's cognitive ability in his understanding of suicide, which he explains as follows: "a person's self-killing is intentional just in case her death has her rational endorsement in the circumstances in which she acts so as to bring about her death" (2011, p. 28). Two questions now arise. First, might depression as a mental illness compromise a person's rational endorsement and, thereby, her moral agency? If so, then, situations in which a person's moral agency is compromised are not appropriate instances for moral appraisal. Hence, the idea that a person is a wrongdoer who dies by suicide, or who attempts to do so or who, otherwise, suffers from suicide ideation is mistaken. Second, might a person rationally endorse death in the grip of severe depression and remain morally blameless in doing so? Acknowledging the latter possibility requires understanding how horrendous severe depression can be. It seems that Styron would answer *yes* to both questions.

Styron, writing for *The New York Times* in 1988 after Primo Levi's suicide, observed that ignorance powerfully perpetuates the social stigma of suicide in the following passage from his article:

> [s]uicide remains a tragic and dreadful act, but its prevention will continue to be hindered, and the age-old stigma against it will remain, unless we can begin to understand that the vast majority of those who do away with themselves – and of those who attempt to do so – do not do it because of any frailty, and rarely out of impulse, but because they are in the grip of an illness that causes almost unimaginable pain. It is important to try to grasp the nature of this pain.

Styron's memoir, *Darkness Visible*, was published just a couple of years later, in 1990. In his memoir, Styron noted that the response to his *New York Times* article was "enormous" and that he "had apparently underestimated the number of people for whom the subject had been taboo, a matter of secrecy and shame" (1990, pp. 33–34). Styron's courage to tell his story and, in his words, "to have invaded [his] own privacy" (1990, p. 34) is illuminating. His story reveals a way of understanding the link between severe depression and suicide, and, ultimately, it shows a pathway toward addressing the ignorance foundational in the accusation of moral wrongdoing. I will now turn to Styron's account of depression.

Styron and the Self as Other

For starters, Styron (1990) recognized the societal failure to differentiate between depression which impacts everyday life and depression which constitutes a mental illness. To argue that this difference is only a matter of degree risks overlooking the fact that the former tracks a healthy response to events in life, while the latter tracks a life-threatening illness "which can be as serious a medical affair as diabetes or cancer" (1990, p. 9). I will be referring to depression as a potentially life-threatening illness.

With humility, Styron (1990) referred to his experience of depression as an illness as just that—his experience. He acknowledged that "depression is too complex for unqualified conclusions to be drawn from the experience of a single individual" (1990, p. 34). It may be that there are as many varieties of depression as there are persons who experience depression. Nevertheless, first-person accounts of depression, like Styron's, offer insights into an illness that are simply lost in the symptomatic understanding of depression as captured by the *Diagnostic and Statistical Manual of Mental Disorders* (DSM-5, 2013).

What is especially insightful is Styron's account of how depression transforms into suicide ideation. In general terms, Styron explained such a transition as he experienced it in the following way:

> [...] the grey drizzle of horror induced by depression takes on the quality of physical pain. But it is not an immediately identifiable pain, like that of a broken limb. It may be more accurate to say that despair, owing to some evil trick played upon the sick brain by the inhabiting psyche, comes to resemble the diabolical discomfort of being imprisoned in a fiercely overheated room. And because no breeze stirs this caldron, because there is no escape from this smothering confinement, it is entirely natural that the victim begins to think of oblivion. (1990, p. 50)

In Styron's account, two characteristics are evident—namely, a lack of freedom, or imprisonment, and a feeling of entrapment, or of suffocating. Either imprisonment or a suffocating entrapment could be enough on their own to compromise moral agency, and yet Styron included both conditions in his description of depression. Certainly, if one were suffocating in a fiercely overheated room, then breaking a window, for example, might become a desirable plan of action, even if one would otherwise deem the action as morally wrong.

What is less clear, however, is the extent to which a person's agency can become fragmented while in the grip of depression. Nevertheless, in explaining what seems to be a rather insignificant event, Styron disclosed a break, or a fragmentation, in his ability to evaluate different reasons for acting. In recounting events in his memoir, Styron explained that he was invited to a prestigious award ceremony in Paris, but that he had made other plans for lunch when it was understood that he was to attend the luncheon in his honor following the ceremony (see especially pp. 6–17). Although it seems like a mundane event—perhaps relatable to many members of Styron's audience irrespective of their personal experiences with depression—Styron attributed his oversight to be a result of his illness. He wrote that "confusion, failure of mental focus and lapse of memory" are "sinister hallmarks" of depression (1990, p. 14). Interestingly Styron was still able to act for reasons and, thereby, to exercise his agency even while burdened by these sinister hallmarks of depression. Styron's account highlights the fact that acting under these conditions impedes one's ability to read social cues, to recognize a moral situation as a moral situation and, ultimately, to make decisions that one would, in fact, rationally endorse. Hence, Styron's seemingly mundane example provides an illustration of depression as compromising his moral agency. He almost failed to keep a promise; and he needed to break another one. Everyday tasks became painful experiences such that Styron remarked "the sufferer from depression [...] [is] like a walking casualty of war, thrust into the most intolerable social and family situations" (1990, pp. 62–63).

It is clear, then, that memory lapse and a general lack of focus is enough to compromise moral agency by intruding upon previous commitments and obligations. But what is less evident is how, exactly, moral agency *is* compromised. One thought could be that moral agency is simply lost; and that idea seems fitting. The idea that moral agency may become lost while experiencing depression coincides with a few of the more common symptoms of depression—such as a loss of motivation, a loss of self-esteem, and sometimes a loss of appetite and of sleep. In fact, Styron (1990, p. 56) wrote that "loss in all of its manifestations is the touchstone of depression – in the progress of the disease and, most likely, in its origin."

Yet, Styron did not describe his experience of depression as a loss of something like moral agency. Rather, Styron (1990, p. 14) attributed his decision to make other plans during what was to be a lunch in his honor as stemming from a "bifurcation of mood." A bit later in his memoir, Styron recounted how he felt upon deciding to end his life. Tellingly, a bifurcation of mood is present here, too, as if he is no longer himself but, instead, watching himself play out different scenes of an ongoing play. Such a distancing from himself is even apparent in his description of this time, in which Styron wrote:

> A phenomenon that a number of people have noted while in deep depression is the sense of being accompanied by a second self – a wraithlike observer who, not sharing the dementia of his double, is able to watch with dispassionate curiosity as his companion struggles against the oncoming disaster, or decides to embrace it. (, p. 64)

This idea of a second self is of interest here because it signifies a break, or a fragmentation, of moral agency.

In one telling memory, Styron recounted a time when he deliberately threw away a journal that had been significant to him, and, as he did so, he recalled:

> I felt my heart pounding wildly, like that of a man facing a firing squad, and knew I had made an irreversible decision. [...] and during the next several days, as I went about stolidly preparing for extinction, I couldn't shake off a sense of melodrama – a melodrama in which I, the victim-to-be of self-murder, was both the solitary actor and lone member of the audience. (1990, pp. 64–65)

In Styron's account, neither the actor nor the audience member is a moral agent—or an individual who can recognize a moral situation as a moral situation and who is able to evaluate alternative courses of action. Yet although moral agency is clearly compromised here, it appears misguided to say that it is lost or diminished. Moral agency is compromised in more than just its degree. The idea of a "second self" does not imply that somehow another self comes into being and takes control because there is nothing holistic that surfaces or remains. Just like a shattered vase cannot hold water since it lacks unity—so, too, Styron's account reveals a lack of unity or internal integration. The self, in its distinct fractions, becomes an unrecognizable *other*—no longer capable of evaluating alternative courses of action from one distinct perspective. Depression is a disorienting affair.

Styron repeated this notion of a "second self" in describing his path toward recovery. Despite his hospital stay and support from his wife, and even despite Styron's insistence that "time is the real healer" (1988) of depression, he claimed that, in part, by incidentally listening to music that had reminded him of his mother, he had, in fact, rescued himself (1990). The idea of rescuing oneself reestablishes an internal integration that is foundational to moral agency.

The idea of a second self or, as I am calling it, the fragmentation of moral agency, is also a theme in Styron's novels. Styron admitted as much in his memoir when he wrote:

> [...] after I had returned to health and was able to reflect on the past in the light of my ordeal, I began to see clearly how depression had clung close to the outer edges of my life for many years. Suicide has been a persistent theme in my books [...]. In rereading, for the first time in years, sequences from my novels – passages where my heroines have lurched down pathways toward doom – I was stunned to perceive how accurately I had created the landscape of depression in the minds of these young women [...]. (1990, pp. 78–79)

Consider Styron's masterpiece *Sophie's Choice* (1979), for instance. It should not be surprising to discover that the Holocaust had socially imposed those characteristics that Styron employed to describe his depression—namely, the loss of freedom accompanied by a suffocating entrapment. The Holocaust indeed has eradicated any doubt that one's environment can become so horrendously evil so as to demand a psyche break or a distancing from oneself. A bifurcation of mood, therefore, is not only a symptom of depression, but it is also an understandable response to uncompromising and suffocating circumstances. Evidence of a bifurcation of mood notably appears in the character of Sophie who is overwhelmed by guilt. Because guilt concerns past thoughts and actions, experiencing guilt entails that a person confronts a previous (or second) self.

To gain a clearer understanding of Sophie's overwhelming guilt, it is necessary to confront her impossible choice. Sophie is forced to choose which of her two children will immediately perish at the hands of the Nazis. Such a choice is unthinkable to her. Failing to make a choice, however, will mean that both children immediately perish. Making such a choice paradoxically robs Sophie of her moral agency since neither choice nor even the option of not choosing aligns with anything that resembles her intentions or desires. In making this impossible choice, Sophie simultaneously becomes both a victim and an accomplice in the horrors perpetrated.

Sophie's guilt as an accomplice to such horrors arises not only from a sense of shared responsibility in the murder of her child but also from a betrayal of her profound parental love. Ironically, earlier in the novel, Sophie chooses not to take a role in the resistance against the Nazis out of fear that, in doing so, she would be further endangering the lives of her children. Her parental love makes the possibility of helping in the resistance efforts unthinkable to her, even though she aligns herself with their aims. Her moral agency is fragmented in this regard as well.

Moreover, Sophie's final so-called choice to end her life is foreshadowed throughout Styron's novel. Once again, due to her parental love and corresponding guilt, Sophie's choice in this matter is also inescapable. As Jeffrey

Berman notes "Sophie presumably chooses suicide, but depression makes the choice for her" (2019, p. 57). Her moral agency is fragmented here, too, since she has betrayed herself.

Styron notably crafted a union between Sophie and Nathan which highlights their similarities. Nathan, who has been diagnosed with paranoid schizophrenia, clearly suffers from a bifurcation of mood. Sophie and Nathan share the same fate insofar as they both make the same impossible choice to end their lives. Yet, by the time they meet their fate in the novel, Styron has well-prepared his audience to recognize their lack of freedom in doing so. Choice in this context for Sophie, as in her two previous choices, is a misnomer.

Compassion in Place of Judgment

The idea that exercising moral agency must entail more than simply intentionality appears to be lost on those who are quick to link suicide with moral wrongdoing. The social stigma surrounding suicide does not allow for the possibility that an illness can fragment one's sense of self—making it impossible for a person to identify with either their lone actor or their lone audience member of their melodrama. In this way, then, suicide becomes an impossible choice. To help illustrate how suicide (in such contexts) fails to reflect a person's moral agency and to highlight how powerful depression can be, Styron made the following observation:

> [t]hrough the healing process of time – and through medical intervention or hospitalization in many cases – most people survive depression, which may be its only blessing; but the tragic legion who are compelled to destroy themselves there should be no more reproof attached than to the victims of terminal cancer. (1990, p. 33)

The fragmentation of moral agency, as I understand it in Styron's account of depression, entails that he no longer experienced freedom as open to a range of possibilities. Rather, the possibilities either vanish or present themselves as scripts in which the author is neither the actor nor the audience member. Styron's account of his suicide ideation in the grip of severe depression thereby presents a gestalt shift. The audience of Styron's memoir is challenged to move away from the tendency to identify some specific reason as to why a person who suffers from depression might desire to end their life and, instead, to shift toward understanding what living with severe depression demands of persons who suffer from it. Additionally, through his writings, which also entail the topics of war and slavery, Styron has powerfully demonstrated situations of suffocating imprisonment and the fragmentation of moral agency in the impossible choices of his characters.

Conclusion

In conclusion, I began by noting that the social stigma against suicide appears paradoxical. It is paradoxical because to attribute moral wrongdoing to persons assumes that such persons are moral agents and, yet, that is precisely what appears to be at issue in cases involving severe depression. Through employing Styron's first-person account of depression, I have shown that it is possible for a person's moral agency to be compromised in at least two ways. First, moral agency may be lost or diminished through the sinister hallmarks of depression, such as memory lapse and a general inability to focus or to concentrate. Second, I have noted that Styron's account of depression reveals a break, or a fragmentation of moral agency, that also compromised his ability to act as a moral agent. If accurate, then the common philosophical understanding of moral agency as a threshold concept is too simplistic. While it may be true that, at some stage of cognitive and social development, persons are held morally accountable for their actions, there is a clear need to recognize the possibility that a person's capacity for moral agency can become shattered, or fragmented, as well as diminished in degree. Hence, Styron's account helps to show that the social stigma surrounding suicide is not only unjust, but it is also unfounded.

The possibility that moral agency may be fragmented has further implications beyond simply combating social stigma, however. Specifically, I believe that the possibility that moral agency may become fragmented has implications for understanding barriers to receiving care. For example, it is widely believed that feeling shame and fearing social isolation might prevent those with mental illnesses—including depression—from seeking out the care they need (see, for instance, Jones, 1998). While shame and the fear of social isolation might deter *some* persons from seeking care, Styron's account of depression shows us that the conditions of mental illness can be far more complex than such reasoning suggests. Shame presupposes the ability to attribute and to reflect upon one's thoughts and actions—which may be impossible for some to do while in the grip of a mental illness. For instance, in Styron's account (1990), neither the actor nor the audience member felt shame in burying his journal in the garbage. Fear of social isolation also would not likely occur for someone who is already internally isolated, as illustrated by

Styron initially declining his lunch invitation. The suggestion, then, that if only social stigma were eliminated, then shame and the fear of social isolation would be eliminated as well, and, consequently, more people will be inclined to seek out care is much too simplistic. While, again, social stigma needs to be eliminated and while it may be a barrier to receiving care for some persons, simply eliminating social stigma is not enough. More needs to be done to address barriers to receiving care among persons whose moral agency has been fragmented. Just as it is commonly acknowledged that a heart attack sufferer would be unable to transport themselves to a hospital or clinic, so too, it ought to be acknowledged that those suffering from a mental illness also need assistance in gaining proper access to care even in the absence of social stigma.

In closing, the title of Styron's memoir, *Darkness Visible*, is itself holding together two seemingly incompatible concepts. Thinking about how the self can become other also challenges us to hold together two seemingly incompatible concepts. Nevertheless, if we are to avoid being blindsided by the prevalence of depression and suicide in our society, then it is a challenge that we must take up.

References

American Psychiatric Association. (2013). *Diagnostic and statistical manual of mental disorders, 5*. American Psychiatric Publishing.

Berman, J. (2019). *Mad muse: The mental illness memoir in a writer's life and work*. Emerald Publishing.

Camus, A. (1955). The myth of Sisyphus. In A. Camus (Ed.), *The plague, the fall, exile and the kingdom, and selected essays* (pp. 489–545). Random House.

Cholbi, M. (2011). *Suicide: The philosophical dimensions*. Broadview Press.

Frankfurt, H. (1971). Freedom of the will and the concept of a person. *The Journal of Philosophy, 68*, 5–20. https://doi.org/10.2307/2024717

Galynker, I. (2017). *The suicidal crisis: Clinical guide to the assessment of imminent suicide risk*. Oxford University Press.

Jones, A. H. (1998). Mental illness mad public: Ending the stigma? *The Lancet, 26*(352), 1060. https://doi.org/10.1016/S0140-6736(98)08418-9

Oshana, M. (1998). Wanton responsibility. *The Journal of Ethics, 2*(3), 261–276.

Posner, K., Brodsky, B., Yershova, K., Buchanan, J., & Mann, J. (2014). The classification of suicidal behavior. In M. K. Nock (Ed.), *Oxford handbook of suicide and self-injury* (pp. 7–22). Oxford University Press.

Styron, W. (1990). *Darkness visible: A memoir of madness*. Random House.

Styron, W. (1979). *Sophie's choice*. Random House.

Styron, W. (1988, December 19). Why Primo Levi need not have died. *The New York Times*. https://www.nytimes.com/1988/12/19/opinion/why-primo-levi-need-not-have-died.html. Accessed 1 Aug 2020.

Robyn R. Gaier is currently a Lecturer of Philosophy at Youngstown State University in Ohio. She earned a doctorate in Philosophy from Saint Louis University, Missouri, and a Master of Arts degree in Philosophy from Ohio University in Athens. She has published articles in the Journal of Ethics in Mental Health, the Association for the Advancement of Philosophy and Psychiatry Bulletin, and the Southwest Philosophy Review. Her primary research interests include topics in applied ethics, ethical theory, and moral psychology.

Part III

Suicide Prevention Strategies of Modern Fictional Literature

Ecological Metaphors: Suicide Versus Life in Paulo Coelho's *Veronika Decides to Die*

Fazila Derya Agis

Contents

Introduction ... 217
Theoretical Framework and Analyses: Ecolinguistics and Cognitive Semiotics ... 219
Negative Nature Metaphors Related to Depression ... 220
Positive Nature Metaphors Related to Hope ... 226
Conclusion ... 232
References ... 235

Introduction

The author of *Veronika Decides to Die*, Paulo Coelho (1947), was recovered to a mental health hospital three times by his parents; in the 1970s, he used to be a hippie, being against the country's military governance; at the age of 39, he became a pilgrim by walking through the Road to Santiago de Compostela, sacred for Catholics as a pilgrimage site. He founded the Paulo Coelho Institute both for children and the elderly (Biography.com Editors, 2019).

Regarding Paulo Coelho's book titled *Veronika Decides to Die* (1998) and its movie version that appeared in 2009, directed by Emily Young (2009), the 24-year-old Slovene Veronika gets bored of living and takes sleeping pills to

F. D. Agis (✉)
Independent Scholar, Ankara, Turkey

J. Ros Velasco (ed.), *Suicide in Modern Literature*,
https://doi.org/10.1007/978-3-030-69392-3_14

commit suicide although she has a well-paying job, an affectionate family, and an excellent university degree. In the novel, she reads a question in a magazine article: "Where is Slovenia?" In the movie, the magazine is dedicated to the theme "Green is the New Black." This special issue of the magazine in the movie makes one think of prominent environmental issues including climate change, endangered species, racism (as nature has been destroyed by wars), and social inequalities as rich people may live in huge villas, while Veronika lives in a convent room.

Accordingly, in the book, she decides to write a reply to the magazine, suggesting that she will have committed suicide because nobody knows where her own country is. She gets saved and wakes up in the most famous mental health hospital in Slovenia, thus in Villete; the chief psychiatrist, Dr. Igor, tells her that she does not have much time in this world, since the pills have damaged her heart. In the movie, Dr. Igor is known as Dr. Blake, and they call 911 to save the life of Veronika, since the movie depicts a Slovene woman working as an accountant at a famous firm called Freeman Stanley in New York, and an aneurysm occurs in her heart, forming a scar. Furthermore, Veronika's surname is Deklava in the movie; this underlines her Slovene origin in the United States. Eduard, the son of a diplomat, once assigned to Brasilia, wanted to be a painter and Veronika a pianist; however, their parents wanted them to make money and did not allow them to get any degrees in these subfields of fine arts.

In the novel, Veronika encounters a clinically depressed woman called Zedka (known as Claire in the movie) as her roommate, another woman called Mari, suffering from panic attacks due to her divorce and job loss, and a schizophrenic man called Eduard with whom she falls in love. Veronika decides to live her last days by doing whatever she has never done: She thinks that she can express her hatred by hitting people and her love by getting naked, playing the piano in the hall, and by making love with Eduard, as she discovers that he observes her through the window. In fact, Veronika's life is not about to end, but the unusual head psychiatrist, Dr. Igor (Dr. Blake in the movie), persuades her that she will die; as she decides to enjoy the rest of her life instead of being depressed, one day she escapes with Eduard from the mental health hospital, and she passes the whole day with him. Finally, both Eduard and she start to appreciate life and get well, after understanding that she will not decease.

In this study, the metaphors used both in the novel and the movie related to the environment that lead to the appreciation of nature will be analyzed from an ecolinguistic point of view as suggested by Arran Stibbe (2015) and cognitive semiotics as explained by Per Aage Brandt (2011).

Theoretical Framework and Analyses: Ecolinguistics and Cognitive Semiotics

Brandt (2011) suggests that the space and time relations between events and the objects that appear in these events lead to metaphorical concepts; accordingly, the remote objects become signs. "Green with envy" is such an expression where the concept of green is not regarded as a color in a specific place where an event leading to envy in a person occurs at a specific time; the rival of a person can be successful at an exam, but this person can fail it, and at this point, she/he becomes green with envy metaphorically as a sign for inevitable excessive jealousy. Therefore, an icon occurs: A green face can symbolize a jealous person as an emoji. Icons are related to Lakoff and Johnson's (1980) conceptual metaphor theory since a signifier and a signified are present (Brandt, 2011): An abstract concept, envy, is associated with a concrete concept, a green face in this case. For Brandt (2011, p. 51), "*three* temporally distinct forms of iconic representations" exist: (i) "*portraits*" as past events' photos, (ii) "maps" as guides in specific events in the present, and (iii) "plans" for the future as preventive measures. As "conventional codes," "monuments" are used for referring to the past, "signals" appear for attracting the attention as warnings, and "writing" involves messages for the future (Brandt, 2011, pp. 52–53). Besides, as knowledge based on casual facts, "natural signs" such as rain, sunshine, and snow can lead to "traces" in the past, "symptoms" in the present time, as exposure to them may lead to illnesses, for instance, and "omens" for the future as in the following sentence (2011, pp. 52–53): If one runs, sweats, and drinks cold water, she/he will suffer from a sore throat. Accordingly, metaphors are related to vital lessons humans must take, and they involve iconic symbols to teach people about the dire or joyous effects of our actions. In Lakoff and Johnson's (1980) theory, source domains, thus metaphorical concepts' qualities determine the effects of a target domain concept; however, in ecolinguistics, one encounters "source frames" associated with "target domains" (Stibbe, 2015, p. 64).

The interpretation and understanding of metaphors require cultural frames where a situation is decrypted through facial expressions, object uses, and weather conditions in literary works as they are based on cultural expressions. Thus, "a frame" can be defined as "an area of life"; when words that remind us of this frame are mentioned, socially acceptable cognitive framing occurs via a "manifestation" as the story is expressed through word games, i.e., metaphors (Stibbe, 2015, p. 17). Thus, a metaphor can be regarded as "a story that uses a frame to structure a distinct and clearly different area of life" (Stibbe,

2015, p. 17). "Appraisal patterns" make one "evaluate" life in a positive or a negative manner; the language use determines who a character in a story is; if some parts of a story are not crucial, an "erasure" takes place; however, crucial parts of life are emphasized through words of "salience" (Stibbe, 2015, p. 17). The "source frame" is the metaphorical concept defining the "target domain" depicted in the metaphorical framing as in "Climate change is a time bomb" where "a time bomb" is in the metaphorical source frame of a terrorist attack and "climate change" is the target domain referred to as a trouble (Stibbe, 2015, pp. 206, 64–66). In this source frame, the bomb, the bomb exploders, the explosion method, the aftermath of the explosion, and the dead and injured due to the bomb explosion are present, since climate change may result in deaths and severe health conditions due to indifferent people who have never cared about the environment (Stibbe, 2015). Besides, a "conviction" is questioning the truth underlying linguistic statements (Stibbe, 2015, p. 17).

This study questions how Veronika can teach humans to love and appreciate nature via her ideologies, framings, evaluations, identity, convictions, and narratives of erasure and salience from an ecological linguistic perspective. In this section, negative and positive nature metaphors are analyzed for constructing a literary theory of suicide prevention.

Negative Nature Metaphors Related to Depression

In the beginning, Veronika expresses the negative ideology that life is boring and it is not worth living via her actions in the novel. She had lost her tolerance: "She carefully cleaned the room that she rented in a convent, turned off the heat, brushed her teeth, and lay down" (Coelho, 1998, p. 1). It was November 11, 1997. Accordingly, for framing her suicide attempt, one can refer to the concept of boredom as a source frame and a suicide attempt as its solution; for this reason, metaphorically, "The month of November/The autumn is boredom" and "Darkness is boredom" as it is dark outside in the afternoon. She takes "four packs of sleeping pills" (Coelho, 1998, p. 1): "Death is help against boredom" metaphorically, in this case. However, Veronika has a good job as a librarian and can afford a room in a convent. In the source frame, we see Veronika's boredom and the desire to die despite all her possessions; reframing the boredom problem, Veronika lives in Ljubljana, the capital city of Slovenia after the cold war period: After the Cold War that ends communism, she does not realize suddenly that she has an excellent degree, a job, and health as blessings for the cultural reshaping process of her country Slovenia apart from ex-Yugoslavia. Therefore, in the target domain, one finds her boredom as a result of a strange question. A magazine titled *Homme* (*Man*) affects her: She starts to read an article on a computer game by Paulo Coelho whom she has already encountered in a *café* at the Grand Union Hotel. However, "underneath an illustration of the computer game, the journalist began his article by asking: 'Where is Slovenia?'" (Coelho, 1998, p. 2). She is feeling imbalanced after the division of Yugoslavia since her new country has become a problem, a source of boredom in the target domain with its citizens with a certain low income around the globe in the source frame. Consequently, "Social inequality is boredom" metaphorically. She feels confined in a small despised country: "[...] it was outside, inside, in the mountains around her and in the square at which she was looking out: Slovenia was her country" (Coelho, 1998, p. 2). The statement of boredom related to social inequality entails another statement: "Discrimination is boredom." In the source frame of discrimination, race, low pays, and wars occur, whereas in the target domain, the boredom, caused by such an economic discrimination. Both the social inequality and discrimination statements are real, and they lead to a depressed world unaware of people's sufferings: "Darkness is depression." In the source frame, ignorance and social indifference can be depicted as darkness for the metaphor above, whereas this darkness may result in depression at which it aims in the target domain. As a result, Veronika's suicide note consists of these sentences: "[...] Slovenia was one of the five republics into which the former Yugoslavia had been divided" (Coelho, 1998, p. 6). Besides, the French game manufacturer invited journalists from Germany, France, Italy, Spain, and Britain, but not from Slovenia to its party. Additionally, the French journalist is criticized for despising Slovene female clothing traditions. Veronika links her depression to racial and economic discrimination related to the history of Slovenia: Yugoslavia, established after the World War I, "broke up under Nazi occupation during World War II with the creation of a Nazi-allied independent Croat state, but was reunified at the end of the war when the communist-dominated partisan force of Josip Broz Tito liberated the country" (Office of the Historian, n.d.).

The multiculturalism of Yugoslavia has shaped Veronika's personality, but she suffers from an identity crisis based on her Cold War experiences as she wants to get recognized as a Slovene librarian; however, she thinks that nobody wants to appreciate her country, and she despises herself although:

> Yugoslavia broke away from the Soviet sphere of influence in 1948, became a founding member of the Non-Aligned Movement in 1961, and adopted a more de-centralized and less repressive form of government as compared with other East European communist states during the Cold War. (Office of the Historian, n.d.).

Regardless of her historical identity crisis, Veronika can see, hear, and smell: She is healthy. According to Coelho (1998, p. 9), looking through the window of her room, she sees the statue of France Prešeren (1800–1849), who was an influential Slovene poet and wrote "Farewell to Youth" (1830) as a poem and "Sonetje nesreče" ("Sonnets of Unhappiness") (1834) (see Cooper, 2020). The statue is an iconic symbol for sadness in terms of cognitive semiotics; however, the poet's poems make him a metaphor for sadness in Slovenia: "France Prešeren is historical and cultural sadness." She does not want to see any wrinkles on her face; as well, she is not strong enough to change the corruption, inequalities, and wars on earth: "Aging, corruption, inequalities, and wars are boredom." In the source frame, oldness, corruption, social inequalities, and wars appear as reasons for hopelessness, and they end up with boredom without any cures. "Snow is boredom" despite its whiteness since it refers to the cold weather irritant for many poor humans around the globe; snowflakes are dropping on the top of Prešeren's statue, when Veronika decides to commit suicide in the dark weather, ignoring snowflakes' different shapes and luminous whiteness, associated with hope in the novel.

Moreover, Veronika is healthy and wealthy, but "Repetition is boredom":

> Veronika had decided to die on that lovely Ljubljana afternoon, with Bolivian musicians playing in the square, with a young man passing by her window, and she was happy with what her eyes could see and her ears could hear. (Coelho, 1998, p. 10).

Veronika sees the same scene every day, and this leads to her desire to die due to her boredom.

She is recovered to Villete, the lunatic hospital surrounded by nature with its huge garden after her suicide attempt. Slovenia was founded on June 25, 1991 (Office of the Historian, n.d.), "the year of the country's independence" as depicted in the novel by Coelho (1998, p. 12). Slovenia was recognized as an independent country successive to the collapse of the Socialist Federal Republic of Yugoslavia in January 1992 (Office of the Historian, n.d.).

In Villete, the chief psychiatrist, Dr. Igor, conducts an experiment, believing that Vitriol causes madness (Coelho, 1998). He is writing a dissertation on this. He conducts experiments most probably with some ex-patients included in a group called "Fraternity" (1998, p. 75), just like Mari. "Vitriol is a poison" metaphorically. Besides, "Vital consciousness is vitriol's cure" from a metaphorical perspective. Vitriol has different meanings in its source frame: (i) "*Visita Interiora Terrae Rectificando Invenies Occultum Lapidem*" which translates into "Visit the interior of the earth, and by rectifying what you find there, you will discover the hidden stone (philosopher's stone)," as mentioned by the fifteenth century's famous philosopher Basilius Valentinus in *L'Azoth des Philosophes* (*The Azoth of the Philosophers*) (1659, p. 144; Adept Initiates, 2020, my emphasis)—"everyone will find the truth within themselves" (Ekşisözlük, 2015); (ii) "a sulfate of any of various metals (such as copper, iron, or zinc)" (Merriam-Webster, 2020a), or (iii) "bitterly harsh or caustic language or criticism" (Merriam-Webster, 2020a). Therefore, as the Latin sentence uttered by Basilius Valentinus implies, "The earth is a treasure" for the plants it has, and it serves the humans through its energies as suggested by Aldo Leopold (1989, p. 216): "Land, then, is not merely soil; it is a fountain of energy flowing through a circuit of soils, plants, and animals." The hidden stone is a treasure, and here "Talents are treasures" metaphorically: Every human has a talent, and she/he must not feel depressed for anything, for this reason. However, Valentinus (1659, p. 28) posits that extreme cold and heat may provoke evil ideas: "Social equality is tranquility" against boredom, for this reason. Besides, humans' emotions must be balanced in front of difficulties based on social inequalities. Furthermore, "Vitriol is a lot of criticism" and "Vitriol is a danger" as a lot of unjust criticism can be dangerous enough to hurt a person and make her or him dislike life: The source frame of vitriol involves poisoning, dangers, and a secret treasure, while the target domain involves strength against harsh criticism. Accordingly, Veronika must try to discover her full potential to restart to appreciate nature and life as long as "Vitriol is bitterness," as explained by Coelho (1998, p. 74). Coelho (1998, p. 90) proposes that nobody is perfect as everybody is injected against tuberculosis and carries this "tuberculosis bacillus"; "Vitriol is an injection, a microbe, or a virus," because it is just a poison that makes humans understand that they are not perfect. Moreover, "Fraternity is equality" metaphorically since every human can be depressed although they have the potential to think positively: "Everybody is a gold mine" as they have diverse talents, just like Veronika who rediscovers herself, playing the piano to the moon one night (Coelho, 1998, p. 81). She has started playing the piano at the age of 12 for the constant support of her piano teacher, encouraging her to become a pianist (Coelho, 1998, p. 94).

Veronica discovers the truth about her, playing the piano: She is talented; her name is a metaphor for this rediscovery since it means "true image" as in the seventeenth century, Veronica Giuliani, an Italian saint, found Jesus Christ's image on the towel with which she wiped his image's face (Behind the Name, 2017). "*Vera*" is the Italian and Latin singular feminine adjective meaning *true* ("*vero*" in Italian and "*verus*" in Latin) and "*eikon*" is a Greek word meaning *image* (CharliesNames, n.d.). Besides, "Nike" is the goddess of victory in Ancient Greece (Cambridge Dictionary, 2020). Thus, "Veronika is the winner" after gathering all these Latin and Greek words in the source frame. Furthermore, veronica is an herb type with flowers (Merriam-Webster, 2020b). Considering the whole meaning of the name, "Veronika is the victory of nature."

At this point, one can start to analyze how Veronika promotes love toward nature. One night she starts to play a sonata to nature, to the moon, used as a metonymy standing for nature, as it illuminates forests in the darkness of the night. "The moon is hope" as an ecolinguistic metaphor; the moon's source frame involves natural light, nature, and illumination, and it aims at describing hope against the metaphorical darkness of despair. Veronika has hopes, and she plays a sonata: "she turned to the moon and played a sonata in homage to it" (Coelho, 1998, p. 71). She likes playing the piano despite her mother who discouraged her to become a pianist since it does not bring much money. Her piano teacher admired her when she was a child. According to Coelho (1998, p. 131), the lunatics and the moon are related; *luna* means *moon* in Latin; the changes in moon's shape led to the naming of mentally ill people as "lunatics" (Lexico, 2020). Veronika likes the new moon that will grow, and the full moon inspires poets (Coelho, 1998, p. 63). She played the *Moonlight Sonata* by Ludwig van Beethoven to Eduard, alluding to her and Eduard's madness (Coelho, 1998, p. 145). Veronika evaluates her life by playing the piano; she gets undressed in front of Eduard; her nakedness is a metaphor for her willingness to live longer despite her limited time on earth linked to her action of committing suicide (Coelho, 1998 ad Young, 2009). Her reevaluation of the concept of life after framing nature and light as lovable objects leads her to think that life is beautiful after a meditation session (Coelho, 1998, p. 98), and she must do everything she has not done before, including falling in love. The rain and the dark night in the movie (directed by Young in 2009) in this scene stand for depression as metaphors; however, the moonlight may heal it: "The moonlight is a cure" metaphor formulates hope, thus moonlight as a cure for depression and sadness. Veronika reevaluates the rest of her life, as "evaluation" is the decision-making process on some positive and negative fields of life (Stibbe, 2015, pp. 83, 104). She starts to think positively about life, being inspired by the moonlight with this conclusion: "Everyone is indeed crazy, but the craziest are the ones who don't know that they're crazy [...]" (Coelho, 1998, p. 96). According to her, Eduard must not pass "the whole day waiting for night to come" (Coelho, 1998, p. 96). "The night/darkness is depression," whereas "The day/light is happiness." Thinking about these concepts, Veronika reevaluates her identity on the brink of death, and she decides to follow the light that aims at showing the positive sides of events instead of the negativity around the globe that causes boredom. She regains a joyful identity and erases darkness from her life through her positive and thoughtful words (see Stibbe, 2015, especially pp. 145–160 for linguistic "erasure").

Concerning Dr. Igor's unethical behavior toward Veronika without getting her informed consent, "Using a drug known as Fenotal, he had managed to simulate the effects of heart attacks" (Coelho, 1998, p. 208). Fenotal is a sedative (Ndrugs.com, 2003–2020). However, Veronika is unconscious and ignorant about the joy of living before this experiment. This "salience" description (see Stibbe, 2015) underlines that Veronika starts to think positively as a result of this experiment, ignoring the negativity in life as she will die in a few days.

In addition, serpents are metaphors for the evil in humans: "Serpents are demons": They are events that harm humans psychologically or physically; the God has given the ability to cope with the evil as indicated in the beginning of Coelho's (1998, front matter, my addition) work that cites the following from *Luke* 10:19 in the *Bible*: "Behold I give unto you power to tread on serpents [...] and nothing shall by any means hurt you." This reminds us of Lynn White's (1967, p. 1205) description that nature is created to serve humans as in the paradise description in the *Holy Bible, New International Version* (1973–2011) from where Adam and Eve were banished by obeying a serpent for tasting the fruit of a forbidden tree (*Genesis* 3:1–20). However, according to Saint Francis, all the creatures are friends, and he "preached to the birds as a rebuke to men who would not listen" (White, 1967, p. 1207). In Coelho's (1998, p. 182) novel, Eduard reads a book about this story, and Saint Francis used to be "a young man like himself." Furthermore, Coelho (1998) refers to the same Adam and Eve scene, but he questions why God placed the tree in the paradise although he did not allow them to eat its fruits. As there is the fight between the evil and the good on earth, animals can be used as metaphors depicting these opposite concepts. In the end, Veronika accepts, "Nothing in this world happens by chance" (Coelho, 1998, p. 2) despite "Dark weather is boredom" and "Rain is depression," as it rains as she plays the piano for Eduard in the movie (Young, 2009), and "Ice is self-hatred" as she commits suicide on a cold day, since "The moonlight is hope" metaphorically. One finds these metaphors both cognitive semiotically as represented in the movie (directed by Young, 2009) and ecolinguistically through word uses in the book (written by Coelho, 1998).

Moreover, another character, Mari, is sensitive: She feels concerned about the poverty and poor children forced into human trafficking in El Salvador (Coelho, 1998, p. 114) and recommends Veronika to watch documentaries on animals who fight for a space to live in; besides, for Veronika, only "ferocious animals, armed attackers, earthquakes" were pernicious, but not lunatics in a refectory (Coelho, 1998, pp. 99, 110). Thus, "Natural disasters and angry animals are demons"; however, humans create them by building huge buildings instead of planting trees and providing habitats for various species in the forests. "Natural disasters are wars" metaphorically. As people's homes get devastated as in a bomb explosion, poverty rates increase, and food safety is not guaranteed in both horrible types of events' frames; both situations aim at the devastation of a whole land together with its people. Therefore, "Nature is an angel that must not be disturbed, but protected" from a metaphorical perspective also in Veronika's story, as "The noise of toilets flushing was like some horrendous force of nature, capable of demolishing an entire building and sweeping everyone down into hell" (Coelho, 1998, p. 122). "Green nature is the door to the paradise," whereas "Threats to nature are streets going down to the hell." Nature devastation may lead to poverty, dirty water, health issues, and pandemics.

Consecutively, positive metaphors regarding the environment transfer Veronika into a happy person as depicted in the successive section.

Positive Nature Metaphors Related to Hope

As Veronika decides to kill herself, she thinks about the darkness of the air: "the sun was setting fast" (Coelho, 1998, p. 9). However, in Villete, after breakfast, patients can sit in the garden "to take the sun [...] there wasn't any sun-the temperature was below zero, and the garden was covered with snow" (Coelho, 1998, p. 37). Veronika's reply to this situation is as follows: "You're the ones who are crazy; there isn't any sun" (Coelho, 1998, p. 37).

After these negative ideas, seeing Zedka's case who gets injected insulin and gets into coma, Veronika remembers, "People struggle to get out of a coma, not to go into one" (Coelho, 1998, p. 48). This medical technique was employed "around 1930," and then forbidden, though (Coelho, 1998, p. 50).

Successively, Veronika says, "Look at me; I was beginning to enjoy the sun again, the mountains, even life's problems, I was beginning to accept that the meaninglessness of life was no one's fault but mine" (Coelho, 1998, p. 96). She wants to feel "hatred and love, despair and tedium" (Coelho, 1998, p. 96). "The sun is hope," since the sun rises in the beginning of a new day, and brightens everywhere, and then the darkness disappears. The sun's social and cultural global source frame includes light, vitamin D, and health, and these qualities target at hope within the framework of ecolinguistics as suggested by Stibbe (2015). As well, children go out to play, when the sun shines in the book by Coelho (1998, p. 39).

As the garden of the mental health hospital is full of flowers and trees fed with sunlight and rain, these metaphors within the source frame of nature prevail in the work by Coelho (1998), aiming at provoking happiness in the target domain in terms of Stibbe's (2015) ecolinguistics: "Green is happiness," "Wilderness is happiness," and "Gardens are hope." Thus, "Green is the new black" metaphor appears as a warning to protect the environment in the movie version of the novel, as "Black is depression," whereas "Green is hope."

Furthermore, Dr. Igor's suggestion to Mari evokes love for nature as a work of art by God:

> It is if you force yourself to be the same as everyone else. It causes neuroses, psychoses, and paranoia. It's a distortion of nature, it goes against God's laws, for in all the world's woods and forests, he did not create a single leaf the same as another. (Coelho, 1998, p. 169).

"Nature is medicine / a psychiatrist" and "The uniqueness of animate objects is hope," as both relieve people by making them analyze God's unique works of art, thus plants that serve as food and medicine.

However, according to Zedka, "The 'insane' always believe in first impressions" (Coelho, 1998, p. 40). Accordingly, prejudices are deceitful. The observation of the characteristics of plants, animals, and humans can prevent this biased approach, as they form a team for the survival of the whole earth according to Aldo Leopold, and humans shall cooperate with plants and animals as the members of the same "biotic community" (1989, pp. 204, 210, 225). Considering this, Coelho refers to Sufism as a therapy method imposing nature as a mental illness cure and a metaphorical food type for the souls and minds: Accordingly, "Nature is a mental nutrient," as it has oxygen, colors, and vitamins in its source frame aiming at mental relief in the target domain. This makes one conceive that humans must not approach nature as "conquerors," who try to find treasures on the lands they discover, but as "biotic citizens" who respect the survival of other species (Leopold, 1989, p. 223). Environmental pollution may lead to depression due to the lack of fresh breathable air. That is why Coelho (1998, p. 181) mentions that Eduard reads a book about Columbus, depicting him as a treasure hunter for a queen; Columbus is regarded as a nature devastator by Alfred Crosby (2003) as the exchange of goods between the Americas, Africa, and Europe caused new pandemics.

Regarding Sufism, this mental purification method teaches the appreciation of nature to all the humans: "All the creations are but not detached from their Creator, hence being one with the Creator requires not only a gnostic view of the environment around us but also the struggle to be one with nature" (Ansari, 2012). In Coelho's (1998, p. 99) work, one day a Sufi master comes to the hospital to give hope to the patients: "Sufism is the spiritual tradition of the dervishes"; they whirl in a trance without any teachers who boast, as Mari explains. The humility and equality of all the dancers in a trance refer to their admiration for God.

> Sufism in the beginning was primarily an individual endeavor. The Sufis would usually live in isolation practicing self-mortification and were distinguished by a cloak of wool (*Suf*), a tradition of Muhammad, which is believed to be the origin of the word Sufi. (Nizamie et al., 2013, p. 216).

For this reason, Veronika asks, "Wool?" (Coelho, 1998, pp. 99, 160). A group of Mohammed's followers rejected every type of worldly wealth and comfort and spent their time praying and:

> Fasting on a stone bench in front of Muhammad's mosque. These people of the bench (*Ashab-e-suffa*), 45 to over 300 in number, were given to much weeping and repentance and are believed to be the origin of the Sufism. However, the name Sufi was given to such ascetics only around the second century of death of Muhammad. (Nizamie et al., 2013, p. 216)

Sufis were not subjected to any neurobiological experiments in relation to their mental-religious experiences during their trances (Nizamie et al., 2013). However, dopamine, as well as serotonin, may increase positive emotions during mental-religious trances (Nizamie et al., 2013). Thus, Nizamie et al. (2013) claim that Sufism should be involved in psychiatric therapies. Dr. Igor appears as a professional psychotherapist who also gives importance to spirituality and diversity by choosing Sufism as a way of psychotherapy. Rumi introduced Sufism to the world in the thirteenth century; Sufis look for spiritual meanings for life in nature (Qudosi, 2009).

Rumi invites sinners, believers, and many others from various countries and faiths to practice Sufism to understand God's work, considering all humans are brothers and sisters with these words underlining that hopelessness is useless in this world of miracles: "Come, come, whoever you are. Wanderer, worshiper, lover of leaving. It doesn't matter. Ours is not a caravan of despair. Come, even if you have broken your vows a thousand times. Come, yet again, come, come!" (2020, my correction). According to Shah (2018, p. 257), "[...] Sufism is a series of therapeutic measures aimed at changing our habitual personality so that we get a new personality not crippled by alienation, angst, and so on and realize the highest potential of human spirit." Thus, Coelho (1998) recommends Sufi practices as ways of depression, schizophrenia, and despair therapies. A rose changes Veronika's attitudes and behavior: She says to Mari, reevaluating life positively, "Some madman decided it was possible to grow flowers in winter, and nowadays, throughout Europe, we have roses all year round" (Coelho, 1998, p. 100). Flowers appear as symbols for hope for impossibilities in the target domain, as they involve freshness, beauty, perfume, and colors in their source frame: "Flowers are hope," "Hope is the environment," "Medicine is nature," "Depression is darkness," and "Happiness is sunshine," when humans consider their joy under the sun, their timidity, fear, and silence in the dark weather together with the natural cures they obtain via various farming methods. A Sufi master accepts the patients to his therapy session and tells them to sit forming a circle; he has many flowers in a vase, but he puts only a rose in the middle of the circle (Coelho, 1998, p. 100). As Mari orders Veronika not to criticize the master, she confesses that she has only "the present" (Coelho, 1998, p. 100), since she thinks she will die soon: In fact, nobody is sure about the future; she thinks she will die and accepts that day as a gift. Coelho (1998) calls the Sufi master Nasrudin, because Nasrudin signifies somebody madly in love with God, and this divine love renders her/him "an 'idiot'" (Wikibooks, 2020). The master warns Veronika to concentrate on the rose in the middle for finding out who she really is. The master warns her that others' ideas on her do not reveal who she is, but only she can know who she really is: "It's what you're, not what others make of you" (Coelho, 1998, p. 102). She succeeds in concentrating on the rose, as the master plays the flute: "Veronika gave herself up to the experience; she stared at the rose, saw who she was, liked what she saw, and felt only regret that she had been so hasty" (Coelho, 1998, p. 103). The plant of rose has its sweet perfume, its own taste for its edibility, spring time, and freshness in its source frame, and it aims at expressing love, kindness, and hope linked to a respect toward the Creator in its target domain: Thus, this metaphor appears in the movie and the novel: "A rose is the power of life and love." Besides, the soft music flute notes and the dim light lead to relaxation (Coelho, 1998, pp. 102–103).

This situation provokes hope in Veronika whose ideology transfers into the fact that every day is precious, and she starts to share the same ideology as that Horace expressed in *Odes* (1.11) in 23 BC: "*carpe diem quam minimum credula postero*" ["pluck the day, trusting as little as possible in the next one"] (qtd. in The Editors of Encyclopaedia Britannica, 2019). She starts to evaluate Mari's, thus an ex-lawyer's concept of diversity and respect toward others and nature: "It was a shame that Allah, Jehovah, God-it didn't matter what name you gave him-did not live in the world today, because if he did, we would still be in paradise [...]" (Coelho, 1998, p. 105). Mari claims that God committed the legal crime of "administrative negligence" by placing the tree whose fruit should not have been eaten in the paradise among other trees with similar peculiarities in the Eden: "God expelled the couple, and their children paid for the crime too" (Coelho, 1998, pp. 106–107). Mari imposes a Stibbean (2015) ecolinguistic "conviction": Laws made by humans are unreliable since Jesus was crucified due to bad laws humans made (1998, p. 108). Therefore, only a human being knows about herself or himself, but the others just gossip about her or him. Also, laws protecting the environment should be made for protecting nature where plants that relieve humans with their perfumes and colors exist. At this point, the declaration that the Chinese must obey the white for being inferior to them by a Californian court in the nineteenth century is a sample discrimination in the human-made laws that must also include the legal rights of trees for existing on earth (Stone, 1972).

Veronika becomes an ecologist after a Sufi meditation practice; however, she always thinks about natural beauties:

> When she used to dream of getting married, she imagined herself in a little house outside Ljubljana, with a man quite different from her father-a man who would be content just to be with her in a house with an open fire and to look out at the snow-covered mountains. (Coelho, 1998, p. 44).

In this case, "Snow is security," as she plans to get married to a man who can satisfy her economic needs. However, in the end of the novel, after the meditation with a rose, she plays the piano to Eduard, the schizophrenic, and decides to escape with him from the mental health hospital for being in love with him. Before her escape, she refers to nature, talking to Dr. Igor. She has two wishes: First, she wants to get a medication to feel pleasure during the rest of her life, and second, she wants to feel the beauty of nature and its offerings:

> I want to leave here so that I can die outside. I need to visit Ljubljana castle [...] I need to talk to the woman who sells chestnuts in winter and flowers in the spring [sic] [...] And I want to go out without a jacket and walk in the snow [...]. (Coelho, 1998, pp. 138–139).

Moreover, she wants to feel the rain, kiss and hug her mother, and go to a dance club with the man she loves: "I want to give myself to one man, to the city, to life, and finally, to death" (Coelho, 1998, p. 140). Accordingly, "Chestnuts and flowers are hope" in the book, whereas "The sea is hope" in the movie, where Veronika wants to eat tacos, go to the Irish pub, and go to the beach to see the sea (Young, 2009). Eduard realizes that the sun's beams are getting "stronger" (Coelho, 1998, p. 209). "The strength of sun rays is the increase in hope" from a metaphorical perspective. The darkness of the night and the grey weather depicted in the movie (directed by Young, 2009) disappear, and the morning comes in the end of the movie (directed by Young, 2009): "Depression is darkness" and "Hope is sunlight" as two opposing weather metaphors. In the morning, after the couple's escape, Dr. Igor finishes the last chapter of his dissertation: "An Awareness of Death Encourages Us to Live More Intensely" (Coelho, 1998, pp. 207–208). Besides, the Virgin Mary is above the two snakes on Dr. Igor's physician ring in the book, alluding to the power of hope based on the belief in God. As well, Mari leaves in the movie, after having found a new job.

The message, leading to the erasure of depression, but to the salience of joy both in Eduard and Veronika, consists of the metaphor of "Hope is the sun" where spirituality, leading to hope, erasing sadness, makes one forget about all the negativity in life and prevails positive thinking as on a summer holiday under the sunlight. Therefore, Eduard cannot discover the *Koran* or any books by Aristotle on the shelves of the library of the mental health hospital but finds out this poem, emphasizing the importance of the following metaphors: "Hope is the sun," "Joy is whiteness," and "Belief is an ointment," as one can go out, walk around, and visit many places, when the weather is sunny, and accordingly, she/he can become happy and relaxed without falling into the trap of any dark negative ideas, observing nature and can start to appreciate God for the plants and the animals He created on earth, and live a happy life through these experiences before passing away, as expressed by Coelho:

Then I said in my heart,
As it
happeneth to the fool
so will it happen even to me....
Go thy way, eat thy bread with joy,
and drink thy wine with a merry
heart;
for God hath already accepted thy
works.
Let thy garments be always white;
and let not thy head lack ointment.
Live joyfully with the wife whom
thou lovest
all the days of the life of thy vanity,
which he hath given thee under the
sun,
all the days of thy vanity:
for that is thy portion in life,
and in thy labor wherein thou
laborest under the sun....
Walk in the ways of thine heart,
and in the sight of thine eyes:
but know thou, that for all these
things
God will bring thee into judgment.
(1998, p. 153, my correction).

Conclusion

To conclude, Stibbe (2015) suggests an ecolinguistic method for interpreting the meanings of metaphors that are based on sociocultural frames based on people's daily experiences; these metaphors aim to deliver a message in the target domain as in the cases of ecological metaphors related to the psychological states of Veronika and Eduard through their recovery stages: "Mental illnesses are darkness" and "Hope is sunshine" metaphorically. However, Veronika, regretting to have committed suicide, escapes from the mental health hospital with a schizophrenic or catatonic guy who regrets to have mourned extremely deeply after losing the traces of his girlfriend after a bike accident in the book written by Coelho (1998), but after the death of his girlfriend in the movie (directed by Young, 2009). This scene alludes to the importance of being positive and hopeful in life. Therefore, "Happiness is an escape from the darkness of problems."

During the healing processes of both characters both in the novel and the movie, four elements suggested to be healthy by Hippocrates (see Gill, 2019) are emphasized via the descriptions related to the weather; but the characters learn to enjoy difficult times, depicted by rain and snow in the novel and the movie, accepting that life may not be smooth sometimes, as well. Thus, in the beginning, "Despair is rain / snow," because there may be numerous problems, hindering felicity, but in the end, the metaphor is reevaluated, its negativity is erased, and its joyfulness becomes salient: "Abundance is snow / rain," as white snowflakes are joyful as their shapes are divergent and numerous raindrops lead to the growth of many plants humans need.

Therefore, succinctly, analyzing the work by Coelho (1998) and its movie version (Young, 2009), three ways can keep humans mentally healthy against the roles that society wants to impose upon them by force: First, one must enjoy the weather and do some activities in nature; second, one must try to communicate with plants and animals; and third, one must seek answers to her or his personal problems by observing natural events.

Finally, the following metaphors become salient: "The sea is the hope for a bright future," "Darkness is hopelessness," "Rain is hope," "The sun is love," "Love is sunshine," "Cold weather is depression," "Hot weather is joy," "Sunbeams are angels," "The night is evil," and "Nature is relief." Besides, "The long beach, blue horizons, and a blue clear sky are hope for a good future" in the movie.

Accordingly, one can reach the conclusion that the ecolinguistic metaphors used in Coelho's (1998) work obey the four-humor theory developed by Hippocrates (see Gill, 2019): "Love / joy / excitement is the summer," "Depression is the autumn," "Recovery is the spring," and "Depression is the winter."

The summer is hot and full of the yellow sun rays; the autumn is rainy, and when people are sad, they cry; besides, when it becomes cold, people usually start to feel unhappy, as they shiver; the spring is full of green sceneries, as flowers blossom; it rains, but the air is fresh; the grey winter is cold and frightening for the poor who cannot afford to pay for the heating systems. Although the abovementioned metaphors are related to this way of thinking, in the end of Coelho's (1998) work, Veronika and Eduard decide to live their life, enjoying all types of weather conditions, as "Yellow is energy," "Black is precaution for protecting the earth and the environment," "Red flowers are crucial changes," as in the case of a meditative red rose, and "Hope is water / rain / snow," since sun rays are useful for all the species in the summer, humans must be careful about climate change and the extinction of some species in the autumn, blossoming flowers make the air fresher in the spring, and both snow and rain provide various species with water in the winter and for the rest of the year. All the seasons help humans, animals, and plants that form a biotic team as proposed by Leopold (1989) survive. For this reason, the theory of Hippocrates must be evaluated, people must be careful about erasing their negative habits from their lives for becoming healthy without any yellow or black bile diseases, by making it salient to enjoy fire, water, air, and soil equally without consuming them excessively for keeping every type of species healthy.

As the four-humor theory of Hippocrates as explained by Gills (2019) warns humans to respect the environment in reality, one can see that the descriptions of depressive moods of mentally ill people and a photo related to the past in the mental health hospital depicting the summertime in Ljubljana in 1910 (Coelho, 1998, p. 93) appear as "iconic representations" during "conceptual imagination" processes for being "portraits" warning people to enjoy their lives, the poem Eduard finds in the library (1998, p. 153) is a "map," a guide for all the human beings to think positively and live happily without committing any sins for not stealing the human rights of others, and the symbolic escape "plan" of Veronika and Eduard is a warning that humans must also protect the environment for living in a clean healthy world in the future in terms of Brandt's (2011) cognitive semiotics.

As "conventional codes," the statue of France Prešeren is used to show the origins of Veronika whose country is in the stage of renovation after the Cold War, atmospheric events are "signals" as they warn the readers about the fact that nature has a balance that must not be disrupted, and the anonymous poem as a form of "writing" found by Eduard in the library is a message for the future generations who should try to live happily enjoying every difficult or easy moment of their lives in accordance with Brandt's (2011, p. 53) cognitive semiotics. This poem involves messages on suicide prevention. The environmental protective ideas are related to the metaphor of a red rose used in a Sufi meditation: It teaches to respect all the people regardless of their creed, gender, disabilities, and socioeconomic classes together with different species' right to life, as all need the soil and its products, the fresh air with which many plants provide them, and the sun as a vitamin and energy resource as members of the same biotic team, as Leopold (1989, pp. 214–215) describes. Consequently, based on "casual knowledge," a rose is a cultural "trace" related to the past, meaning that all the human beings are equal before the Creator although their religions may be different; this red rose and the other flowers are "symptoms" for the need to protect the environment symbolically, and they are all "omens" for the future where nature must be protected in various countries around the world through global collaboration.

References

Adept Initiates. (2020). Decoding the alchemical cypher of V.I.T.R.I.O.L (Vitriol). *Adept Initiates*. https://adeptinitiates.com/alchemical-cypher-vitriol/. Accessed 25 June 2020.

Ansari, M. T. (2012). Sufism and nature. *Dawn*. https://www.dawn.com/news/730244/sufism-and-nature. Accessed 29 June 2020.

Behind the Name. (2017). Veronica. *Behind the Name*. https://www.behindthename.com/name/veronica. Accessed 25 June 2020.

Biography.com Editors. (2019). Paulo Coelho: Biography. *Biography*. https://www.biography.com/writer/paulo-coelho. Accessed 20 June 2020.

Brandt, P. A. (2011). What is cognitive semiotics? A new paradigm in the study of meaning. *Signata, 2*, 49–60. https://doi.org/10.4000/SIGNATA.526

Cambridge Dictionary. (2020). Nike. *Cambridge Dictionary*. https://dictionary.cambridge.org/dictionary/english/nike. Accessed 25 June 2020.

CharliesNames. (n.d.). Veronica. *CharliesNames*. https://charlies-names.com/en/veronica/. Accessed 25 June 2020.

Coelho, P. (1998). *Veronika decides to die*. Harper Collins.

Cooper, H. R. (2020). France Prešeren: The slovene poet. *Encyclopedia Britannica*. https://www.britannica.com/biography/France-Preseren. Accessed 24 June 2020.

Crosby, A. (2003). *Columbian exchange: Biological and cultural consequences of 1492, 30th Anniversary Edition*. Praeger Publishers.

Ekşisözlük. (2015). Vitriol. *Ekşisözlük*. https://eksisozluk.com/vitriol%2D%2D115049. Accessed 25 June 2020.

Gill, N. S. (2019). Hippocratic method and the four humors. *Thought.Co*. https://www.thoughtco.com/four-humors-112072. Accessed 30 June 2020.

Holy Bible, New International Version. (1973–2011). Genesis. *Bible hub: Search, read, study the bible in many languages*. https://biblehub.com/niv/genesis/3.htm. Accessed 28 June 2020.

Lakoff, G., & Johnson, M. (1980). *Metaphors we live by*. The University of Chicago Press.

Leopold, A. (1989). *A sand county almanac and sketches here and there*. Oxford University Press.

Lexico. (2020). Lunatic. *Lexico*. https://www.lexico.com/definition/lunatic. Accessed 25 June 2020.

Merriam-Webster. (2020a). Vitriol. *Merriam-Webster*. https://www.merriam-webster.com/dictionary/vitriol. Accessed 25 June 2020.

Merriam-Webster. (2020b). Definition of Veronica (entry 1 of 3). *Merriam-Webster*. https://www.merriam-webster.com/dictionary/veronica. Accessed 25 June 2020.
Ndrugs.com. (2003–2020). Generic drugs: Therapeutic equivalent brand and generic drugs: Fenotal uses. *Ndrugs*. https://www.ndrugs.com/?s=fenotal. Accessed 28 June 2020.
Nizamie, S. H., Uk Haq Katshu, M. Z., & Uvais, M. A. (2013). Sufism and mental health. *Indian Journal of Psychiatry, 55*(Supplement 2), 215–223. https://doi.org/10.4103/0019-5545.105535
Office of the Historian. (n.d.). Milestones: 1989–1992: The breakup of Yugoslavia, 1990–1992. *Office of the Historian*. https://history.state.gov/milestones/1989-1992/breakup-yugoslavia#:~:text=It%20was%20also%20fundamentally%20inconsistent,dissolved%20into%20its%20constituent%20states. Accessed 25 June 2020.
Qudosi, S. (2009). Sufis are Islam's eco guardians. *Green Prophet*. https://www.greenprophet.com/2009/10/sufis-are-islam's-eco-guardians/. Accessed 29 June 2020.
Rumi, J. (2020). Rumi quotes. *Goodreads*. https://www.goodreads.com/quotes/79822-come-come-whoever-you-are-wanderer-worshiper-lover-of-leaving. Accessed 29 June 2020.
Shah, M. M. (2018). Mysticism, Sufism, and practical spirituality. In A. K. Giri (Ed.), *Practical spirituality and human development: Transformations in religions and societies* (pp. 257–276). Palgrave Macmillan.
Stibbe, A. (2015). *Ecolinguistics: Language, ecology and the stories we live by*. Routledge.
Stone, C. D. (1972). Should trees have standing? – Towards legal rights for natural objects. *Southern California Law Review, 45*, 450–501.
The Editors of Encyclopaedia Britannica. (2019). Carpe diem. *Encyclopaedia Britannica*. https://www.britannica.com/topic/carpe-diem. Accessed 30 June 2020.
Valentinus, B. (1659). *Azoth, ov [ou] le moyen de faire l'or caché des philosophes*. Chez Pier Moet.
White, L. (1967). The historical roots of our ecological crisis. *Science, 155*, 1203–1207.
Wikibooks. (2020). Sufism/Nasrudin. *Wikibooks*. https://en.wikibooks.org/wiki/Sufism/Nasrudin. Accessed 29 June 2020.
Young, E. (Director). (2009). *Veronika decides to die*. Umbrella Entertainment.

Fazila Derya Agis received her Ph.D. from Ankara University in Italian Literature and Language in 2018. She is an interdisciplinary scholar, working in the field of Environmental Humanities today. She also has a Medical Humanities background: in 2012, she earned her M.S. degree from the Middle East Technical University in

Social Anthropology. Also, she has conducted intensive research and published on conceptual metaphors and cognitive linguistics. She earned an M.A. in English Linguistics from Hacettepe University in 2007. She has a TESOL certificate from Arizona State University and a Graduate Certificate in Literary Translation from the University of Bari. She completed her undergraduate degree with the highest honors in Italian Language and Literature at Ankara University in 1999. She has taught at Girne American University and the University of the People, and she was a visiting scholar at the Hadassah Brandeis Institute at Brandeis University in the summer of 2010.

Intertextuality and the Opposition to Suicide and Assisted Suicide in the Netherlands: The Case of Joost Zwagerman

Wouter Schrover

Contents

Introduction 239
Escape from Everyone and from Myself 241
Against Suicide Assistance 245
Concluding Remarks 248
References 249

Introduction

In 2001, the *Termination of Life on Request and Assisted Suicide Act* was passed by the Dutch parliament. Under this law, doctors in the Netherlands may perform euthanasia or assist in the suicide of persons who are in a state of unbearable and hopeless suffering—for example, patients suffering from severe medical conditions, such as cancer or motor neuron disease. At the same time, there is appreciation of the importance of suicide prevention, which is directed at mentally distressed persons with a death wish. Although assisted suicide and suicide prevention seem worlds apart, they are in fact related, namely, when it comes to the question of whether psychological

W. Schrover (✉)
University of Amsterdam, Amsterdam, The Netherlands
e-mail: w.schrover@uva.nl

J. Ros Velasco (ed.), *Suicide in Modern Literature*,
https://doi.org/10.1007/978-3-030-69392-3_15

suffering can be regarded as a medical condition that is hopeless and unbearable.

Dutch novelist, poet, and essayist Joost Zwagerman (1963–2015) addresses this question in his work. This chapter discusses Zwagerman's oeuvre with regard to suicide and the provision of suicide assistance in the context of psychological suffering. More specifically, I will demonstrate how Zwagerman argues against assisted suicide in cases of such suffering and will argue that his own life experiences contributed to his stance. In my discussion, I therefore also use publications—partly published after the author's own suicide—in which the relationship between oeuvre and biography is the focus of attention.

Section "Escape from Everyone and from Myself" covers Zwagerman's weighing of the plight of persons with a suicide wish on the one hand against that of surviving relatives of those who commit suicide on the other hand. My discussion of the author's ideas about depression and suicide provides the framework for understanding his views on suicide assistance for depressed persons, which is the subject of section "Against Suicide Assistance". I will show how Zwagerman rejects the provision of assisted suicide—yet there is some ambivalence.

A novel, essays, poems, and interviews by and with the author will be considered in this contribution. Zwagerman's work abounds with intertextual references to other writings about suicide, references which he uses to arrive at his own views. For this reason, in my analysis, my focus will be on intertextuality, more specifically on what literary theorist Marko Juvan calls *citationality*:

> The idea of citation applies to the conventional, marked introduction of an alien utterance into a text, its obvious presence and otherness. The word 'citation', in addition, etymologically points to the meaning of 'calling upon', or 'evoking', which implies a strategic stance towards others' discourse. (2008, p. 48)

In what he cites and what he does not cite, Zwagerman certainly appears to operate strategically. I intend to lay bare this strategy in this contribution. In doing so, I will give each citation in English, even when the original is in Dutch (the translations are my own).

Studying the work of Zwagerman calls for some clarification for readers outside the low countries. Zwagerman's relevance lies in the fact that he is a well-known author in Belgium and above all in the Netherlands: His novels are well read, while his poetry and essayistic works earned him widespread critical acclaim. Moreover, six of his novels were translated into German; translations of books or parts thereof are also available in Czech, Estonian,

Hungarian, Japanese, French, and English. Zwagerman compiled several anthologies of essays and stories, among which *The Penguin Book of Dutch Short Stories* (2016). He coupled an extensive oeuvre with a strong media appearance, both as an art commentator and opinion maker (Heynders, 2010). Although Zwagerman is relatively unknown outside the low countries, his writings about suicide are relevant to an international audience for at least two reasons. Firstly, his oeuvre reveals certain aspects of the Dutch debate around suicide and assisted suicide. And secondly, the intertextual references in Zwagerman's work concern an international corpus of texts. Thus, this chapter provides a case study on how both national and international influences shape Dutch reflections on death.

Escape from Everyone and from Myself

Toward the end of the 1990s, Joost Zwagerman's father, Jaap (1936–2016), attempted suicide. It was this experience that led Zwagerman to write about the relatives after a successful suicide in his novel *Zes sterren* (*Six Stars*) (2002) and a book of essays and interviews, *Door eigen hand. Zelfmoord en de nabestaanden* (*By Their Own Hand. Suicide and the Relatives*) (2005). Both publications focus on the complicated emotions of the relatives, while also expressing the idea that the suicide actually wants to harm them.

In the opening essay of *Door eigen hand*, Zwagerman refers to *A Tale of Love and Darkness* (2005), an autobiographical work by Israeli author Amos Oz. In the final chapter of this book, Oz poignantly describes his mother's death from suicide at the age of 38. Zwagerman cites at length from the book's last pages, in which Oz makes clear what he would have done to keep his mother from committing suicide if he had been present at the time. According to Zwagerman, the mother's suicide was a decisive event in the life of the young Oz: "After that event, the twelve-year-old child had a radically different outlook on life" (2005, p. 9). Zwagerman does not explain what this change entails. Rather, he uses the case of Oz—together with two similar cases from Dutch literature—to claim that the ideal of acceptance of another person's self-imposed death does not do justice to the range of feelings the death might elicit in relatives, such as powerlessness, guilt, incomprehension, and also the feeling of being deliberately abandoned (2005).

According to another collection of essays by Zwagerman, *Het vijfde seizoen* (*The Fifth Season*) (2003), this feeling of being deliberately abandoned is somehow grounded in the reality of suicide. In the essay "He Looked Like Suicide, He Walked Like Suicide," the author discusses the suicide of rock star

Kurt Cobain (2003). He refers to a 1933 article by Karl Menninger, "Psychoanalytic Aspects of Suicide," in which the American psychiatrist distinguishes three elements of suicide, namely, the elements of dying, of killing, and of being killed (1996). Zwagerman is of the opinion that all three contributed to Cobain's suicide, yet it is the second element that is of concern here. He suspects that Cobain wanted not only to punish his fans with his suicide but also his parents and the "patjepeeërs" ("plebeians") (2003, p. 182) in the music industry. Moreover, Zwagerman illustrates the element of killing by referring to the suicide of Anna Karenina in the eponymous late-nineteenth-century novel by Leo Tolstoy (2015). More specifically, the essay quotes the passage in which Karenina says to herself: "I will punish him [Count Vronsky, WS] and escape from everyone and from myself" (chap. 31, qtd. in Zwagerman, 2003, pp. 181–182). Interestingly enough, Zwagerman neither reflects critically on the tenability of Menninger's theory nor does he dwell upon the fictionality of Tolstoy's narration. Instead, he asks the reader to uncritically accept Menninger's views as well as their corroboration by means of a fictional example. This is all the more remarkable as—as appears from the novel *Zes sterren* (2002)—Zwagerman has read Jean Améry's *Hand an sich legen. Diskurs über den Freitod* (*On Suicide. A Discourse on Voluntary Death*), in which the Austrian author adopts a critical stance toward the element of killing in Menninger's theory (1976).

Looking back on Zwagerman's suicide, author Jeroen Brouwers—in his authoritative work on Dutch writers who have committed suicide, *De laatste deur* (*The Last Door*)—rather cynically remarks: "Who would you have wanted to kill, Joost? Who would you have wanted to kill or punish?" (2017, p. 730). Brouwers is also critical of Zwagerman's use of an example from a work of fiction. Yet Arielle Veerman, Zwagerman's ex-wife, who received many hate mails from her erstwhile beloved during and after their divorce, states in *De langste adem* (*The Longest Breath*), her personal memoirs of their relationship: "His death was a flight, [...] it was also revenge. It was the retribution of a fighting spirit striking its final blow. After all, he knew better than anyone what his act would do to his loved ones" (2020, p. 133). Veerman seems to interpret Zwagerman's deed through the lens of his own work.

The notions of abandonment and punishment are brought up in *Zes sterren* as well. In this novel, it is the middle-aged Siem Merkelbach, editor-in-chief of a magazine for tourists, who commits suicide. His brother condemns his action; he thinks it is an act of cowardice and selfishness, of desertion and betrayal (2002). Ex-wife Tilly believes it is an act of aggression and a manifestation of hostility, "aimed at the one who deserted him" (2002, p. 199). Here, we see Menninger's idea of the element of killing at work in the novel. Both characters perceive the suicidal act as a deliberate attempt to harm the surviving relatives, in much the same way as Veerman would later think of Zwagerman's suicide.

Siem's nephew and co-editor at the magazine, Justus, is the extra- and autodiegetic narrator of *Zes sterren*. By means of a *narration ultérieure* (prior narration), Justus tells about his uncle's suicide and the emotional turmoil he experienced as a consequence (Herman & Vervaeck, 2019). The end of the book contains a quotation, part of the paratext, from "Dream Song 235" by American poet John Berryman: "It all depends on who you're the father of if you want to kill yourself" (2002, p. 211; see also Berryman, 1969, p. 254). These lines do not so much represent the view of the suicide as it does that of the relative. They aptly describe Justus' perspective in *Zes sterren*, because to him Siem is a father figure whose death he has to grapple with (Freriks, 2003). Early in the process, Justus is overwhelmed by a sense of guilt: "If Uncle Siem had indeed betrayed me, then abandonment and betrayal were nothing compared with the prior shortcomings for which I could be blamed. [...] Guilt prevails over self-pity" (Zwagerman, 2002, p. 62). A few months later, however, Tilly tries to convince Justus that he is blameless: "It was meant to be comforting, I understood. And she seemed to mean it. At the same time, I was placed outside the course of things with one stroke of a pen" (2002, p. 203). Thus, Justus hovers between the idea that he is somehow complicit in the death of his uncle and the belief that he was not important to him at all. What is clear, however, is that Justus is very much preoccupied with the suicide of his surrogate father.

In a poem called "Hamsteren" ("Hoarding") Zwagerman refers to another line from Berryman's "Dream Song 235": "Save us from shotguns & fathers' suicides" (Berryman, 1969, p. 254; Zwagerman, 2020, p. 276, in which "fathers'" is, remarkably, misspelled as "father's"). In this poem, the lyrical subject—who might well be identified with the poem's author—reflects on his father's suicide attempt. "Hamsteren" revolves around the verb *to hoard*. A parallel is drawn between the medication his father hoarded to kill himself with and the attitude of the lyrical subject after the botched attempt: "After that, a decision of will: / from now on I hoarded fathers" (2020, p. 277). The Berryman quotation serves as a shorthand to the central idea of the poem, which is that of the profound effect father's suicide attempt has on the lyrical subject and the responsibility the latter feels to keep his father alive. Once again, it becomes clear that in Zwagerman's work two ideas are closely related: On the one hand, the idea that someone planning to commit suicide deals irresponsibly with the feelings of the relatives and, on the other hand, the idea that the relatives might feel responsible for an act of suicide. Moreover, as I will show below, in Zwagerman's work, there sometimes is an identification between the categories of surviving relative and the suicidal mind as well.

The Berryman quotation in the last paragraph is also the title of one of the essays in *Door eigen hand.* In that essay, it is used to illustrate what Zwagerman calls the hereditary burden of suicide. He mentions authors such as Berryman and Hemingway to illustrate his view that children of suicides have an increased risk of committing suicide themselves. To corroborate this view, Zwagerman refers to *Night Falls Fast. Understanding Suicide*, in which Kay Redfield Jamison, a professor of psychiatry, concludes that all the studies on this subject together "make a strong case for a strong genetic influence on suicide and suicidal behaviors" (1999, p. 173). Zwagerman adds to this that, according to Redfield Jamison, the outcome of a suicide attempt is not decisive for the impact it has on the relatives: "Whether the suicide is 'successful' or not, the relatives don't feel any less hereditarily burdened by it" (2005, p. 65).

Because of his father's attempted suicide, Zwagerman identified with the plight of relatives. But in his interactions with "kandidaat-zelfmoordenaars" ("candidate suicides"), among whom his father, he also identified with *their* death wishes, "if only to plug the hellish gap between you and the other" (2005, p. 36). Even before Zwagerman lapsed into severe depression himself, he authored texts that provide insight into the suicidal mind. In *Zes sterren*, Justus imagines what the last hours of his uncle's life must have been like (2002). *Roeshoofd hemelt* (*Flushhead Heavening*), originally published in 2005, is an epic poem in which the thoughts and feelings of a suicidal psychiatric patient, roeshoofd (without capital), are represented (Heynders, 2010; Van Gemeren, 2018). The next lines give an impression of roeshoofd's state of mind (Zwagerman, 2020, p. 185): "how to suppress appetite for thick bleach / ten sips of methylated spirits and you're free / from afar you can hear flasks singing thinly / o drink from me drink from me drink from me." Roeshoofd thirsts to drink bleach and methylated spirits, as they might be able to end his life. Personification (flasks singing), apostrophe (o), and repetition (drink from me) together contrive to suggest the temptation to drink poisonous liquid.

In one of his essays, Zwagerman argued that the perspectives of others do not enter into the suicide's considerations. Citing Al Alvarez' *The Savage God. A Study of Suicide*, he viewed the mental world of someone who commits suicide as a closed world: "Once a man decides to take his own life he enters a shut-off, impregnable [...] world where every detail fits and each incident reinforces his decision" (Zwagerman, 2005, p. 62; see also Alvarez, 1971, p. 144). Although Zwagerman believes relatives have every right to feel betrayed by a suicide, even to morally condemn him or her (2005), he also empathizes with persons who take their own lives. And he especially feels for those who are, in his words, hereditarily burdened—a group he considered himself to belong to. This is in fact the group in which relatives and (potential) suicides converge.

In several obituaries, it was mentioned that Zwagerman's writings about suicide were a form of staving off. Professor of modern Dutch literature Jaap Goedegebuure of Leiden University, for example, claimed that these writings were manifestations of an "urge for self-preservation, knowing that his father had entered an area he himself was anxiously trying to fence off. Until [...] he could no longer resist the urge to kick over the fence and cross the boundary" (2015). In 2013, Zwagerman himself had also acknowledged that his writings were "an exploration and a warding off in one" (2013, p. 511). To no avail, as would later become clear.

Against Suicide Assistance

Section "Escape from Everyone and from Myself" shows that Zwagerman sketches a very bleak picture of suicide: Not only does he believe it causes untold harm to the relatives (this is indeed is what he focuses on) but also that those who are planning to commit suicide live in an enclosed world from which escape is hardly possible—suicidal persons are incapable of making sound decisions about their lives. These ideas contribute greatly to Zwagerman's opposition to providing suicide assistance to depressed persons. In this section, I will show how this opposition takes shape in Zwagerman's work.

As already mentioned, the *Termination of Life on Request and Assisted Suicide Act* makes it possible for doctors to assist in the suicide of patients burdened with unbearable and hopeless suffering. While most people in the Netherlands believe that the regulation of assisted suicide should remain the domain of the medical profession (Onwuteaka-Philipsen et al., 2017), others argue that doctors should give up their monopoly: They plead for life-terminating medicines to be freely available to those who want to die. The main argument proponents of this position put forward are the right to self-determination and the inappropriateness of medical doctors acting as gatekeepers of death, as one critic calls it (Spaink, 2001). There is an organization, De Einder (The Horizon), that clandestinely makes lethal drugs available to individuals who wish to take their own lives.

Justus, the main character of Zwagerman's novel *Zes sterren*, who feels distinct ambivalence about his uncle's suicide, at some point defends the above position. To his psychiatrist he says:

> People have strong feeling regarding the right of self-determination for the sick […] at age, and the consolation of a 'gentle ending'. But as soon as a citizen in the prime of life wants to do away with himself, people become hysterically committed to life. […] You will be kept alive, at all costs. (2002, p. 84)

The author of these words in fact believes this attitude is justified—for reasons mentioned in the previous section—and he vehemently opposes the practices of De Einder: In case of depression, suicide prevention should always prevail (Zwagerman, 2007).

In order to support his belief that suicide assistance for psychological reasons is unwarranted, Zwagerman frequently refers to publications by people who suffered or have suffered from depression. An example of this intertextual strategy is where he quotes a passage from William Styron's autobiographical account of his depressions, *Darkness Visible*: "It is of great importance that those who are suffering a siege […], be told – be convinced, rather – that the illness will run its course and that they will pull through" (1990, qtd. in Zwagerman, 2005, pp. 24–25). In this case, Zwagerman refers to a general statement in a book that is predominantly concerned with the particular experiences of its author; he thus strategically relates experiential knowledge to presumed truths. Zwagerman adopts the same approach when he mentions *Kameraad scheermes* (*Comrade Razor*) (2003) by Dutch author Rogi Wieg. Perceiving this work to be autobiographical and not elaborating on the complex relation between the real-life experiences of the author and his fictionalized account of these experiences (see Van der Meer, 2018), Zwagerman claims that in *Kameraad scheermes*, Wieg argues that a depressed person who claims to want to commit suicide because life has become unbearable for him should never be supported by doctors in bringing his desire to fruition.

A major reference in Zwagerman's writings about suicide is *The Noonday Demon. An Anatomy of Depression* (2001), in which Andrew Solomon—combining a journalistic approach with reflections on personal experiences—maps the territory of depression. In one of the essays in *Door eigen hand*, Zwagerman makes Solomon appear a kindred spirit by referring to the statement in *The Noonday Demon* that "it is, I believe, better to save too many people than to let too many people go" (2001, p. 247; Zwagerman, 2005, p. 33). In fact, Solomon's position is much more nuanced than this quote suggests, as he believes weighing life and death against each other is not that straightforward: In particular, he puts the positive connotation of the verb "to save" into perspective. He regards suicide as a fundamental human right and gives an example of a "wish to die I would be particularly inclined to honour" (2001, p. 269). Moreover, Solomon draws a comparison between assisted suicide in case of physical illness on the one hand—after having already applauded "euthanasia options famously available in the Netherlands" (2001, p. 271)—and psychiatric illness on the other; the comparison leads to the conclusion that the right to suicide should not be restricted to the former. Zwagerman's account of Solomon's position is therefore rather selective, and it has the effect of strengthening his own argument at the expense of Solomon's.

Door eigen hand also contains an interview in which Zwagerman reads quotes about suicide to Solomon and asks him to respond—intertextuality serves as a thread here. One quote is from Dutch author and journalist Betsy Udink, who in the autobiographical account of her depression is fiercely opposed to assisted suicide for depressed patients. Solomon, however, believes that "there is such a thing as terminal mental illness. That means that the right to end life must be expanded" (qtd. in Zwagerman, 2005, p. 57). Thus, in this interview Solomon turns against the image Zwagerman presents elsewhere in his book.

Rogi Wieg, the author of *Kameraad scheermes*, was a close friend of Joost Zwagerman's. He suffered severe depressions for many years. In 2014, Wieg asked his doctor for euthanasia, a request that was honored (which is legal under current Dutch law); he eventually died in July 2015. When Zwagerman heard Wieg would die a self-chosen death, he could not accept this and kept e-mailing and text messaging his friend. According to Wieg's widow, Zwagerman later apologized for his behavior (Verbraak, 2015). In the last interview before his own untimely death, Zwagerman told the interviewer:

> After years of being institutionalized in clinics and hospitals, it was concluded that he [Wieg, WS] was leading an unbearable, hopeless and psychologically devastated existence. I can well imagine that now. But not so well then, because I reminded myself of the promise I made to him years ago: hold me back, hold me back. (Kellerhuis, 2015)

After being opposed to assisted suicide and euthanasia for patients with psychiatric illness for a very long period, he eventually—in fact, just before his own death from suicide—accepted it.

A constant in Zwagerman's position on suicide, however, is his antipathy toward the view represented by Justus' monologue in *Zes sterren* about self-determination. For instance, while debunking utterances by, among others, Romanian-French philosopher E.M. Cioran, Zwagerman argues that he does not have any sympathy for the "libertarian-heroic considerations and pronouncements about the philosophical nobility of self-chosen death" (2005, p. 66). He quotes Cioran saying that the idea of suicide contains an immense wealth: "I am a slave to no one, I can decide for myself" (2005, p. 67). Cioran discerns no freedom if life is the only option; instead, the possibility to choose or not to choose death in a situation of utmost despair causes, as he says in the same text Zwagerman quotes, "a rush of freedom" (Siebelink, 2011, p. 109). Zwagerman, however, does not believe the depressed person is really free; he or she is rather subjected to his own longing for death (2005).

This was also how Zwagerman's suicide was perceived in the media. Columnists spoke of a "terrible mistake" (Truijens, 2015) and a "desperate act" (Schinkelshoek, 2015). On television, Belgian author David van Reybrouck said: "I think Joost is already regretting it" (qtd. in Hanssen, 2015). However, there were dissonant voices too. Historian Léon Hanssen referred to the work of Dutch author Carry van Bruggen (1881–1932), who in her book-length essay *Prometheus* argued that the longing for death is a fundamental cultural force (Hanssen, 2015; Van Bruggen, 1919). Hanssen concluded that in life we are "driven by impulses that we can hardly motivate. But choosing death requires a superhuman will that can only be exerted once" (2015). Hanssen, as does Cioran, sees suicide as an expression of the ultimate freedom of humankind.

Yet given Zwagerman's unrelenting pleas for life, both in his publications and in the interviews he gave, most people find it hard to believe that he freely chose death. Exploring his ideas and evaluating the intertextual references in his work (e.g., Peeters, 2015; Schinkelshoek, 2015; Truijens, 2015; Veerman, 2020), they try to make sense of his death. But the opposite is also true: In the reception of his oeuvre, Zwagerman's suicide functions as an interpretive key. Jeroen Brouwers, for example (in *De laatste deur*), posited an autobiographical reading of *Zes sterren* (2017). Literary critic Rémon van Gemeren published a monograph in which Zwagerman's writings are considered the articulation of the desire to escape from reality (2018). As another critic, Carel Peeters (2015), mentioned, this desire—a recurring motif in Zwagerman's work—actually was his most fragile dream while at the same time being his greatest nightmare. Although Zwagerman eventually succumbed to his desire and chose death, the paradox itself will always remain present in his work.

Concluding Remarks

Zwagerman's position on suicide and assisted suicide is largely established intertextually: Publications he refers to are either evaluated positively or negatively and thus shape his argument in important ways. What is remarkable is that publications that Zwagerman assesses positively often contain an element of experiential knowledge. Lived experiences offer something extra in Zwagerman's view, especially where depressed persons' opposition to assisted suicide is concerned. Yet another aspect of the intertextual strategy employed is its selectivity, the fact that knowledge and views are represented in a decontextualized and sometimes one-sided way.

Zwagerman's biased approach is less surprising if one considers his publications as autobiographical in nature, in other words: Not so much a contribution to debates about depression as an expression of his own obsessions. And this is actually how his essays were perceived, especially after his death from suicide. In this way, they become understandable as attempts to gain insight into and control of one's own plight (see Van der Meer, 2018). This does not mean that there is no room for ambiguity in Zwagerman's work: His novel *Zes sterren* is in fact representative of widely differing opinions about suicide, while his poetry articulates both the lure and the horror of suicide. The tension between lure and horror is a determining factor in Zwagerman's oeuvre, which is the reason why he unconditionally rejected assistance in suicide for clinically depressed persons—that is, until the very last interview he gave. Zwagerman offered an idiosyncratic perspective by bringing together two discourses that are for the most part separate: The discourse of suicide prevention in which the value of life over death is assumed and the discourse of euthanasia and assisted suicide that focuses on self-determination and preventing unbearable and hopeless suffering. He acknowledged that the assisted suicide movement poses an important question to those who work in or write about suicide prevention, namely, whether suicide in depression is always undesirable. Zwagerman actively engaged with this question: From an international perspective his views might not be surprising (see Miller & Appelbaum, 2018), but in the Netherlands, he had to relate to completely different views in the public debate about euthanasia and assisted suicide. What was characteristic of Zwagerman's position is that he advocated keeping the reach of suicide prevention as large as possible, in opposition to the many advocates of euthanasia and assisted suicide who, he felt, regarded life in a too lighthearted fashion.[1]

References

Alvarez, A. (1971). *The savage god. A study of suicide*. W.W. Norton.
Améry, J. (1976). *Hand an sich legen. Diskurs über den Freitod*. Klett-Cotta.
Berryman, J. (1969). *The dream songs*. Farrar, Straus, & Giroux.

[1] The author would like to thank Anne-Fleur van der Meer for her feedback on an earlier version of this text.

Brouwers, J. (2017). *De laatste deur. Zelfmoord in de Nederlandstalige letteren.* Atlas Contact.
Van Bruggen, C. (1919). *Prometheus.* Nijgh & Van Ditmar.
Freriks, K. (2003). Hommage en demasqué. Over *Zes sterren.* In E. Lettinga (Ed.), *Standplaats Zwagerman* (pp. 125–131). De Arbeiderspers.
Van Gemeren, R. (2018). *Leven in een doodgeboren droom. De wereld van Joost Zwagerman.* Prometheus.
Goedegebuure, J. (2015, September 10). Gedachte aan zelfmoord werd wurgkoord. *Het Financieele Dagblad.* https://fd.nl/profiel/1118075/gedachte-aan-zelfmoord-werd-wurgkoord. Accessed 30 Jul 2020.
Herman, L., & Vervaeck, B. (2019). *Handbook of narrative analysis.* University of Nebraska Press.
Hanssen, L. (2015, September 18). Zelfdoding leert wat het leven waard is. *Trouw.* https://www.trouw.nl/nieuws/zelfdoding-leert-wat-het-leven-waard-is~b4f5455a/. Accessed 30 Jul 2020.
Heynders, O. (2010). Politics in poetry: Epic poetry as a critique of Dutch culture. *Literator, 31*(3), 79–99. https://doi.org/10.4102/lit.v31i3.59
Juvan, M. (2008). *History and poetics of intertextuality.* Purdue University Press.
Kellerhuis, T. (2015, September 29). Joost Zwagerman: het laatste interview. *HP/De Tijd.* https://www.hpdetijd.nl/2015-09-09/laatste-interview-joost-zwagerman-zelfmoord-beschouw-ik-als-no-go-area/. Accessed 30 Jul 2020.
Van der Meer, A. (2018). *Ladders naar het licht. Depressie en intertekstualiteit in hedendaagse autobiografische literatuur.* Eburon.
Menninger, K. A. (1996). Psychoanalytic aspects of suicide. In J. T. Maltsberger & M. J. Goldblatt (Eds.), *Essential papers on suicide* (pp. 20–35). New York University Press.
Miller, F. G., & Appelbaum, P. S. (2018). Physician-assisted death for psychiatric patients – Misguided public policy. *New England Journal of Medicine, 378*(10), 883–885. https://doi.org/10.1056/NEJMp1709024
Onwuteaka-Philipsen, B., Legemaate, J., Van der Heide, A., Van Delden, H., Evenblij, K., El Hammoud, I., Pasman, R., Ploem, C., Pronk, R., Van de Vathorst, S., & Willams, D. (2017). *Derde evaluatie wet toetsing levensbeëindiging op verzoek en hulp bij zelfdoding.* ZonMw.
Oz, A. (2005). *A tale of love and darkness.* Harvest Books.
Peeters, C. (2015, September 19). Het verlangen te verdwijnen. In memoriam. *Vrij Nederland.* https://www.vn.nl/joost-zwagerman-18-november-1963-8-september-2015/. Accessed 30 Jul 2020.
Redfield Jamison, K. (1999). *Night falls fast. Understanding suicide.* Alfred A. Knopf.
Schinkelshoek, D. (2015, September 10). Stilte om Zwagerman. *Nederlands Dagblad.* https://www.nd.nl/opinie/commentaar/597776/commentaar-stilte-om-zwagerman. Accessed 8 Aug 2020.
Siebelink, J. (2011). *Conversaties.* De Bezige Bij.
Solomon, A. (2001). *The noonday demon. An anatomy of depression.* Vintage.

Spaink, K. (2001). *De dood in doordrukstrip*. Nijgh & Van Ditmar.
Styron, W. (1990). *Darkness visible: A memoir of madness*. Random House.
Tolstoy, L. (2015). *Anna Karenina*. Andesite Press.
Truijens, A. (2015, September 12). Een verschrikkelijke vergissing, Joost en Lucas. *de Volkskrant*. https://www.volkskrant.nl/nieuws-achtergrond/een-verschrikkelijke-vergissing-joost-en-lucas~bd9ceb86/. Accessed 30 Jul 2020.
Veerman, A. (2020). *De langste adem. Een leven met Joost Zwagerman*. Prometheus.
Verbraak, C. (2015, October 3). Ik vond alles fijn aan hem, behalve zijn ziekte. *NRC Handelsblad*. https://www.nrc.nl/nieuws/2015/10/03/ik-vond-alles-fijn-aan-hem-behalve-zijn-ziekte-1540197-a793049. Accessed 30 Jul 2020.
Wieg, R. (2003). *Kameraad scheermes*. De Arbeiderspers.
Zwagerman, J. (2002). *Zes sterren*. De Arbeiderspers.
Zwagerman, J. (2003). *Het vijfde seizoen*. De Arbeiderspers.
Zwagerman, J. (2005). *Door eigen hand. Zelfmoord en de nabestaanden*. De Arbeiderspers.
Zwagerman, J. (2007). *Hollands welvaren. Nederland 2004–2008*. De Arbeiderspers.
Zwagerman, J. (2013). *Americana. Omzwervingen in de Amerikaanse cultuur*. De Arbeiderspers.
Zwagerman, J. (2016). *The Penguin book of Dutch short stories*. Penguin UK.
Zwagerman, J. (2020). *Verzamelde gedichten*. De Arbeiderspers.

Wouter Schrover obtained a BA degree in Literary Studies at Leiden University and an MA degree in Literature at Vrije Universiteit Amsterdam (VU). At the latter university, he also defended his Ph.D. (2015) about the representation of euthanasia and assisted suicide in contemporary narrative fiction. He currently works as a policy advisor at the Academic Affairs Department of the University of Amsterdam (UvA). His main research interests are thanatology and fictionality, especially in relation to Dutch literature and culture. His key publications include "Fiktionalität und Ethnologie" (Walter de Gruyter, 2020), "Reading Literature through Medical Sociology: The Doctor-Patient Relationship in Thomas Rosenboom's *Public Works* and a Poem by Neeltje Maria Min" (V&R unipress, 2015), and "Representing Life's End in *Dancing with Mister D.* Literature and the Dutch Debate on Euthanasia and Assisted Suicide" (Cambridge Scholars Publishing, 2014).

Suicide in Contemporary Young Adult Novels

Michelle Falkoff

Contents

YA Literature as a Category 254
Suicide as a Popular Topic 255
Thirteen Reasons Why 256
Suicide in YA Literature Post-Thirteen Reasons Why 259
Takeaways 262
References 263

Ever since the recognition of young adult (YA) literature as its own category, teen readers have sought out books that address difficult and challenging topics. These topics have included physical and sexual abuse, alcohol and drug abuse, racism and anti-Semitism, pregnancy, and self-harm. Access to books about these topics is helpful for teen readers in acknowledging the existence and relevance of these challenges in the lives of teen readers, and both teens and adults have expressed gratitude for books that help readers know they are not alone.

All writers are responsible for treating difficult subject matter with the respect and care it deserves, but writers of young adult novels bear the additional burden of remembering that their audience may not be as well equipped

M. Falkoff (✉)
Northwestern University, Chicago, IL, USA
e-mail: michelle.falkoff@northwestern.edu

J. Ros Velasco (ed.), *Suicide in Modern Literature*,
https://doi.org/10.1007/978-3-030-69392-3_16

to deal with the fallout of authors handling a topic poorly. While we generally understand adults to have the emotional maturity to process difficult topics on their own or to know when it is time to seek outside help, young adults may not be as well situated and may not have either the awareness or the resources to help themselves.

With this in mind, in this chapter, I will briefly discuss the development of the YA category leading up to the present, where numerous books address the topic of suicide in particular. I will then look at Jay Asher's *Thirteen Reasons Why* (2007 [2017]), a novel that sparked a larger discussion of suicide and how to handle it responsibly in YA literature, and then I will talk about books published subsequently and what authors can do to ensure their books help young readers rather than damaging them.

YA Literature as a Category

While different constituencies define young adult literature in different ways, most people understand the category to include books written about and for teenagers. To get a little more granular, YA literature focuses on the experience of being a teenager during that particular window (usually the 13- to 18-year-old range). Books that include the retrospective perspective of an adult are not included in the category, though teens often read those books as well.

Most agree that the YA category began with publication of S.E. Hinton's *The Outsiders* in 1967 (2007). While her book was not the first to focus on the teen experience, it did center teens in a way that felt new at the time, and its popularity established the market for books targeted at teen readers (Eschner, 2017; Michaud, 2014). *The Outsiders* set a high bar for what YA could be: It was honest about how difficult its characters' lives were; it acknowledged class, violence, and alcohol and drug use and abuse; it dealt realistically with the teens' relationships with their parents, or the lack of those relationships where appropriate; it did not guarantee happy endings for all its characters, though it left the possibility of hope for some. Overall, it told a generation of readers that books could speak directly to them without trying to teach them life lessons.

The creation of the YA marketing category continued to include books that dealt with difficult and realistic topics, some of them overtly message-driven (such as *Go Ask Alice* by Beatrice Sparks (1971 [1999]), a book that purported to be the real diary of a drug addict discovered after her death but which was later revealed to be the work of a drug counselor) (Thomas, 2018), most of them highlighting teenagers' ability to solve problems themselves (many of which served as the basis for episodes of ABC's Afterschool Special TV series) (Rossen, 2019). Dark topics continue to be a source of fascination for teen readers, and many books that many now consider classics address these topics.

Suicide as a Popular Topic

Suicide as a topic of literary fascination dates all the way back to Goethe and *The Sorrows of Young Werther* (1774 [2002]), a book whose publication and popularity led to something called "Werther Fever," in which young men started mimicking the main character, first by dressing like him and eventually by recreating his suicide. More recently, the phenomenon of suicide rates increasing after highly publicized suicides has been referred to as the "Werther Effect" (Andrews, 2017; Devitt, 2017). This article takes as its premise that, for authors who choose to write young adult novels about suicide, it is and should be a goal to avoid creating either Werther Fever or a Werther Effect through the publication of their books.

It is not clear precisely where the present literary fascination with suicide began nor what prompted it, though many have explored the question. Some suggest that books about suicide have become more popular because teens feel powerless about everything happening in the world around them and they are unconvinced it is possible to save the world, a la Katniss in *The Hunger Games* (2008 [2011]). Instead, their version of heroism involves taking individual control and deciding when it is time for their lives to end. Others situate the concept of control in a different place: Books about suicide are popular because the best way to understand those feelings is to learn about them, and then teens can process their feelings in a safe place, thereby taking control over the emotions and regaining control over their environments (Hateley, 2014).

The idea that books about suicide have grown popular because readers feel hopeless about the state of the world is disheartening, even if it's true; the current state of activism and engagement around topics relating to the state of the world suggests that the issue might not be hopelessness but rather the quest for understanding (Grady, 2017a). Books have always served as safe spaces to consider hard questions, and while the increase in suicide as a topic may reflect teens' increasing feelings of frustration, it may also reflect increasing awareness of the importance of attending to mental health. Culturally, the growing acceptance and destigmatizing of mental health issues permits conversations that might have been taboo in another time and only by airing out these issues is it possible to have honest discussions about them.

Regardless of the reason, there is little disagreement about one thing: There has been an explosion in the number of books about suicide in the past 15 years. Many feel this is attributable to the success of the novel *Thirteen Reasons Why*.

Thirteen Reasons Why

Jay Asher's *Thirteen Reasons Why* was published in 2007 and sold so steadily the publisher opted not to release a paperback edition until 2011, at which point the book hit *The New York Times* bestseller list (Rich, 2009). A TV series of the same name that started with the events of the first book and then continued on into multiple seasons has been hugely successful on Netflix, though both the book and the show have been the source of some controversy.

In the book, narrator Clay receives a mysterious package that contains a set of audiotapes from Hannah, a girl he liked who killed herself. The tapes contain Hannah's description of the events that led her to take her own life; she identifies thirteen individuals who need to hear her story, most of whom she views as responsible. The book alternates between Clay's thoughts and the information he hears on the tapes, along with occasional interactions between Clay and some other characters, and at the end Clay learns what happened to Hannah and his role in it, which leads him to start treating other characters differently.

The book's central mystery is compelling and the structure effectively moves the plot along. The tapes provide insight into the increasing level of frustration and pain Hannah feels as a result of not getting the support she needs from her family, friends, or community. In the end, readers have a clear understanding of why Hannah made her choice, as well as some indication of how the tapes affected Clay, if not the other 12 characters.

Thirteen Reasons Why facilitated two important conversations: First, its popularity highlighted the need for frank and public conversation about teen suicide, with teens as an important part of the audience. Second, it raised the issue of whether authors, and authors of young adult novels in particular, have an elevated level of responsibility to readers when taking on difficult topics such as suicide. Critical discussion of the book, and later the TV series based on it, often centered on the intersection between these two conversations.

Positive feedback about *Thirteen Reasons Why* emphasizes its role in facilitating more open dialogue about teen suicide, but critics of the book (myself included) have identified several concerns with Asher's approach to the topic. These include treating suicide as a revenge fantasy, centering the narrative on a lesser male character, and excluding a discussion of mental health. These concerns were exacerbated by the television series, which did not resolve any of these issues and added an additional level of violence.

Suicide as a Revenge Fantasy

Thirteen Reasons Why is structured as a mystery novel, with the protagonist functioning as a kind of passive detective, working his way through the tapes to solve the crime. But mysteries are satisfying because they allow us to identify a responsible party (or parties, in this case). The idea that other people are responsible for an individual's decision to take her own life is problematic as a general matter; as the plot of a novel, it runs the risk of being irresponsible.

Asher has said his goal in writing the book was to show how even the smallest of interactions can be meaningful, which means people need to spend more time thinking about how their behavior affects other people. It is a laudable goal, and there is a utility in showing how the aggregation of a series of events can damage someone so deeply they are unable to rebound once they hit a certain tipping point, as happened to Hannah in the novel. But there is a difference between what motivated Hannah to take her own life and where responsibility for that decision lies, and the book does not acknowledge that distinction. Clay's quest to solve the mystery of Hannah's motivation is not one over which he has any autonomy; he is listening to the tapes to find out who Hannah blames. This shifts the book from mystery novel to revenge fantasy: Hannah is reaching out from beyond the grave to name the people responsible for her death. The revenge fantasy runs the risk of romanticizing suicide and deemphasizing the finality of death.

Decentering Suicidal Characters

The decision to make Clay the narrator complicates the book as well. Clay is a usefully utilitarian narrator in that he cared about Hannah even though he did not know her all that well, and readers are able to contextualize the tapes through his experience of listening to them. That said, Clay is ultimately a peripheral character in Hannah's story, and centering him as a means of evaluating Hannah's choice raises the issue of how best to tell the story of this kind of decision and how to address its aftermath.

In having the bulk of the narrative come through Hannah's tapes as filtered by Clay's experience of listening to them, we go through the process of getting to know both characters at once. But while our access to Hannah's voice allows us to get to know her well throughout the course of the novel, establishing both who she is and the ways in which others failed to see her properly, Clay is able to largely shield himself behind the tapes, and he provides us little information about who he is beyond his feelings for Hannah. This makes sense in that Hannah is the most important character to the story, but it is problematic in that the book ends up being not about Hannah and her choices but about how those choices affect Clay. By centering Clay, Asher takes what is really a girl's story and places it in the hands of a boy, and a peripheral boy at that, which has a diminishing effect Asher likely did not intend. Much of Hannah's difficulty came from the way the people around her failed to get to know her fully; the process of having Clay deepen his understanding of her as a means of understanding her decision to kill herself could come across as vindicating that decision.

Ignoring Mental Health Issues

Another concern involves the absence of any real discussion of mental health in the novel. Hannah rarely if ever considers her own mental health as she moves through her narrative, and at no point does anyone in the novel, including Clay, suggest that counseling might be appropriate for Hannah. Even when she finally reaches out to an adult at the school and suggests that she is struggling, he all but tells her to get over herself and does not recommend any possible means for her to get help. This is not necessarily inaccurate; it is unfortunately all too conceivable that there are teens who have been wronged in numerous ways by the adults around them. The issue is whether teen readers are, as a group, positioned to recognize what is missing from the novel when its own characters, charged with caring for one another, are incapable of doing so themselves.

Escalating the Violence Onscreen

Criticism of the story increased upon its adaptation as a Netflix series. The basic plot remained the same, which means Hannah's revenge fantasy served as the show's structure and Clay remained the protagonist. The show exaggerated the violence beyond that depicted in the novel, changing Hannah's method of suicide from pills to wrist-slashing and showing it onscreen, along with graphic rape scenes (Grady, 2017b). There were initially insufficient content warnings before the show began and a lack of resource materials made available afterward, though Netflix addressed these concerns after complaints (Kelley, 2017). The show's creators also did not add any discussion of mental health (Greenstein, 2017). Despite these concerns, the show was hugely successful and has completed its fourth and final season.

Suicide in YA Literature Post-*Thirteen Reasons Why*

In the years since *Thirteen Reasons Why* was published, many YA authors have addressed the topic of suicide in their books in ways that serve as reactions, corrections, and additions to the existing literature. I am one of those authors: My experience of reading Asher's book was complicated enough that I decided to work through my feelings by writing about them. I was particularly concerned about the idea of suicide as a mystery to solve, but I was also put off by the idea of Clay, a person so peripheral to Hannah's life, as the focus of the book. I appreciate that some families are still loath to address mental health issues (I eventually wrote a whole other book about that topic), but I was not comfortable with a book addressing suicide that failed to acknowledge the dangers of that approach.

With all those things in mind, I wrote *Playlist for the Dead* (2015), a novel about a boy named Sam whose best friend Hayden commits suicide and leaves behind music for the Sam to help him understand. Sam takes this to mean there is a mystery to solve, but my goal was to show that suicide does not work that way. I wanted to explore a relationship with some depth (like a best friendship), as opposed to a relationship still in the burgeoning stages; I also wanted to address the complexity of Hayden's family life, as well as his parents' resistance to acknowledging his depression. Whether I pulled off any of these things is an open question and not one I am capable of evaluating; for purposes of this article, I am more interested in my own impulse to write through my concerns in this way and the fact that I was not alone in doing so.

To be more specific, in the month my book was published, five other YA novels about suicide were released, each of which addresses suicide in a different way (Glass, 2015). This does not include the numerous books that came out before, which I will not discuss here, not to mention the many books that came out afterward, though I will touch on a few of them.

Gayle Forman, *I Was Here*

The most famous author to release a book during this month-long period was Gayle Forman, author of *I Was Here* (2015). The book is about a girl named Cody whose best friend Meg commits suicide for reasons Cody seeks to discover by going on a road trip. On the road trip, Cody learns that there were many aspects of Meg's life that she hid from Cody; upon her return, she learns that Meg suffered from depression. Cody eventually accepts that Meg's suicide is not a mystery to solve and starts trying to move forward.

While Forman's book and mine are very different in execution, we appear to have had similar reactions to reading *Thirteen Reasons Why*—Forman and Asher are friends and have done suicide-awareness benefits together, and she acknowledges his book in one of her interviews (Zoella Book Club, 2016). Forman's book focuses on the complexities of friendship (female rather than male, in her case), as well as the way some families treat mental illness as stigmatizing.

Cindy Rodriguez, *When Reason Breaks*

Rodriguez's debut novel (2015) centers on two girls in the same English class who both suffer from depression. Both become obsessed with Emily Dickinson and are mentored by their teacher. The two girls are not friends as the book opens, but they grow closer as the narrative progresses, and the central mystery of the book concerns which of them will attempt suicide before the novel ends. Rodriguez is careful to address both girls' mental health issues with nuance, and she also addresses a frequent concern with the absence of adults in YA novels by having a teacher serve a helpful and important role (Butler, 2015).

Cynthia Hand, *The Last Time We Say Goodbye*

Hand's novel shifts the focus away from friendship and onto the family. In *The Last Time We Say Goodbye* (2015), Lex, the narrator, struggles with guilt over ignoring a text message her brother sent right before he committed suicide. While the book effectively shows how grief can cause the lines between fantasy and reality to blur, it also incorporates discussion of mental health at all points, including discussions of both Lex's and her brother's experiences with therapy.

Jasmine Warga, *My Heart and Other Black Holes*

In *My Heart and Other Black Holes* (2015), Jasmine Warga writes about Aysel, a girl who struggles with depression and who visits a website designed to bring suicidal teens together so they can help each other take their own lives. There she meets Roman, and they eventually fall in love and decide it is worth continuing to live. The book is careful not to romanticize depression, though the author has discussed the importance of not pitying people who suffer from it. Critics and readers alike responded well to the sophisticated and non-condescending way Warga handled the topic while managing to end on a hopeful note (Herrington, 2015).

Jennifer Niven, *All the Bright Places*

In contrast, one of the more popular books released after *Thirteen Reasons Why* received a lot of criticism for how the author handled certain aspects of the novel. *All the Bright Places* (2015) is about two teens who meet and become friends during a suicide attempt. Violet is devastated by the death of her older sister, for which she feels responsible; Theodore suffers from depression and bipolar disorder and obsesses about suicide even while trying to convince Violet to move past her sadness. While Violet eventually starts to find happiness, in part through her budding relationship with Theodore, his condition deteriorates. Near the end of the novel he attempts suicide again, and this time he succeeds. Though Niven treated the characters' relationship with care, providing depth absent from *Thirteen Reasons Why*, some critics found it irresponsible to end with one of the characters succeeding in taking his own life, particularly when the way it fits into the story might have romanticized that decision in the eyes of some teen readers.

Emily X.R. Pan, *The Astonishing Color of After*

A more recently published novel serves as an exemplar of the ways writers both talented and responsible can take on the complexity of suicide for younger audiences. In the lyrically written *The Astonishing Color of After* (2018), narrator Leigh's mother commits suicide, leaving behind a cryptic note. Leigh spends much of the book trying to understand what the note means and why her mother made her choice, but ultimately she accepts that there will be no easy resolution of the question. Leigh's quest to understand her mother does help her become closer to her father, moving the focus of the book away from the idea of suicide as mystery and toward an emphasis on the value of openness.

Karen McManus, *One of Us Is Lying*

Karen McManus's wildly successful mystery novel *One of Us Is Lying* (2017) is not explicitly about suicide, and it is something of a spoiler to discuss it here, but suffice to say she takes the idea of suicide as a puzzle to solve and turns it inside out. That did not stop critics from expressing concern about representations of suicide and depression in the novel (Orsini, 2019), though there has not been the kind of public conversation about whether the book does harm that has dogged *Thirteen Reasons Why*. This might suggest that readers are growing desensitized to suicide as a topic; at a minimum, it indicates that the connection between suicide and mystery remains one that resonates with readers.

Takeaways

The challenges *Thirteen Reasons Why* faced as both a book and a TV show, as well as the concerns raised by critics of *All the Bright Places*, highlight the difficulties inherent in authors addressing suicide in literature for teen readers. Books that address the depth and complexity of teenage life are necessary, and treating them with sensitivity and care is crucial, as is avoiding didacticism and condescension. But it is not always clear what an author's responsibility is to readers, particularly younger readers, and the line between being helpful and harmful might be hard to locate.

As a baseline, it is important to emphasize that *Thirteen Reasons Why* made clear how much YA audiences wanted to read about and discuss the issue of suicide. For this reason alone, the book has made an invaluable contribution to YA literature. The fact that it spawned a plethora of novels on the topic is beneficial for a number of reasons.

First, only through increasing our collective knowledge and openness to addressing how suicide affects teens can we help them learn how to engage with the topic responsibly. By expanding the available literature, we broaden the range of areas where teens can find resources and support. Showing teens that discussing suicide is not taboo but useful insofar as it helps them understand their own feelings or those of other people and shows that, to paraphrase the musical-turned-young-adult-novel *Dear Evan Hansen* (2018), they are not alone.

Second, the more books about difficult topics there are, the less necessary it is for every book to be all things to all readers. There is room for books addressing all kinds of relationships, from crushes to families; there is room for books with differing levels of realism.

Finally, the ways in which books written earlier raise concerns about authorial responsibility have led to increased conversation about what those responsibilities are and how writers can address them. Most of the books about suicide published in the years after *Thirteen Reasons Why* come with content warnings or resource lists, either in the books themselves or in the promotional materials around them. Authors are doing more and more research to make sure their approaches to topics like suicide are responsible and authentic and avoid harm. We may not be able to provide answers to the hard questions, but in the process of identifying the questions, we can avoid suggesting problematic answers. And if the number of emails I have received from readers is any indication, they are grateful to us for trying to help.

References

Andrews, S. (2017, April 22). The Werther effect: A spike of emulation suicides after a highly publicized suicide following Goethe's novel 'The sorrows of young Werther'". *The Vintage News*. https://www.thevintagenews.com/2017/04/22/the-werther-effect-a-spike-of-emulation-suicides-after-a-widely-publicized-suicide-following-goethes-novel-the-sorrows-of-young-werther/. Accessed 3 Aug 2020.

Asher, J. (2017). *Thirteen reasons why*. RazorBill. (Original work published in 2007).

Butler, L. L. (2015). Review: When reason breaks by Cindy Rodriguez. *Disability in Kidlit*. http://disabilityinkidlit.com/2015/02/20/l-lee-butler-reviews-when-reason-breaks/. Accessed 3 Aug 2020.

Collins, S. (2011). *The hunger games*. Scholastic. (Original work published in 2008).

Devitt, P. (2017). 13 reasons why and suicide contagion. *Scientific American*. https://www.scientificamerican.com/article/13-reasons-why-and-suicide-contagion1/. Accessed 3 Aug 2020.

Emmich, V., Levenson, S., & Pasek, B. (2018). *Dear Evan Hansen*. Poppy.

Eschner, K. (2017). 'The outsiders' was groundbreaking, but it didn't create YA fiction. *Smithsonian Magazine*. https://www.smithsonianmag.com/smart-news/why-outsiders-didnt-create-ya-fiction-180962967/. Accessed 3 Aug 2020.

Falkoff, M. (2015). *Playlist for the dead*. HarperTeen.

Forman, G. (2015). *I was here*. Simon and Schuster.

Glass, T. (2015). Dealing with suicide and depression in teen literature. *The Hub*. http://www.yalsa.ala.org/thehub/2015/01/23/dealing-with-suicide-depression-in-teen-literature/. Accessed 3 Aug 2020.

Von Goethe, J. W. (2002). *The sorrows of young Werther*. Dover Publications. (Original work published in 1774).

Grady, C. (2017a). The YA dystopia boom is over. It's been replaced by stories of teen suicide. *Vox*. https://www.vox.com/culture/2017/10/18/15881100/ya-dystopia-teen-suicide-13-reasons-why-hunger-games. Accessed 3 Aug 2020.

Grady, C. (2017b). Critics say 13 reasons why has artistic merit. Suicide prevention experts say it's dangerous. *Vox*. https://www.vox.com/culture/2017/5/1/15501102/13-reasons-why-controversy-suicide-contagion. Accessed 3 Aug 2020.

Greenstein, L. (2017). 13 reasons why hurts vulnerable teens. *NAMI*. https://www.nami.org/Blogs/NAMI-Blog/May-2017/-13-Reasons-Why%E2%80%9D-Hurts-Vulnerable-Teens. Accessed 3 Aug 2020.

Hand, C. (2015). *The last time we say goodbye*. HarperTeen.

Hateley, E. (2014). Young adult fiction can be a safe space to discuss youth suicide. *The Conversation*. https://theconversation.com/young-adult-fiction-can-be-a-safe-space-to-discuss-youth-suicide-30562. Accessed 3 Aug 2020.

Herrington, S. (2015). Jasmine Warga's unromanticized depression. *Interview Magazine*. https://www.interviewmagazine.com/culture/jasmine-warga-my-heart-and-other-black-holes#_. Accessed 3 Aug 2020.

Hinton, S. E. (2007). *The outsiders*. Viking Press. (Original work published in 1967).

Kelley, S. (2017). Netflix pledges to add more trigger warnings to '13 reasons why'. *Variety*. https://variety.com/2017/digital/news/13-reasons-why-trigger-warnings-netflix-1202404969/. Accessed 3 Aug 2020.

McManus, K. (2017). *One of us is lying*. Delacorte.

Michaud, J. (2014). S.E. Hinton and the Y.A. Debate. *The New Yorker*. https://www.newyorker.com/culture/cultural-comment/hinton-outsiders-young-adult-literature. Accessed 3 Aug 2020.

Niven, J. (2015). *All the bright places*. Knopf.

Orsini, J. (2019). Why one of us is lying by Karen McManus is problematic. *Book Riot*. https://bookriot.com/why-one-of-us-is-lying-by-karen-mcmanus-is-problematic/. Accessed 3 Aug 2020.

Pan, E. X. R. (2018). *The astonishing color of after*. Little Brown.

Rich, M. (2009, March 9). A story of a teenager's suicide quietly becomes a bestseller. *The New York Times*. https://www.nytimes.com/2009/03/10/books/10why.html. Accessed 3 Aug 2020.

Rodriguez, C. (2015). *When reason breaks*. Bloomsbury.

Rossen, J. (2019). Traumatic episodes: A history of the ABC afterschool special. *Mental Floss*. https://www.mentalfloss.com/article/577502/abc-afterschool-special-history. Accessed 3 Aug 2020.

Sparks, B. (1999). *Go ask Alice*. Simon and Schuster. (Original work published in 1971).

Thomas, F. (2018). A queer reading of Go ask Alice. *The Paris Review*. https://www.theparisreview.org/blog/2018/01/22/queer-reading-go-ask-alice/. Accessed 3 Aug 2020.

Warga, J. (2015). *My heart and other black holes*. Balzer + Bray.

Zoella Book Club. (2016). Gayle Forman: An exclusive interview on I was here. *WHSmith*. https://blog.whsmith.co.uk/zbc1016-gayle-forman-an-exclusive-interview-on-i-was-here/. Accessed 3 Aug 2020.

Michelle Falkoff is the author of *Playlist for the Dead*, *Pushing Perfect*, and *Questions I Want to Ask You* (Harper Collins, 2018). Her fiction and reviews have been published in *ZYZZYVA*, *DoubleTake*, and the *Harvard Review*, among other places. She is a graduate of the Iowa Writers' Workshop and currently serves as Director of Communication and Legal Reasoning at Northwestern University School of Law.

"Our Precarious Selves": Suicide and Autoimmunity in Yiyun Li

Andrew Bennett

Contents

Suicidality: Dear Friend, from My Life I Write to You in Your Life 268
Surviving Suicide: When Reasons End 274
References 279

What does mourning feel like? How does one sense and make sense of grief? How can one register the specific permutations and ramifications of sorrow, anguish, and suffering, of "anger, pity, unforgivingness, even condemnation" (Li, 2018a, p. 51) in the case of a suicide? What are the dimensions and effects of such grief, what are its qualities? And then, on the other hand, we must surely ask the other set of questions: What does it feel like to want to die, to kill yourself, or to do so? How do those feelings and that logic work? The Chinese-American writer and former immunological researcher Yiyun Li directly addresses both series of questions in two recent books—her memoir from 2017, *Dear Friend, from My Life I Write to You in Your Life*, and her most recent novel, *Where Reasons End*, from 2019. She does so, I will suggest, by configuring suicide and suicidality, as well as the repercussions of the act, within the terms of a certain autoimmunity.

A. Bennett (✉)
University of Bristol, Bristol, UK
e-mail: A.Bennett@bristol.ac.uk

J. Ros Velasco (ed.), *Suicide in Modern Literature*,
https://doi.org/10.1007/978-3-030-69392-3_17

Suicidality: *Dear Friend, from My Life I Write to You in Your Life*

Written during and after two periods as an inpatient on a psychiatric ward and more than one suicide attempt, Li's hybrid book *Dear Friend* is many things: A meditation on reading and writing, a memoir of the author's emigration from a post-Tiananmen China to the center of global capitalism, a journal-like account of her move away from science to creative writing, and a series of autobiographical essays on memory and mourning, on hope and despair, on mental illness, and on the nature of authorial reticence and, or within, the autobiographical impulse. In other words, the book is, not least, an example of that relatively rare thing, a serious and thoughtful first-person account of suicidal despair and its implications and consequences, its affects and associated thought-processes: *Dear Friend* engages with the phenomenology of suicide in ways that offer often elusive but nevertheless periodically clarifying insights into that difficult and often highly conflicted and friable state of mind. "Is writing not my way of rehearsing death?", she asks herself (2018a, p. 114).

"I came to this country as an aspiring immunologist," Yiyun Li comments early on in her memoir on her move from China to the USA in 1996 to study for a Ph.D. at the University of Iowa (2018a, p. 14). *Dear Friend* records, among other things, the two years that Li spent descending into and being "confined by" suicidal depression in 2012–2014 (2018a, p. 200). And it is an account that repeatedly links the immune system and the biological mechanism of autoimmunity with the impulse toward suicide and with the act itself. Early on in the memoir, Li raises (without naming it) the unavoidably recursive paradoxicality—the deconstructionism, as we might think of it—of the immune system: Its autoimmunity.[1] The job of the immune system, Li writes:

> [...] is to detect and attack nonself; it has memories, some as long lasting as life; its memories can go awry selectively, or, worse, indiscriminately, leading the system to mistake self as foreign, as something to eliminate. The word *immune* (from the Latin *immunis*, *in* + *munia*, services, obligations) is among my favorites in the English language, the possession of immunity – to illnesses, to follies, to love and loneliness and troubling thoughts and unalleviated pains – a trait that I have desired for my characters and myself, knowing all the while the

[1] See Naas (2008, p. 124), on autoimmunity, that "illogical logic," in Derrida's phrase, as "another name, in some sense the last, for what for close to forty years Derrida called 'deconstruction'."

futility of such a wish. Only the lifeless can be immune to life. (2018a, pp. 14–15)

Integrated into her lucidly nontechnical explanation of immunity—smuggled into it, so to speak—Li's description of autoimmunity as the capacity of the system's memories to "go awry selectively, or worse, indiscriminately, leading the system to mistake self as foreign, as something to eliminate" (2018a, pp. 14–15) gestures toward the structural role of autoimmunity in immunity and emphasizes its paradoxical, indeed deconstructive integrity: No immunity without autoimmunity.[2] Perhaps it is this, indeed, that attracts Li to the word "immune," what makes it her "favorite" word. Both the Latin *immunis* and its derivatives in English involve specific exemptions from duties or obligations, whether ecclesiastical, legal, fiscal, or other. Immunity involves a certain freedom from responsibility. For Li, this includes the responsibility entailed by love—freedom from its constraints or constrictions, we might surmise, from its limitations, from one's duty or obligation toward the feeling itself, or from the loved one toward whom the feeling is directed. And in this sense, as her statement intimates, the kind of immunity that Li welcomes and embraces ultimately involves immunity to life—and therefore to oneself and to one's self, indeed, in as much as one's self becomes, or is interpreted as, not oneself. Li recognizes that the paradoxical desire for a shield against, or for immunity from, illnesses, "follies," love, loneliness, "troubling thoughts," and "unalleviated pains" constitutes a desire for autoimmunity, since the desire for a release from all ties of obligation, duty, or indeed connection (including the connection of love) ultimately involves immunity from or protection against the self—from the desires, aggravations, excitements, investments, wishes, memories, and thoughts by which the subject is constituted. To be free from loneliness, from troubling thoughts, or from unalleviated pains is to be free of selfhood, but also and therefore to be liberated from life itself, in this logic of autoimmunological thinking, since human life—being *humanly* alive—is precisely constituted by such phenomena, by experiences, feelings, affections, memories, or thoughts.

As it happens, Li's thinking of immunity and autoimmunity in *Dear Friend* chimes in critical ways with Jacques Derrida's meditations on autoimmunity in his late work—in texts such as *Specters of Marx* (1994), *Acts of Religion*

[2] Compare Nass' comment that autoimmunity seems to "name a process that is inevitably and irreducibly at work more or less everywhere, at the heart of every sovereign identity" (2008, p. 124). And see the wry comment by Noel R. Rose and Ian R. Mackay that "autoimmune disease will remain a problem as long as variation and natural selection remain laws of nature" (2014, p. 8).

(2013), and *Rogues* (2005).[3] In a series of detailed considerations of the individualistic philosophical foundations of the intrinsically ego-based nature of democracy and democratic institutions, Derrida argues that the "living ego" (*le moi vivant*) that necessarily underlies such institutions can itself be conceived of as paradoxically autoimmune: "To protect its life, to constitute itself as unique living ego, to relate, as the same, to itself," Derrida proposes in *Specters of Marx*, the autonomous, stand-alone, or sovereign ego is "necessarily led to welcome the other within" (1994, p. 141). Linking the problem to the death drive and to the apparent perversity of a kind of universal sadomasochism, Derrida argues that for the ego to function at all, it must "take the immune defenses apparently meant for the non-ego, the enemy, the opposite, the adversary and direct them at once *for itself and against itself*" (1994, p. 141). Derrida returns to the question of autoimmunity in *Rogues*, analyzing it as a central organizing metaphor for a thinking of democracy as a political category or idea based fundamentally on the sovereignty or *ipseity* of the self—but on a sovereignty or ipseity that is always incalculably compromised, irreducibly conflicted, itself not itself (as is verified by the phenomenon of the unconscious, through which it is constituted).[4] When Derrida talks in *Rogues* of the unconscious as a "vital" or "privileged" source for the "implacable law of the self-destructive conservation" of the subject or of what he calls "egological ipseity," he is pointing in the first place to the principle of autoimmunity, of a mechanism that turns (or just is) self-destructive because its primary function is its own conservation—which entails, in fact, its own destruction (2005, p. 55).

This might throw light on the rhetorical and conceptual strategies and maneuvers in Li's *Dear Friend*, as well as on her later novel, *Where Reasons End*. As much a description of her own psychological state and of her relationship to herself as it is a description of the mechanism that helps all vertebrates survive, the immune system in Li's brief account in *Dear Friend* also and at the same time links with a key concern of her books: The nature of, and impulse toward, suicide. "As a body suffers from an autoimmune disease, my mind targets every feeling and thought it creates," she writes, in "a self dissecting" that "itself finds little repose" (2018a, p. 52). After all, as Li comments, "One always knows how best to sabotage one's own life" (2018a, p. 25).[5]

[3] On Derrida and autoimmunity, see Nass (2008) and Zalloua (2018).

[4] For a discussion of the question of suicide and sovereignty, see Bennett (2017, pp. 11–16).

[5] Li comments further on "the dissecting part" in an interview from 2017: "I realised [...] whatever I felt, whatever I thought, my own mind was targeting at itself. So I would call it an autoimmune condition of my own mind. And that was almost an unresolved problem—I'm attacking myself, so I thought the only

The immune system that Li describes early on in her book also works as a metaphor for the unnamed impulse to survive (which means not to survive), in effect, life—a metaphor for what we might think of as the indifference or dispassion, the disinterest or unconcern, that allows one to survive what Hamlet refers to in his famous suicide speech as the "slings and arrows of outrageous fortune" (Shakespeare, 2006, III.i.57). At one point in her meditation on "this war against myself" (2018a, p. 152), Li refers to the "autoimmune condition of the mind" (2018a, p. 67) and talks about her desire, in the past, to be "nothing," to be therefore "invisible and replaceable," suggesting that this is "one way to battle" that condition—to close in on oneself, in other words, to remain "everything to oneself," not to share or divide or complicate oneself. And yet, to protect oneself in this way, to protect oneself from outside hostility or attack, is, paradoxically, also to open oneself up to a recursive "autoimmune" self-destructiveness. Explicitly and otherwise, in fact, the book repeatedly returns to autoimmunity as a definition of the self's strategies for surviving the world and other people. "One's intuition is to acquire immunity to those who confirm one's beliefs about life," Li writes in a sentence that then closes off any other alternative, "and to those who turn one's beliefs into nothing" (2018a, p. 15). The sentence that follows reinforces the idea that one must defend oneself not only against those who would "confirm" or support but also against those who would threaten one's sense of self: Li remarks of "those who turn one's beliefs into nothing" that they are "the natural predators of our hearts"; while of those who "confirm" one's beliefs, she comments that they are "made into enemies because we are, unlike other species, capable of not only enlarging but also diminishing our precarious selves" (2018a, p. 15). But why would you choose to turn those who would *confirm* your beliefs into your enemies? In addition to insisting on a double bind (those who are against you are against you, out to destroy you, but so are those who are for you or with you), the riddle hints at the recursive suicidality of autoimmunity, of the self turning against the self. The danger is equally in the self's "enlargement" as in its diminishment—the self, after all, being the problem. Thus, in a comment that recalls a memorable line from George Eliot, Li says she wishes she could "erase that troublesome *I* from my narrative" (2018a, p. 33) and claims that she writes precisely in order to become a "non entity" (2018a, p. 46).[6] The precarity of selfhood, it seems, is to be valued even if it can lead ultimately to the elimination of the self, even to suicide.

thing I could do while I was in the middle of it was, I could maybe use all this condition—why don't I just attack myself a little more, by writing?" (2017, mins. 18:49–19:26).

[6] Although George Eliot is not mentioned among the "Partial list of books" that Li includes as an appendix to her memoir (books read, books that have influenced her as a writer, books that she recommends),

A few pages after declaring the need to "acquire immunity" from others, Li explores another dimension of her autoimmunological thinking when she writes of the "emptiness in me": "There is this emptiness in me. All the things in the world are not enough to drown out the voice of this emptiness that says: you are nothing" (2018a, p. 18). The emptiness, in other words, fills the "me," fills it with nothing. And yet it is, at the same time, what makes up this "me," what forms me. It is not nothing in that it is the nothing that is me. And the message of this emptiness that is (in) me is: *Itself.* Its message is that you (which is me) are nothing, that you are/I am empty. Some days, Li says, she "battles" this emptiness until "we both fall down like injured animals": "That is when I wonder: What if I become less than nothing when I get rid of this emptiness? What if this emptiness is what keeps me going?" (2018a, p. 18). The emptiness is at least a thing—albeit a thing that is empty. To do battle with it, autoimmunologically, is to risk destroying not just the emptiness but the self upon which it relies and which relies on it. In this sense, it is (or it may be) precisely the battle with the emptiness that "keeps me going." To overcome the emptiness would be to overcome myself. There is nothing, in fact, but this battling (this battle with or against nothing). And this would then be one of the paradoxes of suicidality in Li's account: It is not the nothing that is the problem but the sense that there is nothing but the nothing, the sense that without it and without the battle with it, one is not.

For Li, then, the immune system can be a metaphor for the way that the psyche or self is impelled to develop a sense of indifference in order to survive the manifold misfortunes and setbacks of life and the way that that sense of indifference can also lead ultimately, and in its extreme form, to a rejection of the life that it is designed, however, to support. Li's sense of the necessary indifference that one must build toward life in order to live chimes with Freud's analysis of the dangers to consciousness of (over-)stimulation in his famous essay on the death drive: "*Protection against* stimuli is an almost more important function of the living organism than *reception of* stimuli," Freud remarks (1984, p. 299). In a remarkable prefiguration of a kind of psychic autoimmunity,[7] Freud speculates that it is not only external stimuli that are the problem but more tellingly internal stimuli (thoughts, memories, fears, anxieties), such that to protect itself from the internal stimuli by which con-

the use of the word "troublesome" in this context is surely a pointed echo of a notable moment in *Middlemarch* (1871–1872), where the detached authorial third-person omniscient narrator comments that "I know no speck so troublesome as self" (Eliot, 1994, p. 419).

[7] We can call it a "prefiguration" because, according to Paul Ehrlich's influential principle of *horror autotoxicus*, from the early twentieth century right up until the 1950s or 1960s, what we now call autoimmunity was thought to be biologically contradictory or impossible (see Silverstein, 2001).

sciousness is unceasingly assailed, there is "a tendency to treat them as though they were acting, not from the inside, but from the outside" (1984, p. 301).[8] What Freud calls a "shield" against stimuli is ultimately a shield against what is "internal" as much as against the external. As such, it is a shield, a defense, against life itself.

The principle or mechanism of autoimmunity presupposes an *autos*, a self, against which the biological or psychic system acts. But Li suggests that the concept or very ontology of selfhood is also a societal or cultural question (such that, in that sense, the self is never in any simple sense simply itself). She returns repeatedly to the idea of the "precarious" self as a category that translates poorly between Chinese and English, European, or especially American languages and cultures, noting the West's massive, seemingly all-encompassing investment in the self as unique, singular, individual, and as politically, spiritually, and ethically fundamental—the self as, in effect, the grounding principle of democracy, Christianity, personal responsibility, and value itself. Li explains that, having grown up surrounded by the totalitarian ideologies of collectivism and anti-individualism in Communist China, she "hates" to use the "melodramatic" English word "I." The Chinese language, she argues, has less invested in subject pronouns and allows for a more fluid interchangeability of the singular and plural first-person pronouns (2018a, p. 27). Li therefore insists that she is not an autobiographical writer, explaining that one cannot be such a writer "without a solid and explicable self" (2018a, p. 26).[9] And yet, at the same time, Li's book is in fact insistently just about the insistent "I," an *I* that it rages against and that turns in on itself, contradicting itself indeed in this and other arguments. In this sense, the book may be said to perform (perhaps as an articulation of a certain cross-cultural or emigrant paradoxicality) the recursive damage of the immune system gone haywire, gone rogue, as it turns against itself in a way that directly reflects on the condition of suicidality: "for months after the hospital stays," she tells us, "I tried to explain to those around me that anyone can be, and should be replaceable"—"What does this *I* matter to *you* when it means so little to myself?," she recalls herself thinking, or saying, autoimmunologically—in a memoir that is, in line with its generic affiliation, about nothing other than the autonomous, unique, singular self (2018a, p. 27). And even in this resistance to the "I," we can see emerging what Li describes as a "humble and

[8] This is the origin, for Freud, of the critical psychoanalytic principle of "projection."

[9] She is "absolutely not" an autobiographical writer, Li remembers telling a reader, and yet since "One writes about what haunts one," no one is in fact "exempt from being autobiographical" (2018a, p. 101).

presumptuous though innately human" desire to use the word, to invent oneself in at least a minimal way as "distinctive and irreplaceable" (2018a, p. 27).

Surviving Suicide: *When Reasons End*

"The intense emotions around suicide," Li writes in *Dear Friend* as she lists some of them as "anger, pity, unforgivingness, even condemnation," demand "what no one has the right to claim: an explanation, and the authority to judge the explanation" (2018a, p. 51). Just months after the publication of Li's extraordinary memoir—a memoir, it should be noted, that is as much about her literary influences (including Kierkegaard, Turgenev, Katherine Mansfield, Elizabeth Bowen, Stefan Zweig, Elizabeth Bishop, Philip Larkin, and especially the Irish writer William Trevor) as it is about herself and about her suicidal depression[10]—Li's 16-year-old son killed himself.[11] Her next novel, *Where Reasons End*, written in the aftermath of her son's death, links itself explicitly with the memoir by referring to the "year of my disintegration" five years earlier (2019a, p. 63). And yet the question of suicide is switched around, turned on its head, so to speak, in a novel that persistently and urgently addresses the "inexplicable tragedy" of suicide from the other side (2019a, p. 5). *Where Reasons End* is about the mixed and manifold phenomenology of mourning, guilt, and grief and of the sense of blame, anger, exasperation, longing, and enduring love that follows a suicide.

Where Reasons End, we might say, both records and invents the unbearable anguish of the suicide survivor. In the novel, Li's cultural-national-ethnic background emerges as part of a complex negotiation of identities that both joins and divides the Chinese-born mother from the person that she refers to, at one point, as her "ABC" (American-born Chinese) son (2019a, p. 141). In what are often unspoken or at least only indirect ways, the transnational crisis or matrix of the relationship emerges in particular in relation to the question of language, to words and to word choices. "Words are falcons," the mother says at one point, "our minds the trainers"; "No, our minds are the targets,"

---

[10] But reading can itself be autoimmunologically suicidal: "Not having the exact language for the bleakness I felt," Li says of Katherine Mansfield's journals, "I devoured her words like thirst-quenching poison" (2018a, p. 149).

[11] See Li (2019b); when her son killed himself, it turns out the 44-year-old Li was writing both a short story about a 44-year-old mother whose daughter has killed herself (the story was published as "When We Were Happy We Had Other Names" in *The New Yorker* on October 1, 2018 [2018b]) and a separate novel, also about a 44-year-old mother whose daughter has committed suicide, entitled *Must I Go* (Li, 2020), which was eventually published in August 2020 (see Westenfeld, 2020, para. 5, for Li's comments on this *coincidence* of novel and life).

the son replies, "the prey" (2019a, p. 123). Words are reflexively, even obsessively, discussed in a book that is as much about motherhood, emigration, cultural discontinuity, inheritance, desire, longing, and complex, hybrid cultural identities as it is about death, mourning, and grief. For it is words that join together and pull apart the mother and the son—not least (or only) the words that go to make up this novel.

Presented largely as an uninflected dialogue in 16 chapters (a division that pointedly aligns the book's trajectory with the temporality of two 16-year-old decedents, fictional and biographical, that it evokes and recalls), there are no speech marks or even dashes to indicate the start and stopping points for any of the book's innumerable speech events. Written in the wake of the suicide in 2017 of Li's son, Vincent, the novel presses at the always permeable border crossing or no-man's-land between life-writing and fiction by imagining the endless "quibbling" (2019a, p. 25) of a mother and her son, Nikolai, in the months paradoxically, impossibly *after* the boy's suicide.[12] Hence, perhaps, the book's subtitle, or clarification: "A Novel." The book is a fiction, just as, according to the novel's own irrefutable internal logic, the 16-year-old dead boy who speaks in it is a fiction within a fiction. As the boy says at the novel's close: "Here is where you are, not where I am. I am in fiction […] I am fiction now" (2019a, p. 168). The mother makes up a world of stories, making a dialogue of, doubling up, her own singular voice. Since there is no other way to communicate with the dead boy, the mother makes up stories "to talk with Nikolai" herself (which is also, or only, to talk with herself) (2019a, p. 56). There is no way to talk with the suicided son except in this made-up way, and the book knows it. In fact, in spite of the searing autobiographicity of her novel, Li is a writer for whom, as Rachel Cusk puts it (2019), fiction "only works through the emphatic denial of its links to personal experience" (including in Li's case "the denial of native language itself"). In this sense, there is an insistent de-personalization or impersonalization involved in Li's work. Writing involves impersonating someone other than the "I" who speaks or writes—which is perhaps what makes the impersonal but clearly autofictional "I" of *Where Reasons End* so striking and so unsettling. But this is also what links the novel so insistently to questions of autoimmunology that we encountered in the memoir.

In fact, Li's novel is, above all, a novel about the inexplicable, unspeakable loss of a son to suicide. "Words fall short," she says, "but sometimes their

[12] The novel's epigraph refers to the "Memory of Vincent Kean Li (2001–2017)" (2019a, n.p.). But the name of the fictional "Nikolai," we are told in a biographically teasing way, is fictional (a fiction within a fiction): It is "not his real name, but a name he had given himself, among many other names he had used" (2019a, p. 6).

shadows can reach the unspeakable" (2019a, p. 167). "These imaginations made it easier for me to feel sad, to weep even," the mother says at one point, "but the tears were a veneer over the unspeakable" (2019a, p. 85). What we might call the "inexplicable unspeakable" is, she says, "a wound that stays open always, always, and forever" (2019a, p. 85). Not being able to know and speak something *is* the wound, a wound that can never close.[13] That, it would seem, just is the nature of (inexplicable unspeakable) grief—"What does not make sense is what matters," Li comments aphoristically in *Dear Friend* (2018a, p. 183). For the mother to abandon her grief would be to abandon the one who is lost, and speech—or writing—must continue in order to go on expressing the unspeakable. At one point, the mother remembers that in the wake of the 2016 presidential election she had decided to read and re-read all of Shakespeare's works for the four years of the presidency (an ambition that she says she abandoned on the death of her son)—as if everything can be found in Shakespeare, everything meaningful, intelligent, and just. And in an interview on *CBC Radio*, Li refers to the moment in Shakespeare's *King John* (2018a, b), when another mother, Constance, can't believe that her son has died.[14] "Grief fills the room up of my absent child," Constance laments: Grief, she says:

> Lies in his bed, walks up and down with me,
> Puts on his pretty looks, repeats his words,
> Remembers me of all his gracious parts,
> Stuffs out his vacant garments with his form;
> Then, have I reason to be fond of grief?
> (Shakespeare, 2018, III.iv.93–98)

This is the situation in which the mother finds herself in *Where Reasons End*. Her room, her life, her head, and her novel is full of her dead son: there is nothing, virtually no one else in the book that she is writing, that she is living, almost no one else in her life. Her suicided son (she has another, as Li does, who is hardly mentioned) is present everywhere. It is her grief that keeps him there, and it is her persistent expression of the inexpressible that allows him to stay. But this, too, makes the novel a work that accords with the logic of immunity (which is also the logic of autoimmunity). To ensure her

[13] "Words provided to me – loss, grief, sorrow, bereavement, trauma – never seemed to be able to speak precisely of what was plaguing me" (2019a, p. 93).

[14] Li (2019b, mins. 42:45-43:30): Talking specifically about her story "When We Were Happy We Had Other Names," which takes its name from *King John*, Li comments that "I was thinking about how much grief is about not believing this thing has happened" (min. 43:20).

immunity from an overwhelming and inexpressible sense of grief, the mother must keep on talking with her son. But to write a novel is necessarily at some point to end it, to end the conversation. You write a novel, as you hold a conversation, in order to complete or conclude it. The further you progress with it, the nearer you come to the end and to the nothingness that underlies it.

The relationship between mother and (dead) son is quibbling, bickering, and querulous—it precisely announces its presence, and the presence of the son, in the opposition of the two in their bickering—"Even arguing for the sake of arguing was better than dead silence," she says (2019a, p. 26). After all, if the son—a 16-year-old boy, we must remember—was simply to agree with, accept, respect, and not mock his mother, he would not be independent, autonomous, whole, or complete. He would not be, would have no self, no *autos* or *ipseity*, no separate existence, and no sovereignty. The gap and the friction that ensues between the two speakers are, paradoxically, both an effect of loss and that which might overcome that loss—even if that overcoming is at the expense of a grounding in or fidelity with regard to the empirical or tangible, to the real (or to whatever it is that is the opposite of the fictional). As Elizabeth Bishop puts it in a poem—"Argument" (1955)—from which Li takes the title of her novel and that she prints in full as a kind of epigraph, "argue argue argue with me / endlessly / neither proving you less wanted nor less dear" (lines 5–7, qtd. in Li, 2019a, n.p.). At once constative (statement of fact), imperative (command made of another person), and performative ("argue with me" argues with you, makes you argue with me), Bishop's lines stumble grammatically and rhetorically: They quiver autoimmunologically over the kinds of speech act that they constitute in a way that engages movingly with the novel to which Li attaches the poem. The endless and endlessly repetitive quarrel with the loved one in *Where Reasons End* is both an argument with that other and at the same time self-contained, internal, and imagined. As constative, imperative, and performative, this way of speaking (in Bishop and in Li) is a way of proving, in effect, that the lost lover or lost son *is* still wanted and beloved, not forgotten—and in that sense in fact not gone because still present in the thought and speech patterns of the grief-raddled writer-mother-lover. It's a form of denial, of course, and in that sense no doubt conventional, familiar, predictable, and necessary. But, at the same time, it is a way of engaging with a loss that can never emotionally, logically be resolved and an articulation of a certain autoimmunity.

The son's response to his mother's evocative declaration that the unspeakable is "a wound that always, always, always and forever" stays open, is to mock: "Oh gosh, he said. An open wound – that makes you sound like a mediocre self-help book," he remarks scathingly (2019a, p. 85). The mother responds by claiming that a self-help book would speak of healing rather than of an always-open wound, at which point the son changes the angle of attack, switching to his habitual critique of his mother as a nonnative speaker of English (see, e.g., 2019a, p. 13).[15] "What bad language you use now," he says:

> There is no good language when it comes to the unspeakable, I thought. There is no precision, no originality, no perfection.
> Oh fine, he said, if you insist.
> Fear not, I said. I would be the last person to write a self-help book.
> Wouldn't a non-self-help book be more interesting?
> A book about not helping oneself? I asked. A self-sabotaging book?
> A book helping non-selves, he said. Like me.
> (2019a, p. 86)

The suicided son invents the genre of the "non-self-help book," seeming to mean a book that helps those who do not have selves—dead people, for example. But the mother misunderstands his invention (or understands it too well) as a different kind of book, a self-sabotaging or autoimmune book—one that uses all its power to undo itself—"You can add 'un' to many words," the dead son says, at one point, "and undo yourself" (2019a, p. 122). But even here, in the word "self-sabotaging," there is a further ambiguity at work, since a non-self-help book might sabotage itself or it might sabotage *the* self (or both: Sabotaging the self in sabotaging itself). It is, I think, the mother's interpretation of the (non-)self-help book that remains, that holds more weight, complying as it does with the autoimmunological principle that drives both the novel and the memoir before it. Writing is commonly conceived of as a form of self-help, particularly for victims of tragedy, for those who have suffered trauma, or for suicide survivors.[16] But an arguably more compelling, more efficacious kind of book would be a book that doesn't help the self, that even satirizes such an endeavor, precisely because it is the self and its ramifications—that contentious, precarious, fictional construct—that is at stake in

[15] The question of speaking/writing in one's nonnative language pervades both of Li's books, and what the son overlooks in his scathing assessment of his mother's nonnative English is that her "private salvation," as she calls it, "is that I disowned my native language" (2018a, p. 139). To "own" a language, she explains, is "to allow oneself to be owned, too" (2018a, p. 140). But it is the "absoluteness" of her "abandonment" of Chinese that Li wants to emphasize and the "determination" with which she carries out the plan: it is, she remarks, "a kind of suicide" (Li, 2018a, p. 140).

[16] For the philosopher Michael Cholbi, the problem of grief *is* the problem of the self: Citing Colin Parkes's assertion that when someone we love dies "a whole set of assumptions about the world that relied upon the other person for their validity are suddenly invalidated," Cholbi argues that the suffering entailed by the loss of a loved one is accounted for by the fact that "another's death poses a threat" to our "practical identities"; as such, grief "raises questions of self-identity and self-definition in especially acute ways" (Parkes, 1996, p. 90, qtd. in Cholbi, 2019, p. 500).

the first place. Such would be a book that questions, indeed, the efficacy or stability of the self or subject as a fundamental ethical and ontological category. "Is it a fatal condition," the author asks herself at one point, "for some people just being themselves?" (2019a, p. 122), as if in response to her son's autoimmunological assertion, earlier on, that he has found "a perfect enemy in myself" (2019a, p. 79). So that when the mother tells her son that "All selves need some help," his response raises an important conundrum: "if a self is seeking help," he asks, "is it because it wants to be better at being itself, or being like others?" (2019a, p. 87). What does it mean, in other words, to be a self that needs help? The self needs help to be what? Not itself? But that, paradoxically, would compromise or alienate precisely that which makes it a self: Its singularity, autonomy, sovereignty, and separateness. And yet, if a self-help book is designed "to help a self to be better at being itself," as the mother responds, then the mathematics, as the son puts it, fail to add up: "How can a book help a million selves when each self is different?", he asks (2019a, p. 87).

Li's autoimmunological reasoning and her autoimmunological writing offer at least one solution to the conundrum of suicide and of suicidality, even if that solution eventuates in a realization that the system constructed to protect the precarious self from auto-destruction (immunity from a seemingly hostile outside world) is also the system that will turn on itself in a disastrous and destructive psycho-autoimmunological response. But her writing also deploys the autoimmunological model as a metaphor for the grief and mourning-work that follows a suicide (including the grief and mourning-work of writing *Where Reasons End*), for an undoing of the precarious self in order to protect it, to nurture, and defend it against a cataclysm that cannot be contained, or reasoned, or expressed.

References

Bennett, A. (2017). *Suicide century: Literature and suicide from James Joyce to David Foster Wallace*. Cambridge University Press.

Cholbi, M. (2019). Regret, resilience, and the nature of grief. *Journal of Moral Philosophy, 16*(4), 486–508. https://doi.org/10.1163/17455243-20180015

Cusk, R. (2019). The case of Yiyun Li. *The New York Review of Books*. https://www.nybooks.com/articles/2019/07/18/case-of-yiyun-li/. Accessed 6 Jun 2020.

Derrida, J. (1994). *Specters of Marx: The state of the debt, the work of mourning, and the new international*. Routledge.

Derrida, J. (2005). *Rogues: Two essays on reason*. Stanford University Press.

Derrida, J. (2013). *Acts of religion*. Routledge.

Eliot, G. (1994). *Middlemarch*. Penguin.
Freud, S. (1984). *Beyond the pleasure principle*. In J. Strachey (Trans.), *On metapsychology: The theory of psychoanalysis* (Vol. 11). Penguin Freud Library.
Li, Y. (2017). Interview with Carmen Machado. *Free Library of Philadelphia*. https://www.youtube.com/watch?v=BRN81NXBFSA. Accessed 6 Jun 2020.
Li, Y. (2018a). *Dear friend, from my life i write to you in your life*. Penguin.
Li, Y. (2018b). When we were happy we had other names. *The New Yorker*. https://www.newyorker.com/magazine/2018/10/01/when-we-were-happy-we-had-other-names. Accessed 3 Aug 2020.
Li, Y. (2019a). *Where reasons end: A Novel*. Hamish Hamilton.
Li, Y. (2019b). Writers & Company Interview ("Yiyun Li Navigates the Loss of a Child in Her Heartbreaking New Novel). *CBC Radio*. https://www.cbc.ca/radio/writersandcompany/yiyun-li-navigates-the-loss-of-a-child-in-her-heartbreaking-new-novel-1.5326406. Accessed 6 Jun 2020.
Li, Y. (2020). *Must I go*. Hamish Hamilton.
Naas, M. (2008). *Derrida from now on*. Fordham University Press.
Parkes, C. (1996). *Bereavement: Studies of grief in adult life*. Penguin.
Rose, N. R., & Mackay, I. R. (2014). Autoimmune disease: The consequence of disturbed homeostasis. In I. R. Mackay & N. R. Rose (Eds.), *The autoimmune diseases* (pp. 3–9). Elsevier.
Shakespeare, W. (2006). *Hamlet*. Thomson Learning.
Shakespeare, W. (2018). *King John*. Bloomsbury.
Silverstein, A. M. (2001). Autoimmunity Versus *Horror Autotoxicus*: The struggle for recognition. *Nature Immunology, 2*(4), 279–281. https://doi.org/10.1038/86280
Westenfeld, A. (2020). Yiyun Li Is expanding our vocabulary for grief. *Esquire*. https://www.esquire.com/entertainment/books/a33432137/yiyun-li-must-i-go-interview/. Accessed 31 Aug 2020.
Zalloua, Z. (2018). *Theory's autoimmunity: skepticism, literature, and philosophy*. Northwestern University Press.

Andrew Bennett teaches English at the University of Bristol, UK. He is the author of *Suicide Century: Literature and Suicide from James Joyce to David Foster Wallace* (Cambridge University Press, 2017).

Epilogue: Leaving One's Comfort Zone to Write About Suicide: Arya's Story

Jeffrey Berman

Contents

Helping Students at Risk 282
Arya 284
Avoiding Landmines 287
The Classroom as a Holding Environment 291
References 292

Whatever doesn't kill me makes me stronger, Nietzsche famously said. The suicide of my college mentor, Len Port on Labor Day 1968, did not make me stronger, but it has compelled me to help my students who struggle with suicidal thoughts. I was a second-year graduate student at Cornell University in Ithaca, New York, when Len telephoned me from Brooklyn, telling me that he was in the process of killing himself. His death left me confused, grief-stricken, and bereft. I wrote my doctoral dissertation on the theme of suicide in Joseph Conrad's life and art: His fictional characters often die by their own hand. I did not realize at the time that by writing about Conrad's abortive suicide attempt—he shot himself in the chest when he was a young man, dejected over a failed romantic relationship—I was trying to understand Len's

J. Berman (✉)
University at Albany, State University of New York, Albany, NY, USA
e-mail: jberman@albany.edu

J. Ros Velasco (ed.), *Suicide in Modern Literature*,
https://doi.org/10.1007/978-3-030-69392-3_18

death. I completed my dissertation, *Joseph Conrad and the Self-Destructive Urge*, in 1971, and it was published in 1977 as Joseph Conrad: Writing as Rescue (Berman, 1977).

I began teaching at the University at Albany in 1973, where I created the first course in the English Department on literature and psychoanalysis. The most innovative aspect of the course was a weekly "Freudian diary" in which students made connections between the fictional stories discussed in class and their own lives. Before handing the diaries back the next week, I read a few aloud, always anonymously, and without class discussion—students who did not want a diary read aloud wrote "no" on it. In their written evaluations at the end of the semester, students said that writing and hearing the diaries read aloud were the most powerful moments of the course. Over the next two decades, I received thousands of diaries, and I began to consider authoring a book on how students wrote about their lives. After receiving students' consent to use their writings, along with the permission of the University Institutional Review Board, which oversees human research, I wrote *Diaries to an English Professor* (Berman, 1994).

The book marked a turning point for me, the first time I wrote about my students rather than fictional characters. It was also the first time I used the first-person pronoun in my scholarly writing, which went counter to my training. *Diaries to an English Professor* included topics that are usually deemed too personal to discuss in a classroom: Parental divorce, eating disorders, sexual abuse, and cutting. I had no personal experience with these topics, but I could relate to the chapter on how my students wrote about a relative or friend's suicide or their own suicidal thinking. For the first time, I wrote about my own experience as a suicide survivor—a person affected by the legacy, or illegacy, of self-inflicted death.

Helping Students at Risk

My experience as a self-disclosing teacher has confirmed one of the main insights reached by other researchers: Self-disclosure begets self-disclosure. The more I disclose about myself to my students, the more they are willing to disclose to me. Many of my self-disclosures have focused on the grief and guilt I experienced when Len committed suicide. My willingness to talk about his suicide emboldens students to talk and write about their own experiences. Most students know a relative, friend, or acquaintance who has attempted or completed suicide—or have themselves thought seriously about committing suicide. I share with students the alarming statistics about the prevalence of suicidal thinking. The figures I cited in *Surviving Literary Suicide* (Berman, 1999), from the 1991 national school-based Youth Risk Behavior Survey, sponsored by the US Centers for Disease Control (CDC), are sobering:

> 27 percent of all high school students thought seriously about committing in 1990; 8 percent of all students actually attempted suicide; and 2 percent of all students sustained injuries in the course of a suicide attempt serious enough to warrant medical attention. (1999, p. 18)

In June 2018, the CDC released statistics indicating that from 1999 through 2016, the suicide rate has increased by more than 30% in half the states. Nearly 45,000 lives were lost to suicide in 2016 and, most disturbing of all, "more than half of people who died by suicide did not have a known mental health condition" (CDC, 2016). A 2007 study evaluating college students' mental health concluded that "44.3% of undergraduates and 41.2% of graduate students reported that mental or emotional difficulties affected their academic performance in the past 4 weeks" (Eisenberg et al., 2007, p. 537).

Suicide results in what Kenneth J. Doka calls disenfranchised grief: One experiences a "sense of loss but does not have a socially recognized right, role, or capacity to grieve" (1989, p. 1). Shame and stigma surround suicide, but writing is a countershame activity, a way to detoxify dark emotions by exposing them to others.

I believe that teachers can play a significant role in suicide prevention: First, by informing students of the prevalence of suicidal thinking; second, by discussing the complex factors that contribute to suicide, including the feeling of hopelessness, which is usually the best predictor of suicide; third, by creating a safe and nonjudgmental classroom where suicide may be discussed openly and candidly, without being either romanticized or stigmatized; and finally, by telling students that help is readily available, beginning with the university counseling center, which has helped countless students in the past. Literature abounds in suicidal characters, and discussions of why they choose to die or live can be illuminating.

Trust becomes the key issue in a self-disclosing classroom. Students realize that no one will criticize their emotions or make a derogatory comment. They learn that acknowledging a vulnerability is a strength rather than a weakness. They discover the commonalities that link them to their classmates, realizing they are not alone in struggling with problems.

I accompany my students on their journey outside of their comfort zone, and we return together safely at the end of the semester. It is always a round-trip journey that ends where it begins, in the classroom, but with a difference.

Students have opened up their lives to classmates and teacher, revealing aspects of their lives often not shared with a relative or best friend.

Arya

Arya had taken two of my literature courses and believed that taking a third course, "Writing about Love and Loss," would motivate her to write about the most devastating event in her life. In her first assignment, a brief discussion of four loves and four losses, she mentioned the deaths of her four grandparents as well as the suicide a year earlier of her first cousin. "Suicide is a concept I had never expected to become familiar with. Nobody expects to become familiar with suicide. The specific loss hit my family like a freight train." Arya wrote a long paragraph filled with the details of her cousin's suicide and a shorter paragraph describing how she had not yet processed the event. "I get nightmares and I close myself off because the idea of talking to anyone seems too much. Most days I find myself wanting to lie in bed and not get up. Thinking about it makes me feel physically ill."

In an early diary, Arya noted that her cousin's suicide sensitized her to a dark subject:

> People often joke about suicide. They use throwaway sayings such as 'I'm gonna kill myself' or 'I wanna die.' I unfortunately used those sayings in the past. One of my losses has opened my eyes to how horrifying these words truly are. It will take a long time before I come to terms with that specific loss.

Arya ended the diary by declaring that although she will never be grateful for her losses, she is grateful for the knowledge and growth the losses have provided. "This change is welcome. I will continue to change and grow as I experience loss. My losses have given me strength, closeness, and newfound trust. For this I am grateful."

In the next three assignments, Arya wrote about a classmate's gratitude for an anonymous organ donor whose heart now beats in her sister's chest; a former student, Isabella, who wrote in my book *Death Education in the Writing Classroom* (Berman, 2012) about how her firefighter father suffered irreparable lung damage during the World Trade Center attack; and about a classmate's relationship with his girlfriend that was destroyed by their clashing religious and ethnic differences. Arya's following diary described her feelings about reading her next essay aloud in class:

> I will be reading my essay to the class on Wednesday. I am nervous and excited. Having to wait over a week gave me anxiety; knowing that my turn was coming scared me. The idea of reading an essay as open and honest as the one I had written was daunting.

Hearing her peers share their writings helped to lessen Arya's fears. "Being able to listen to others be brave inspired me to be the same." During the next class, she read the following essay aloud. I have not changed a word except to use the pseudonym she later requested:

> January 8, 2018 was the day that my assumptive world was shattered to a million unsalvageable pieces. These pieces will never be put back together. My view on life was upended and changed. I had foolishly assumed that my family was exempt from depression and suicide. I had foolishly believed that everyone was happy. I had foolishly assumed that my cousin would never kill herself.
>
> The last time I saw her she was laughing. She had a bright, beautiful, and contagious laugh. Christmas Day was the last time I saw her. The cousins all gathered at our aunt's house to exchange our annual inappropriate secret Santa presents. We all had a few drinks and were engaged in a rather aggressive game of "spoons." My cousins and I are loud and competitive; we take our card games seriously. My last memory of her was her shoving our cousin out of the way to grab the remaining spoon. She had a smile on her face that lit up the entire room. She was beautiful. She was full of spirit. She was unique and kind. Her favorite accessory was a bucket hat. She was also depressed and bipolar. She was not on medication. She was not receiving help. We did not notice, and we failed her. She was eighteen when she took her life.
>
> It is easier for me to write how I feel about this event than it is to discuss it with someone aloud. Is it healthy that I would rather write about it than talk about it? Is it healthy that I have only discussed my feelings about this with three people? That is unknown. I guess I am now sharing my feelings about this with the class. I haven't dealt with my feelings yet. I have acknowledged them, but they sit there idly. My feelings are a ticking time bomb; counting down the seconds until they detonate. I am plagued with nightmares. Often, I can't close my eyes without seeing what she looked like in her casket. When the nightmares are particularly bad, I stay in bed for longer than normal. The bad dreams turn into bad days; talking seems too difficult these days. I am haunted by what she did. It makes me psychically sick. Suicide was foreign, and I was in denial. It has been a year and I constantly have to remind myself that what she did is not my fault. But, how could it not be my fault? There are so many what-ifs? What if I had noticed? What if I had asked how she is feeling? What if I told her she could

talk to me rather than assuming she already knew she could? The only part of this experience that I am sure of is that none of us could have stopped her. She was determined to die.

The afternoon she was discovered I was at work [...] My phone rang with the call from my mom. She was frantic and I could tell she had been crying. She was trying to remain calm; for whose sake? I couldn't tell. She told me I needed to leave work and get to my aunt's house immediately. I asked her what's happening. She repeated that I needed to get to my aunt's house immediately. If I didn't leave right now she would come and get me [...] When I opened the front door my mom was waiting. I didn't have time to prepare myself. "Mary killed herself. She's gone." This is how my mom told me. I couldn't process the situation. I thought I was going to vomit. The only words I could manage were "what?" I hadn't realized that my mind was trembling until I collapsed into my mother's arms [...]

We were told that she hanged herself. We were told that she didn't show up to her friend's party and that while she was missing she set up the rope in her closet and put it around her neck. I was in the car with my mom when I accidentally found out the truth. The ugly truth is that her first attempt failed. Her closet wasn't suitable to hold the rope. She was determined to die; she strangled herself. My 18-year-old cousin strangled herself to death. She used her own hands to ensure that she did not survive. She was determined to die.

I wasn't meant to find out. My mom was talking to her friend and they were discussing what happened. One of the first responders was a family friend; he told the family the truth. I had so many questions, but no answers. How did it feel knowing that my cousin used her own hands to kill herself? I was destroyed. I was terrified. I can't talk about the way they described her when she was found. I am haunted by the description, and I see her ghost in my nightmares.

I tried to hide my feelings from my family. I assumed that I needed to be strong for everyone else. I couldn't stand to watch the rest of them crumble. The wakes and funeral went by in a daze. I felt like a zombie. I was walking and talking. I don't remember much. As my cousin and I sat in the church pew; we promised each other that we would tell the other if we ever got to this point. If it ever got this bad we would call each other. At the time my anger appeared often. I was angry at her. How could she do this to her family. I often think of where I'm at in life; about to graduate college. She will never get this chance. She will never have such accomplishments. She is gone.

> This loss changed everything. I take nothing for granted. It changed the way I think, feel, and act. This experience has given me a new perspective on life. I will never assume that someone is alright. I will never assume that someone's smile equals his or her happiness. My loss has made me aware that I cannot assume the way people are feeling. I will no longer assume that I must hold the weight of their feelings on my shoulders. This loss has made me forever sorry that I couldn't spot what she needed.

Arya's voice wavered but never cracked as she read the essay aloud. She notes in the third paragraph that it was easier for her to write about her cousin's suicide than to speak about it. Why? Writing is a more deliberative process than speaking. The writer can take as much time as necessary to formulate thoughts and feelings. If writers hit an emotional wall or find the composition process too intense, they can walk away from their word processor and return hours or days later when they are emotionally ready. Because writers have more time to express their words than do speakers, they have the time to revise carefully their words. Speakers can "take back" their words but not before the words may inadvertently cause pain to others or themselves.

Arya's feelings may be a "ticking time bomb; counting down the seconds until they detonate," but she writes with remarkable control. One would never sense from her voice, tone, diction, or grammar that any part of the composition process was explosive. There are only a few punctuation errors, mainly in the use of the semicolon. In my written comments, I noted that this was the most powerful essay she had written in any of the courses she had taken with me, "an essay of which to be proud." I noted that the questions she raised in the third paragraph were particularly noteworthy, though I did not attempt to answer them.

Avoiding Landmines

How did the class respond to Arya's essay? Students follow their teacher's lead in responding to essays read aloud, and I take special precautions in self-disclosing writing courses. Leaving the familiarity, security, and certainty of one's comfort zone can lead to personal and educational growth, but it can also lead to unproductive anxiety and stress. A self-disclosing writing course is fraught with dangers—hence the title of my 2001 book, *Risky Writing: Self-Disclosure* and Self-Transformation in the Classroom (Berman, 2001*). Risky writing implies risky teaching. To avoid exposing students to unnecessary risk, I put the following protocols into practice:*

(i) Students have the option of *not* writing on any topic they regard as too personal. Instead, the student can write on another topic related to love and loss.

(ii) We don't discuss an essay's content. After an author reads an essay aloud, classmates identify their favorite sentences, and I point out other sentences that contain a grammatical or stylistic error. Following this, the three students sitting to the author's right raise content questions. For example, if an essay is about a grandparent's death, the questions might involve the author's relationship to the grandparent, whether the grandparent had been ill for a long time, and the impact of the death on the family. These questions are what Irvin Yalom (1995) calls *vertical* self-disclosures, which refer to the content about a secret and involve digging, stripping away, uncovering, and excavating. If a student writes about an abortion, the questions might include whether writing about this topic was hard, why the author decided to write about this, and whether she would share the essay with relatives or friends. Yalom calls these *horizontal* self-disclosures, questions about the disclosure itself, or *metadisclosure*, the interactional nature of personal revelation.

(iii) Authors are not allowed to answer these questions in class, mainly because the questions may be too difficult to answer or place students on the defensive (such as a question about the possible idealization of the dead). Students can answer the questions in a diary, which I read aloud if they give me permission to do so.

(iv) Students do not ask me advice about how to live their lives nor would I offer such advice beyond what is appropriate for a professor. They know that I cannot "fix" their problems. The best I can do is to create an empathic, nonjudgmental classroom in which they write about loves and losses and reach their own conclusions. They teach and instruct each other and leave the classroom feeling a heightened connection to their classmates and teacher.

Arya's classmates singled out several sentences for praise. They commented on her use of repetition in the first paragraph ("I had foolishly assumed"); the questions raised in the third paragraph (the "what-ifs?"); and sentences like "I had so many questions, but no answers." Arya may have hidden her dark feelings from her relatives, but she shares them with her classmates and teacher. She *shows* us rather than merely tells us about her changed perspective at the end. I think everyone was stunned, as I was, by the image of Mary strangling herself to death after the rope broke. Arya conveys the violence of her cousin's death without romanticizing it.

Arya's essay raises many questions, both vertical and horizontal. Why did Mary stopped taking her medication? Why was she reluctant to reach out for help? These questions may remain forever unanswerable. The horizontal questions have answers, but Arya may not have felt ready to answer them. How did she feel writing the essay? Was it hard or easy to write? Hard or easy to read? Is she willing to share the essay with relatives or friends? How did she feel about her classmates' response to the essay? With my response? Authors think about these questions long after the class ends.

In her penultimate diary, Arya expressed her gratitude toward the class. "This class has taught me how to open up without fear and has shown me that others are struggling despite what they appear like on the outside." Although writing about love and loss made her "incredibly nervous," it also served as an outlet to her.

> I knew that I had a lot to get off my chest, and this class challenged me to write about everything I had once feared to say [...] I needed to move on, and this class helped me to do that.

One of the paradoxes of self-disclosing writing is that students will often share their most personal stories with classmates rather than with their relatives or closest friends. This was true of Arya, who sent me the following note after the semester ended:

> Today, as I was speaking with Professor Berman, he asked me if I had shown my parents my writings about my cousin. Last year, right after it happened, I had written a diary about what happened in Berman's Fitzgerald/Hemingway class. I showed my mother that diary, after removing about half of what I wrote. She didn't respond. She told me "what is there to say?" I understood because, what is there to say? Did I show her the essay that I wrote for "Writing about Love and Loss?" Absolutely not. I couldn't. It is way too personal. I am terrified of how she would respond. Her response could range from anger, heartbreak and worry.
>
> My mom is my best friend. I am not exaggerating; my mom and I have an extraordinary relationship. We have always been extremely close, and I have always shared everything with her. This time, however, I could not. It's not that I don't trust my mom; it's just that this paper took a lot out of me. It was difficult to write. I have never been as open and honest as I was when writing this paper. I cried while writing the paper. I cried while reading the paper aloud. I am scared to show her. I probably won't ever show her [...]

> I love my mom with my entire heart. Maybe one day I will find the courage to share these papers with her. Today is not that day.

In her first assignment, in January, Arya hoped that she would be able to write about her cousin's suicide; by the end of the semester, in May, she had written several essays and diaries about Mary. We never discussed "bereavement" theory in class, but in his book *Children and Grief: When a Parent Dies* (1996), J. William Worden outlines a child's four "tasks" in the grieving process, tasks that may apply to other grievers as well: Accepting the reality of the loss, experiencing the pain of the loss, adjusting to a new environment without the loved one, and memorializing the loss (see pp. 13–15). Arya had completed the first three tasks before the semester began; by the end of the semester, she completed the fourth task.

After Arya gave me permission to use her writings, I sent her a copy of the present essay and asked her to describe her feelings while reading it. Here is what she wrote:

> It was bittersweet reading my work in Professor Berman's chapter when he sent me a rough draft of his work. It was sweet because it made me feel accomplished and proud that I was able to write something as honest as I did. I was able to include details and truths without holding back. I was proud of myself for opening up and letting myself heal. It was bitter because of the potential what-ifs. What if my stories trigger someone else? What if people judge [me] for allowing my tragedies to be shared with multiple readers? However, I reminded myself that these what-ifs that made me hesitate are futile because I am not in control of others' minds. I can only hope to help them, and ultimately I believe my stories will help and make an enormous impact on others.

I realize that there are few if any college courses like "Writing about Love and Loss." I remain in a tiny minority of English professors who regularly teach personal writing courses that encourage students to explore dark topics in their lives. Dying and death surround us, but professors are uncomfortable allowing students to write about their experiences with mortality. One of the implicit fears of a self-disclosing writing course, particularly on love and loss, is that the teacher will open a Pandora's box, unleashing unruly emotions that cannot be contained. My own experience, however, suggests a different metaphor: Opening the classroom door to heightened self-awareness and connection with fellow students. Professional journals are beginning to acknowledge the value of death education. In a 2017 issue of *English Journal* devoted to "Death in the Classroom," Brittany Rose Collins (Collins, 2017) observed that studying death in literature "externalizes the interiority that is so messy in early stages of grief, providing a 'safe' and alternate vehicle for affective and intellectual reactions to loss, shaping the schemata through which students view their self-created stories" (p. 48).

The Classroom as a Holding Environment

My experience teaching self-disclosing writing courses suggests that the classroom becomes what the British analyst D.W. Winnicott called a "holding environment" (1965), capable of containing volatile emotions. Sitting in a semicircle rather than in straight rows, as in a traditional classroom, heightens the feeling of community and connection: Students see their classmates' faces, alternately joyful and sorrowful, and they appreciate the difficulty of reading aloud personal essays on loss. As a result of the protocols I put into place, students never respond inappropriately to emotionally charged writings. They recognize the courage and strength required to leave the comfort zone: Even low self-disclosers are willing to share something highly personal with the class.

Students are highly protective of each other in all the self-disclosing writing courses I have taught. Without exception, all the students travel outside their comfort zones, exposing hidden vulnerabilities. They are surprised by and moved by their classmates' revelations. Students are willing to self-disclose only if they are certain they will not be judged, criticized, or attacked by their classmates or teacher. What emerges is not only shared vulnerability but a recognition of strength and resilience.

Those who do not remember the past are condemned to repeat it, the philosopher Santayana observed. In an illuminating 1960 essay, the psychoanalyst Hans W. Loewald (Loewald, 1960) distinguishes between ghosts and ancestors to show how trauma, like depression, evokes the image of haunting:

> Those who know ghosts tell us that they long to be released from their ghost-life and led to rest as ancestors. As ancestors they live forth in the present generation, while as ghosts they are compelled to haunt the present generation with their shadow-life. (p. 29)

Arya, we recall, had referred to being "haunted" by her deceased cousin's "ghost." Like the "talking cure," both the "reading cure" and the "writing cure" can be a first step in transforming ghosts into ancestors.

References

Berman, J. (1977). *Joseph Conrad: Writing as rescue*. Astra Books.
Berman, J. (1994). *Diaries to an English professor: Pain and growth in the classroom*. University of Massachusetts Press.
Berman, J. (1999). *Surviving literary suicide*. University of Massachusetts Press.
Berman, J. (2001). *Risky writing: Self-disclosure and self-transformation in the classroom*. University of Massachusetts Press.
Berman, J. (2012). *Death education in the writing classroom*. Routledge.
Centers for Disease Control and Prevention. (2016). Suicide and self-inflicted injury. *CDC*. https://www.cdc.gov/nchs/fastats/suicide.htm. Accessed 3 Aug 2020.
Collins, B. R. (2017). Associative mourning: Learning to lose through literature. *English Journal, 107*(2), 47–52.
Doka, K. J. (1989). *Disenfranchised grief: Recognizing hidden sorrow*. Lexington Books.
Eisenberg, D., Gollust, S. E., Golberstein, E., & Hefner, J. L. (2007). Prevalence and correlates of depression, anxiety, and suicidality among university students. *American Journal of Orthopsychiatry, 77*(4), 534–542. https://doi.org/10.1037/0002-9432.77.4.534
Loewald, H. W. (1960). On the therapeutic action of psycho-analysis. *International Journal of Psychoanalysis, 41*, 16–33.
Winnicott, D. W. (1965). *The maturational processes and the facilitating environment: Studies in the theory of emotional development*. Hogarth Press.
Worden, J. W. (1996). *Children and grief: When a parent dies*. Guilford Press.
Yalom, I. (1995). *The theory and practice of group psychotherapy*. Basic Books.

Jeffrey Berman is a Distinguished Teaching Professor of English at the University at Albany, State University of New York, where he has been teaching since 1973. He is the author or co-author of 20 books, including Confidentiality and Its Discontents: Dilemmas of Privacy in Psychotherapy (Fordham University Press, 2015), which received the 2017 Book Prize from the American Psychoanalytic Association. His latest books are *Writing the Talking Cure: Irvin D. Yalom and the Literature of Psychotherapy* (State University of New York Press, 2019); the two-volume work *Off the Tracks: Cautionary Tales About the Derailing of Mental Health Care* (Ipbooks, 2019), co-authored with Paul Mosher; and *Mad Muse: The Mental* Illness*Memoir in a Writer's Life and Work* (Emerald, 2019). Berman has written on a wide range of subjects, including literature and psychoanalysis, the pedagogy of self-disclosure, love, and loss, and death education. An Honorary Member of the American Psychoanalytic Association, he was selected by the *Princeton Review* in 2012 as one of the country's top 300 professors.

Index

A
Abandonment, 4, 90, 242, 243, 278n15
Abortion, 77, 90, 288
Abrutyn, S., 144n1
Absurdity, 192, 194, 196, 199
Abuse, 37, 38, 40, 41, 49, 82, 85, 90, 91, 253, 254, 282
Ackley, H., 15, 18, 21
Adolescence, 100
Adorno, T.W., 121
Adultery, 101, 111
Affective disorders, 9, 9n3
Africa, 87, 228
Agencies, 20, 21, 29, 41, 42, 47–65, 61n8, 91, 176, 204–213
Aggression, xi, 4, 57, 186, 192, 196, 242
Agony, 156–158, 161
Ahmed, S., 51n3
Alaimo, S., 51
Alcestis, 4, 5
Alienation, 188, 192, 194, 200, 229
Altruistic suicides, 4, 5
Alvarez, A., 18, 244
Álvarez-Castro, L., 156
Améry, J., 199, 242
Amphetamines, 74, 82
Ancient Greek, 3
Andreasen, N.C., 9n3
Andrews, S., 255
Andriessen, K., 47, 48
Anger, 5, 89, 267, 274, 286, 289
Annihilation, 176, 181
Anomy, 141, 143
Ansari, M.T., 228
Anti-semitism, 253
Anxieties, 7, 19, 82, 272, 285, 287
Apathy, 156
Appelbaum, P.S., 249
Appelius, S., 150n2
Appignanesi, L., 81
Aristotle, 231
Asher, J., 254, 256–260
Astar, R.K., 54
Atkinson, J., 49
Attention-seeking, 48, 57
Australia, 2
Autobiography, 19, 143
Autoimmunity, 267–279, 269n2, 270n3, 272n7
Autonomy, 57, 62, 257, 279

J. Ros Velasco (ed.), *Suicide in Modern Literature*,
https://doi.org/10.1007/978-3-030-69392-3

B
Backman Rogers, A., 53n6, 54
Baker, A.F., 157
Baker, R.W., 73
Bakunin, M., 125
Barad, K., 49–52, 51n3, 60
Barbagli, M., 123, 176
Barbiturates, 82
Bardot, B., 75
Barnaby, P., 103
Barnett, R.V., 49
Baroja, P., 111, 155
Barreca, R., 113
Barris, G., 83, 89
Barroso Martínez, A.A., 33
Bayet, A., 17n2
Belgium, 240
Bellak, L., 6
Bell, M., 19
Benavente, J., 110, 111
Benedetto Croce, 180
Bennett, A., 268, 270n4
Benstock, S., 19
Berman, J., 211, 281–291
Berryman, J., 243, 244
Bertelli, D., 176n6
Berto, G., 174n4
Bertolote, J.M., 47
Betrayal, 4, 78, 210, 242, 243
Bettelheim, B., 7
Beutin, W., 120, 122
Bille-Brahe, U., 47
Bipolar disorder, 261
Bishop, E., 274, 277
Black, C., 36, 39, 57
Blames, 56, 257, 274
Blankenship, R., 120, 122, 130
Blasco Ibáñez, V., 110
Bloom, J.D., 58
Bohr, N., 50
Bonner, R.L., 48
Borderline personality disorder, 81, 82, 82n3
Boredom, 220–223, 225
Botticelli, S., 86
Brancaccio, M.T., 100n6
Brandt, P.A., 218, 219, 234
Brantley, Eric, 40
Braun, V., 123, 124, 126–128
Braunmühl, C., 51n3
Brennan, M.A., 49
Brinks, J.H., 122
Brockington, I., 48
Brodsky, B., 204
Brouwers, J., 242, 248
Brown, L.G., 36, 39
Broz, J. (Tito), 221
Buchanan, J., 204
Butler, J., 50, 51
Butler, L.L., 260

C
Calcraft, L.G.A., 1
Callanan, V.J., 48, 49
Camus, A., 23, 196, 199, 203
Cancer, 112, 126, 189, 207, 211, 239
Canetti, E., 133, 134
Canetto, S.S., 48, 49
Cannibalism, 7
Capitalism, 268
Capuana, L., 95–107
Casey, J.T., 48, 49
Cassirer, E., 200
Catholicism, 186
Cato, J.E., 49
Cervantes, M. de, 110, 164
Chandhuri, S., 58
Childhood, 21n4, 74, 76, 77
Cholbi, M., 206, 278n16
Choo, C.C., 48
Cioran, E.M., 247, 248
Civil Rights, 34, 35
Cline, E., 52, 53n6, 54
Clinical suicidology, v, xiii
Cobain, K., 242

Coelho, P., 217–235
Cold War, 220–222, 234
Coleman, D., 48, 49
Collado-Rodriguez, F., 54
Collins, B.R., 290
Collins, S., 255
Colt, G.H., 23, 24n8
Compassion, 211, 212
Compulsion, 6, 75, 142
Communism, 120, 121, 221
Conrad, J., 281
Contagion, 58, 134, 135
Cooper, H.R., 222
Coppola, S., 53n6
Cowardice, 122, 125, 126, 242
Crazy, 61, 78, 129, 165, 225, 226
Creative writing, 7–9, 268
Creativity, 84, 112, 127, 129
Crime, 23, 24, 27, 75, 99, 101, 230, 257
Critchley, S., 112
Crosby, A., 228
Cuba, 75
Cusk, R., 275

D

Dahlen, E.R., 48, 49
D'Arienzo, S., 176n6
Darkness, 26, 75, 89, 203–213, 220, 221, 224–227, 229, 231–233, 241, 246
Darwin, C., 197
Daspin, E., 74
Davis, M.S., 48, 49
Davis, W., 48
Daydreaming, 7
de Burgos, C., 110
Decadentism, 103
Deconstructionism, 268
Deiritz, K., 120
De Leo, D., 47
Demastes, William, 36
Democracy, 270, 273
Denmark, 2, 150
Dependency, 2, 4, 54, 58
Depersonalization, 191, 195
Depression, 79–81, 83, 119, 123, 128, 174n4, 190, 203–213, 220–229, 231, 233, 240, 244, 246, 247, 249, 259–262, 268, 274, 285, 291
Derealization, 191, 195
Derrida, J., 268n1, 269, 270, 270n3
Desai, S., 82
Descartes, 198, 199
Desertion, 83, 126, 127, 242
Desolation, 64, 181
Despair, 39, 105, 121, 162, 163, 165, 167, 176, 177, 187, 192, 196, 199, 200, 207, 224, 227, 229, 233, 248, 268
Desperation, 61, 105, 106, 196, 199
de Unamuno, M., 110, 156–167
de Urquía, J., 111
Devitt, P., 255
de Zayas y Sotomayor, M., 110
Díaz, J.W., 158
Dicenta, J., 111
Dickinson, E., 42, 260
Dieckmann, C., 120
Dilthey, W., 121
DiMaggio, J., 77
Dimitrov, G., 122
Disillusionment, 192
Disorientation, 176
Dissatisfaction, 119, 138
Dissociation, 195
Distress, 36, 195, 239
Divorce, 34, 218, 242, 282
Doka, K.J., 283
Dolan, J., 36
Donato, M., 110
Donnersmarck, F.H. von, 145
Dopamine, 228
Dorfman, R., 82

Dostoyevsky, F., 191
Dougherty, J., 77
Dreiser, T., 26n9
Drinking, 2
Driscoll, C., 57
Drugs, 48, 49, 82, 88, 225, 245, 253, 254
Durkheim, E., 25, 26, 26n9, 29, 54, 100, 134–150, 158, 167, 174, 177, 185

E

Eating disorders, 282
Eccles, J.C., 198, 199
Ecolinguistic, xiv, 218–220, 224, 226, 227, 230, 232, 233
Economy, 120, 124, 127, 136, 140, 141, 147
Education, 34, 99n6, 109, 115, 157, 284, 290
Egoism, 143, 145
Egotism, xii, 101
Ehrlich, P., 272n7
Eisenberg, D., 283
Elderly, 76, 217
Elias, N., 123
Eliot, G., 271, 271n6
Embodiment, 54
Empowerment, 36, 41, 42
Emptiness, 63, 82n3, 83, 188, 272
Ena Bordonada, A., 110, 112, 114
Engels, F., 146
Engler, W., 120
Epilepsy, 40, 191
Erikson, E., 3
Eroticism, 54, 192
Eschner, K., 254
Eternity, 155–167
Ethical society, 29
Ethical subject, 29
Ethnicity, 35, 75
Eugenides, J., 49, 52, 52n4, 53n6, 54–65
Europe, 18, 228, 229
Euthanasia, 190, 239, 247, 249
Existential crisis, 188–200

F

Faber, M.D., 4, 5
Families, 20, 26, 27, 37, 40, 60, 77, 83, 84, 89, 91, 100, 102, 105, 123–126, 147, 148, 173, 186, 188, 191, 194, 208, 218, 256, 259, 260, 263, 284–286, 288
Fascism, 122
Fear, 38, 48, 77–80, 83, 103, 122, 125, 166, 190, 210, 212, 213, 229, 272, 278, 285, 289, 290
Feminist, vi–viii, 33–43, 49, 50, 58, 86–87
Fenichel, O., 141
Fincham, B., 35
Finland, 52, 150
Fliess, W., 3
Foessel, M., 149
Foolishness, 49
Forman, G., 260
Forte, J., 36
Fortichiari, V., 172n1, 173, 176n6, 177n7
Foucault, M., 50
France, 110, 144, 145, 221, 222, 234
Franco, F., 115
Frankfurt, H., 205, 205n1
Fraser, B., 161
Freedom, 86, 88, 115, 125, 189, 196, 198, 207, 210, 211, 248, 269
Freriks, K., 243
Freud, S., 3, 90, 177, 186, 194, 196, 272, 273, 273n8
Friedman, S., 39
Friend, J., 49
Frustration, 79, 113, 119, 123, 171, 192, 196, 255, 256
Fusaro, E.C., 98

G

Galligan, S.B., 48, 49
Galynker, I., 205
Ganivet, Á., 156
Gates, B.T., 17n2
Gates, H.L., 87
Gender bias, 34
Genius, 26, 104, 157
Gentile, G., 180
George, R.M., 36
Germany, 119, 123, 125, 126, 128, 145, 150, 172, 221
Ghiselin, B., 6
Gifford, S., 83n5
Gilbert, J.R., 115–117
Gilligan, C., 74, 87, 92
Girlhood, 54
Giuliani, V., 224
Glaspell, S., 34
Glass, T., 259
Glory, 49, 166
Goedegebuure, J., 245
Goethe, J.W. von, 255
Goldman, M., 88
González Vicen, F., 165
Goodman, P., 7, 79
Görlitz, x, 121, 124–126
Grady, C., 255, 258
Grashoff, U., 119, 120, 125
Greenson, R., 80
Greenstein, L., 259
Grief, 34, 63, 260, 267, 274–277, 279, 282, 283, 290, 291
Guilt, 2, 4, 21, 78, 122, 123, 157, 158, 210, 241, 243, 260, 274, 282
Gunn, J.F., 2

H

Haenel, T., 186
Haines, J., 2
Hand, C., 260
Handke, P., 187
Hanssen, L., 248
Happiness, 42, 104, 114, 120, 129, 134, 173, 174, 225, 227, 229, 233, 261, 287
Harassment, 128
Haraway, D., 50
Hardy, T., 18n3
Harlow, J., 75
Harris, K.M., 48
Hateley, E., 255
Hefner, J.L., 283
Hegel, F., 180
Heidegger, M., 199
Heiduczek, W., 123, 124
Hein, C., 122–124
Helplessness, 49
Helwig, G., 120
Hemingway, E., 6, 244
Hempstead, P., 43
Hendin, H., 2, 3
Herman, L., 243
Heroism, 25, 26, 155, 158, 165, 166, 255
Herrera Medalle, R., 35, 36
Herrington, S., 261
Herzberg, G., 120
Heß, M., 146
Heteronormativity, 51
Heterosexuality, 49, 58, 60, 61, 64
Heynders, O., 241, 244
Hickey-Moody, A.C., 51
Highmore, B., 63
Higonnet, M., 15
Hinton, S.E., 254
Hippocrates, 233, 234
Hitler, A., 124
Hjelmeland, H., 54n7
Hoffa, J., 75
Hoffman, P.S., 82
Hollywood, 58, 74, 75, 82, 85, 91, 92
Holocaust, 78, 210
Homant, R., 5
Homicides, 2, 5, 16, 19, 75, 77, 106, 176

Hopelessness, 119, 160–163, 167, 222, 229, 233, 255, 283
Hopes, 4, 36, 42, 78, 80, 105, 129, 144, 158, 160–163, 166, 167, 192, 194, 222, 224, 226–233, 254, 268, 290
Ho, R.C., 48
Horeck, T., 85, 90
Hörz, H.E., 120
Hoskin, B., 52–54, 53n6
Hospitals, 5, 57, 77, 112, 116, 128, 209, 213, 217, 218, 222, 227, 228, 230–232, 234, 247, 273
Hostility, 242, 271
Houston, W., 82
Humiliation, 149
Huxley, A., 1, 9

I

Iamblichus, 178, 179
Ibsen, H., 2, 3n1, 83
Idealization, 82n3, 96, 98n3, 288
Identities, 37, 73–76, 78, 82n3, 83, 136, 140, 188, 220–222, 225, 274, 275, 278n16
Iler, D.R., 52
Illness, 40, 49, 100, 119, 134, 186, 189, 193, 206–208, 211, 219, 246, 247, 268, 269
Imitation, 144, 150n3
Immaturity, xi
Immorality, 194, 195
Immortality, 160–163
Impoverishment, vii
Impulsivity, 49
Incarceration, 16, 37, 38, 41
Incomprehension, 241
Individuality, 121
Industrialization, 17, 109, 112, 142, 147
Inequalities, 41, 218, 221–223
Inequity, ix
Inhibition, 6
Injustice, 86, 120, 122, 149
Innocence, 18, 21, 27
Insecurities, 80
Instability, 98, 179, 191
Instinct, 27, 166, 186, 191, 194
Institutionalization, 83
Intentionality, 19, 50, 205, 211
Intimacy, 88, 142, 149
Introspection, 205
Irony, 112–117, 124, 128, 180, 188
Irritability, 82n3
Isherwood, C., 36, 43
Isolation, 6, 20, 37, 38, 49, 54, 58, 64, 128, 174, 175, 178, 179, 212, 213, 228
Israel, G.D., 48, 49
Italian Realism, ix
Italy, 95, 99, 104, 175, 180, 221

J

Jackson, M., 82
Jafari, Sepideh, 54
Jafari, Simin, 54
Jaffe, A., 9
James, H., 17, 22n6
James, W., 22–26, 29, 156n1, 161
Jans, F., 48
Jarausch, K., 122
Jeane, N., 73–92
Jehova's Witnesses, 122
Jiménez Lozano, J., 158
John, E., 73n1
Johnson, M., 219
Joiner, T.E., 2, 3n1, 54, 54n7
Jones, A.H., 212
Juvan, M., 240

K

Kähkönen, L., 74, 75
Kalmar, B., 83n4
Kammann, R., 2
Kanz, C., 120, 122

Kaplan, E.A., 58
Keith, M., 38
Kellerhuis, T., 247
Kelley, S., 259
Kelly, A., 53
Kennedy, J.F., 75–77, 75n2
Kennedy, R.F., 75–77, 75n2
Kerkhof, A.J., 47
Kierkergaard, S., 199, 200
Kirby, V., 50
Kirkpatrick-Smith, J., 48
Klein, M., 186
Klimasmith, B., 24n7
Knizek, B.L., 54n7
Kolakowski, L., 121, 126
Kostova, B.V., 54
Kral, M.J., 47
Krauß, A., 123
Krauss, H., 120
Kress, J.M., 22n6
Kris, M., 90
Kushner, H., 17n2, 18n3

L

Labrador Ben, J.M., 111, 116
Lakoff, G., 219
Langer, S., 200
Langford, R., 49
Langhinrichsen-Rohling, J., 49
Leach, M.M., 48, 49
Ledger, H., 82
Legemaate, J., 245
Legitimation, 23, 122
Lehmann, J.M., 54
Leibniz, 196, 198, 200
Leopardi, G., 180
Leopold, A., 223, 227, 228, 234
Lessona Fasano, M., 172n1
Lester, D., 2–9, 48, 49
Levi, P., 206
Lewinsohn, P., 49
Lewis, J.R., 49
Lewis, R.W.B., 17
Lieberman, L., 18n3, 49
Li, V.K., 275, 275n12
Li, Y., 268
Loewald, H.W., 291
London, J., 26n9
Loneliness, 84, 105, 123, 160, 192, 195, 200, 268, 269
Losses, 2, 4, 5, 23, 49, 52, 63, 73–92, 101, 109, 119, 157, 188, 208, 210, 218, 275, 277, 283, 284, 287–291
Louis XVIII, 146
Love, 5, 38, 39, 49, 54, 61, 73–92, 97, 100–104, 105n8, 120, 125, 126, 128, 129, 157, 159, 162, 162n3, 163, 165, 166, 176, 190, 210, 218, 220, 224, 227, 229–231, 233, 241, 261, 268, 269, 274, 284, 288–290
Low class, 117
Lowell, R., 7, 8
Lower, A., 77
Luther, M., 3
Lutz, B., 120, 122
Luxury, 99, 173
Lynch, A., 134
Lytess, N., 77

M

Maaz, H.-J., 123
MacDonald, M., 17n2
Machado, A., 158, 161
Machon, J., 41, 42
Mackay, I.R., 269n2
Madness, 21, 23, 25, 85, 88, 106, 222, 224
Malaise, 134, 189, 190, 195
Mallory-Kani, A., 53
Maltsberger, J.T., 39
Mania, 157
Mankind, 171–182, 178n8
Mann, J., 204
Mansfield, J., 75

Mansfield, K., 274, 274n10
Manuel, F.E., 3
Manzoni, A., 174n4
Marcuse, Herbert, xiii
Mari, M., 176n6, 218, 223, 226–231
Marino, S., 79
Marriage, 34, 40, 77, 79, 86, 89, 125
Marshall, B.L., 54
Martínez-Quiroga, P., 115, 117
Martin, P., 83
Marx, K., 134–150
Masculine gaze, 50, 58–60, 64
Masiello, V., 104
Materialism, 48, 52, 143, 174
Matheson, R., 181n10
Maugham, S., 6
McCall, G.J., 137
McClelland, D.C., 2, 3, 5
McDermott, A., 86
McDowell, L., 36
McKee, G., 77
McLuhan, M., 179
McManus, K., 262
Meaninglessness, 195, 199, 227
Media, xv, 34, 57, 86, 92, 116, 120, 173, 241, 248
Medication, 80, 231, 243, 285, 289
Mehring, F., 125
Meid, V., 120, 122
Memories, 4, 8, 52, 53, 76, 106, 122, 123, 127, 166, 191, 208, 209, 212, 268, 269, 272, 285
Mende, H.J., 120, 121
Menninger, K., 186, 242
Menon, P., 22n6
Mental illness, 74, 77, 82, 82n3, 90, 144, 185, 186, 204, 206, 207, 212, 213, 227, 232, 247, 260, 268
Me Too, 80
Meyer, C.F., 3
Meyer, K.A., 49
Meyer, M., 3n1
Michaud, J., 254
Michelacci, L., 100
Millard, K., 53
Miller, A., 33, 77–81, 90
Miller, F.G., 249
Mill, J.S., 157
Minois, G., 17n2
Misogyny, 54, 88
Mistreatment, 16, 41, 128
Mocek, R., 120, 121
Modernity, 15–29, 97–101, 103–106, 147, 172
Mogin-Martin, R., 116
Monden, M., 53n6, 54, 57, 58
Monroe, M., 73, 74, 78, 82, 83n4, 85, 87, 90, 92
Monson, C.M., 49
Morselli, E., 99, 100
Morselli, G., 171–182
Mortality rates, 48
Motor neuron disease, 239
Mourning, 267, 268, 274, 275
Mueller, A.S., 144n1
Mulvey, L., 58
Murders, 2, 5, 27, 57, 85, 91, 106, 210
Murphy, T.R., 17n2
Muthesius, S., 126–129

N

Naas, M., 268n1
Narcissism, 60, 92
Narcissus, 84, 86, 91
Nazism, 122
Nelken, M., 109–117
Neuroses, 98, 227
Niederland, W.G., 3
Nietzsche, F., 50, 281
Niezen, R., 144n1
Niven, J., 261
Nixon, R., 54
Nizamie, S.H., 228
Noel, E., 110

Norman, M., 34
Norris, M., 51n3
North America, vi
Norway, 2

O

Oates, J.C., 73–92
Obsessions, 23, 52, 148, 249
Offner, C.B., 180
Onwuteaka-Philipsen, B., 245
Opioids, 82
Oppression, x
Orme, K., 26, 29
Orne, M., 8
Orphanage, 76, 77, 85, 90
Orringer, N.R., 155
Orsini, J., 262
Oshana, M., 205n1
Ouimette, V., 161
Overdoses, 48, 49, 56, 73, 75, 82
Ovid, 84
Oz, A., 241
Ozieblo, B., 36, 38, 40–42

P

Pagliaro, A., 102, 103
Pain, 76, 82, 84, 89, 103, 159, 167, 175, 176, 190, 192, 195, 199, 205–207, 256, 268, 269, 287, 290
Paladin, L., 176
Pan, E.X.R., 261
Panic, 135, 156, 218
Pardo Bazán, E., 97, 110
Parkes, C., 278n16
Pascal, B., 187
Pascual Martínez, P., 110, 110n1, 117
Passions, 24, 89, 95, 98, 104, 135, 136, 142, 145, 157, 160–162, 165–167
Patriarchy, 39, 64
Patriotism, 34
Pavese, C., 6
Peeters, C., 248
Peirce, C.S., 187
Penner, L., 5
Percy, W., 185–201
Pérez Galdós, B., 110
Pérez Zúñiga, J., 110
Performativity, 50, 51
Pessimism, 102
Peuchet, J., 146
Phoenix, R., 82
Pile, S., 38
Piotrowski, Z.A., 6, 6n2
Pischedda, B., 176n6
Plath, S., 6–9
Plato, 175, 199
Plenzdorf, U., 124, 125
Poison, 41, 178, 223
Pöldinger, W., 186
Policies, 119, 122
Pop culture, 87
Popper, K., 198, 199
Pornography, 6
Port, L., 281
Posner, K., 204
Posthumanism, 50n2
Poverty, 37, 40, 41, 75, 106, 226
Powell, A., 49
Powerlessness, 76, 117, 241
Predators, 80, 271
Pregnancies, 89, 90, 253
Prešeren, F., 222, 234
Prestige, 112, 116, 137, 138, 142, 149
Prince, 82, 85, 87
Prisons, 35, 37, 40–42, 124
Private spaces, 38
Privileges, 51, 127
Productions, 8, 79–81, 83, 129, 136
Promiscuity, 61
Properties, 60, 137–141, 144, 146, 147, 149
Proust, M., 172

Public spaces, 142
Punishments, 128, 149, 242
Putnam, S., 160

Q

Qudosi, S., 229
Quijano, A., 166

R

Racism, 54, 190, 218, 253
Range, L.M., 48, 49
Rape, 2, 76, 85, 90, 100, 101, 258
Raphael, L., 28n10
Reagan, R., 76
Rebellion, 23, 105, 175, 176
Redfield Jamison, K., 244
Reeducation, 127, 129
Regret, 98, 103, 156–158, 229, 232
Relaxation, 230
Religion, 27, 134, 135, 161, 179–181, 186, 234, 269
Reminiscences, 158
Rensi, G., 180, 181, 181n9
Responsibilities, 16, 23, 74, 189, 196, 198, 205, 210, 243, 256, 257, 262, 263, 269, 273
Revenge, 77, 78, 242, 256–258
Rich, A.R., 48
Rich, M., 256
Rinaldi, R., 176n6
Rivera, P. de, 114
River, J., 49
Rodriguez, C., 260
Rohde, P., 49
Rokeach, M., 5
Ronningstam, E., 39
Rose, N.R., 269n2
Rossen, J., 255
Rouse, J., 50
Routines, 40, 41, 173, 189
Ruby, H., 83n4
Rumi, J., 228

S

Sachse, C., 128
Sacrifice, 4, 5, 36
Sadness, 98, 102, 222, 224, 231, 261
Sadomasochism, 270
Saint Francis, 225
Sakinofsky, I., 48
Salmela, A., 52
Salvation, 23, 155–167
Sánchez Álvarez-Insúa, A., 111, 116
Sartre, J.-P., 199
Scalessa, G., 101
Scari, R.M., 158
Schiff, J., 53n4
Schinkelshoek, D., 248
Schizophrenia, 74, 82, 83, 123, 211, 229
Schnell, R., 120, 122
Schroeder, K., 120, 126, 127
Scourfield, J., 35
Scudder, H., 87
Secularization, 17
Seeley, J., 49
Self-analysis, xii
Self-assassination, 149
Self-consciousness, 6
Self-destruction, 17, 17n2, 29, 139, 141, 186, 188, 196
Self-determination, 23, 121, 199, 245–247, 249
Self-disclosure, 282, 287
Self-esteem, 40, 191, 208
Self-harm, 253
Selfhood, 17, 269, 271, 273
Self-image, 2
Self-immolation, 28, 29
Self-perception, 191
Self-realization, 120, 188
Self-reflection, 196
Sennett, R., 142, 143
Senselessness, 194
Serotonin, 228
Servén Díez, C., 117
Sexton, A., 6–9

Sexuality, 5, 50, 61–64, 75, 81, 188, 192
Shaftesbury, 135
Shah, M.M., 229
Shakespeare, W., 5, 21n4, 33, 83, 174n4, 271, 276
Shame, 28n10, 34, 88, 122, 206, 212, 213, 230, 283
Sharp, J.P., 36
Sheldon, W., 1, 9
Shelley, M., 175, 178
Shiel, M.P., 178
Shiner, M., 35
Shneidman, E.S., 5
Shostak, D., 52, 53, 60
Shovlin, J., 49
Sickness, 146, 187
Siebelink, J., 248
Silverman, M.A., 7–9
Silverman, M.M., 47
Silverstein, A.M., 272n7
Skinner, B.F., 5
Skomp, E., 58
Slatzer, R., 77
Slovenia, 218, 220–222
Smiley, J., 86
Smith, M., 74, 75n2
Snodgrass, W., 7
Socialism, 120, 121, 124–126, 129, 130, 145–150
Socrates, 3
Solipsism, 179
Solitude, 89, 158–160, 163, 167, 175, 179, 181
Solomon, A., 246, 247
Sophocles, 5, 33
Sorrows, 80, 103, 105, 255, 267
Soule, E.B., 82
Soviet Union, 76, 127
Spain, 34, 109, 111–114, 117, 165, 221
Spaink, K., 245
Spangler, G.M., 26n9
Spanish Republic II, 111
Sparks, B., 254
Spinazzola, V., 95
Spirituality, 198, 228, 231
Stack, S., 48
Stalin, I., 120, 125, 148
Stanislavski, C., 89
State Apparatus, 145
Stein, P., 120, 122
Steinem, G., 76, 77, 83, 83n5, 89
Stephan, I., 120, 122
Stibbe, A., 218–220, 225, 227, 232
Stigma, xi, xiii, 100, 203, 204, 206, 211–213, 283
Stinson, J., 78
Stone, C.D., 230
Stothart, H., 83n4
Strasberg, L., 88
Stress, 5, 6, 82n3, 125, 126, 128, 181, 197, 287
Styron, W., 204–213, 246
Subjectivity, 37, 50
Subordination, 87
Sufism, 227–229
Suicidal behaviors, 4, 5, 185, 244
Suicide assistance, 240, 245–248
Suicide ideation, 204, 206, 207, 211
Suicide prevention, 22, 23, 25, 119, 220, 234, 239, 240, 246, 249, 283
Suicidology, 33, 35, 41, 187
Sullivan, N., 51n3
Sullivan, R., 74
Sundermann, H., 16n1
Support, 36, 41, 80, 120, 124, 126, 140, 209, 223, 246, 256, 262, 271, 272
Sweden, 2
Syria, 178

T

Taboo, 22, 123, 185, 206, 255, 262
Tarde, G., 144n1
Tate, D., 120

Taupin, B., 73n1
Tellini, G., 176n6
Tennyson, A., 85
Terrorism, 176
Terry, R., 8, 81
The Netherlands, 239–249
Therapies, 8, 119, 128, 129, 190, 227–229, 260
Thomas, F., 254
Thon, S., 110, 111n2
Tolstoy, L., 242
Tomás, F., 158
Tragedies, 53, 77, 177n7, 193, 274, 278, 290
Transcendence, 192
Trauma, 39, 52, 54, 76, 77, 278, 291
Truijens, A., 248
Tuana, N., 51
Tuberculosis, 186, 223
Turner, J.H., 136, 137
Tyler, A., 86

U

Udink, B., 247
Ungaretti, G., 177
Upper classes, 99, 115
Utopias, 3

V

Valentine, G., 37
Valentinus, B., 223
Valero Martín, A., 110
Valle-Inclán, Ramón del, 111
van Beethoven, L., 224
van Bruggen, C., 248
Van der Meer, 246, 249, 249n1
Van der Tuin, I., 51n3
Van Gemeren, R., 244, 248
van Reybrouck, D., 248
van Strafelen, H., 180
Veblen, T., 142
Veerman, A., 242, 248
Velotti, P., 37, 40
Verbraak, C., 247
Verdugo Martí, V., 114
Verga, G., 95–107
Verismo, 95, 101
Vervaeck, B., 243
Vespucci, S.C., 86
Vidal y Planas, A., 110
Villani, P., 181n9
Violation, 87
Violence, 55, 57, 65, 85, 90, 91, 254, 257, 258, 288
Volition, 58
Voltaire, 173, 180
Voyeurism, 52, 54
Vulnerabilities, 61, 84, 283, 291

W

Wallace, N., 34
Walton, S., 63
Wander, M., 124
Warfield, K., 60
Warga, J., 261
Warner, S.O., 87
Warren, H.M., 24n8, 85
Wasserman, I., 48
Weakness, 2, 49, 148, 166, 283
Weariness, 191
Webster, B., 81
Westenfeld, A., 274n11
Wharton, E., 18–29, 29n11
White House, 90
White, L., 225
White, M., 58
Whiteness, 54, 75, 80, 222, 231
Wieg, R., 246, 247
Wilcock, R., 178
Wilder, B., 83n4
Wilhite, K., 53
Wilke, U., 120
Will, N.P., 7–9
Winnicott, D.W., 291
Wittgenstein, L., 200

Witz, A., 54
Wolfersdorf, M., 186
Wolff, C.G., 16
Wolfgang, M.E., 5
Womack, K., 53
Worden, J.W., 290
Working class, 105, 128
World War I, 172, 221
World War II, 16, 76, 82, 175, 189, 221

Y

Yalom, I., 288
Young, E., 217, 224, 226, 231–233
Young, S.J., 150
Youth, 60, 63, 64, 80, 88, 104, 121, 127, 222, 283
Yugoslavia republic, 221, 222

Z

Zalloua, Z., 270n3
Zamacois, E., 110
Zavattini, G.C., 37
Zeitgeist, 187, 192, 195, 198
Zimmermann, M.D.S., 120, 122, 123
Žižek, S., 121, 123, 179
Zuccala, B., 102n7
Zwagerman, J., 239–249

The manufacturer's authorised representative in the EU is Springer Nature Customer Service Centre GmbH, Europaplatz 3, 69115 Heidelberg, Germany. If you have any concerns regarding our products, please contact ProductSafety@springernature.com

Printed and bound by CPI Group (UK) Ltd, Croydon, CR0 4YY
30/09/2026
02225659-0010